The YEAR BOOK se
recent international 1
editors who critically 1

Anesthesia: *Drs. ......, ...mer, Saidman, and Stoelting.*

Cancer: *Drs. Clark, Cumley, and Hickey.*

Cardiology: *Drs. Harvey, Kirkendall, Kirklin, Nadas, Resnekov, and Sonnenblick.*

Dentistry: *Drs. Hale, Hazen, Moyers, Redig, Robinson, and Silverman.*

Dermatology: *Drs. Dobson and Thiers.*

Diagnostic Radiology: *Drs. Whitehouse, Adams, Bookstein, Gabrielsen, Holt, Martel, Silver, and Thornbury.*

Drug Therapy: *Drs. Hollister and Lasagna.*

Emergency Medicine: *Dr. Wagner.*

Endocrinology: *Drs. Schwartz and Ryan.*

Family Practice: *Dr. Rakel.*

Medicine: *Drs. Rogers, Des Prez, Cline, Braunwald, Greenberger, Bondy, and Epstein.*

Neurology and Neurosurgery: *Drs. De Jong, Sugar, and Currier.*

Nuclear Medicine: *Drs. Hoffer, Gottschalk, and Zaret.*

Obstetrics and Gynecology: *Drs. Pitkin and Zlatnik.*

Ophthalmology: *Dr. Ernest.*

Orthopedics: *Dr. Coventry.*

Otolaryngology: *Drs. Strong and Paparella.*

Pathology and Clinical Pathology: *Dr. Brinkhous.*

Pediatrics: *Drs. Oski and Stockman.*

Plastic and Reconstructive Surgery: *Drs. McCoy, Brauer, Haynes, Hoehn, Miller and Whitaker.*

Psychiatry and Applied Mental Health: *Drs. Freedman, Kolb, Lourie, Meltzer, Nemiah and Romano.*

Sports Medicine: *Drs. Krakauer, Shephard and Torg, Col. Anderson, and Mr. George.*

Surgery: *Drs. Schwartz, Najarian, Peacock, Shires, Silen, and Spencer.*

Urology: *Drs. Gillenwater and Howards.*

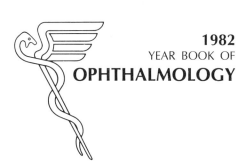

1982
YEAR BOOK OF
OPHTHALMOLOGY

The YEAR BOOK of
Ophthalmology
1982

Edited by
J. TERRY ERNEST, M.D., Ph.D.
Illinois Eye and Ear Infirmary,
Professor of Ophthalmology, Department of Ophthalmology,
University of Illinois, Chicago;
Research to Prevent Blindness, Inc., Eye Research Professor;
Adjunct Professor, Technological Institute,
Northwestern University

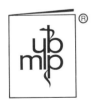

YEAR BOOK MEDICAL PUBLISHERS, INC.
CHICAGO • LONDON

Copyright © September 1982 by YEAR BOOK MEDICAL PUBLISHERS, INC.

All rights reserved. No part of this publication may be reproduced, stored in a retrieval system, or transmitted, in any form or by any means, electronic, mechanical, photocopying, recording, or otherwise, without prior written permission from the publisher.

Printed in U.S.A.

Library of Congress Catalog Card Number: 58-1522

International Standard Book Number: 0-8151-3136-4

Table of Contents

The material covered in this volume represents literature reviewed up to January 1982.

JOURNALS REPRESENTED 7

INTRODUCTION 9

1. LIDS, LACRIMAL APPARATUS, AND ORBIT 11
   Innovations in Oculoplastic Surgery, *by*
   ALLEN M. PUTTERMAN, M.D. 11

2. MOTILITY 43
   The Adjustable Suture, *by* EUGENE R. FOLK, M.D.,
   and MARILYN T. MILLER, M.D. 43

3. VISION, REFRACTION, AND CONTACT LENSES 67

4. CONJUNCTIVA 77
   Acute Hemorrhagic Conjunctivitis, *by* JOEL
   SUGAR, M.D. 77

5. CORNEA AND SCLERA 93
   Refractive Surgery, *by* STEVEN G. KRAMER, M.D.,
   PH.D. 93

6. GLAUCOMA 129
   Advances in the Management of Glaucoma,
   by JACOB T. WILENSKY, M.D. 129

7. THE LENS 173
   **Lens Implantation, Correction of Aphakia,
   and Cataracts,** *by* EDWARD COTLIER, M.D.,
   and YOG R. SHARMA, M.D. 173

8. THE UVEA 199
   Update on Sympathetic Ophthalmia, *by*
   HOWARD H. TESSLER, M.D. 199

9. VITRECTOMY 229
    Treatment of Endophthalmitis, *by* GHOLAM A. PEYMAN, M.D. 229

10. RETINA. 239
    Usher's Syndrome, *by* GERALD A. FISHMAN, M.D. . . . 239

11. NEURO-OPHTHALMOLOGY. 289
    Blepharospasm, *by* JONATHAN D. TROBE, M.D.. 289

12. MEDICAL OPHTHALMOLOGY AND DRUG THERAPY 315
    Opportunistic Infections, *by* LEE M. JAMPOL, M.D.. 315

13. SURGERY 329
    Pars Plicata Surgery for Neonatal Anterior Segment Disease, *by* MORTON F. GOLDBERG, M.D. 329

14. BASIC SCIENCES, INJURIES, AND MISCELLANEOUS 359
    Giants of Visual Science, *by* J. TERRY ERNEST, M.D.. 359

Journals Represented

Acta Dermato-Venereologica
Acta Ophthalmologica
Acta Paediatrica Scandinavica
Albrecht Von Graefes Archiv fur Klinische und Experimentelle
　Ophthalmologie
American Family Physician
American Journal of Epidemiology
American Journal of Medicine
American Journal of Ophthalmology
Annals of Allergy
Annals of Ophthalmology
Annals of Plastic Surgery
Annals of the Royal College of Surgeons of England
Archives of Dermatology
Archives of Ophthalmology
Arthritis and Rheumatism
British Journal of Ophthalmology
British Medical Journal
Canadian Family Physician
Canadian Journal of Ophthalmology
Cancer
Chinese Medical Journal
Clinical Allergy
Clinical Genetics
Hospital Practice
International Ophthalmology Clinics
Investigative Ophthalmology and Visual Science
Japanese Journal of Ophthalmology
Journal of the American Academy of Dermatology
Journal of the American Medical Association
Journal of Clinical Neuro-ophthalmology
Journal Français d'Ophtalmologie
Journal of Nervous and Mental Disease
Journal of Neurology
Journal of Neurology, Neurosurgery and Psychiatry
Journal of Pediatric Ophthalmology and Strabismus
Klinische Monatsblaetter fur Augenheilkunde

Lancet
Leprosy Review
Neurology
Neurosurgery
New Zealand Medical Journal
Ocular Therapy and Surgery
Ophthalmic Research
Ophthalmic Surgery
Ophthalmologica
Ophthalmology
Pediatrics
Plastic and Reconstructive Surgery
Public Health Reports
Radiology
Schweizerische Medizinische Wochenschrift
Southern Medical Journal
Transactions of the American Ophthalmological Society
Transactions of the Ophthalmological Society of New Zealand
Wiener Klinische Wochenschrift

Introduction

Doctor Hughes' retirement as editor of the YEAR BOOK OF OPHTHALMOLOGY after 22 years marks the 81st year of series publications by Year Book Medical Publishers, Inc. The past two decades have seen exponential growth in ophthalmology, with ultrasonography, computer-assisted tomography, rebirth of intraocular lenses, microscopic closed eye surgery, and new drugs for the treatment of viral disease and glaucoma, to name only a few. Doctor Hughes has helped us through the rapid evolutionary changes in our specialty with care and wisdom. As we look to the future, only one thing is sure: changes will occur at a still faster rate. Some may look with trepidation to a horizon apparently filled with ocular holograms, corneal endothelial cell transplantation, and retinal surgery performed on both the outer as well as the inner retina. We shall miss Dr. Hughes' sage comments on the articles he carefully culled from the world's literature.

In 1901, Casey A. Wood edited the Eye section of the first YEAR BOOK.* He selected 370 articles from the literature, and, it is interesting to note, approximately two thirds of these were in a foreign language and had to be abstracted into English. He used the *American Journal of Ophthalmology* and the *Archives of Ophthalmology,* as well as *Lancet* and *JAMA,* but Wood relied heavily on the German *Albrecht Von Graefes Archiv fur Klinische und Experimentelle Ophthalmologie* and the *Klinische Monatsblaetter fur Augenheilkunde* and the French *Annales d'Oculistique* and the *Archives d'Ophtalmologie* (combined in 1978 into the

---

*Beginning in 1901, Casey A. Wood edited the Eye section of the Eye, Ear, Nose, and Throat book, which was volume III of the PRACTICAL MEDICINE SERIES OF YEAR BOOKS. He was followed in 1925 by Charles P. Small and in 1931 by E. V. L. Brown and Louis Bothman. In 1934 the volume was distributed separately from the Series as the YEAR BOOK OF EYE, EAR, NOSE AND THROAT, and in 1940 Louis Bothman took over as sole editor of the Eye section. In 1949, Derrick Vail became editor; under his direction, a volume devoted exclusively to the eye was published as the 1957–58 YEAR BOOK OF OPHTHALMOLOGY. Doctor Hughes became editor beginning with the 1959–60 volume.

Journal Francais d'Ophtalmologie), plus articles from a host of other foreign presses. Over the years, the pendulum has moved toward more and more articles published in English and Japanese.

Today, over 50 journals devoted to ophthalmology alone are listed in *Index Medicus,* and new ones seem to appear with startling frequency. Moreover, at least that many more journals devoted to other fields have articles of interest to the ophthalmologist. A computer may be used to find information about a particular subject, but, if one is not careful, scores of articles will spew out of high-speed printers and one is back at the beginning.

Year Book Medical Publishers, Inc., currently subscribes to almost 500 journals, and the purpose of the YEAR BOOK series remains the same as its founder, G. P. Head, stated it to be over 80 years ago: ". . . (the YEAR BOOK is) . . . an epitome of much of the best literature of the year put into a volume convenient for reference." I will do my best to maintain the fine tradition established by Dr. Hughes and his predecessors, and I anticipate reading (if not editing) the YEAR BOOK OF OPHTHALMOLOGY on its 100th birthday in the year 2000.

J. TERRY ERNEST

1. Lids, Lacrimal Apparatus, and Orbit

Innovations in Oculoplastic Surgery

ALLEN M. PUTTERMAN, M.D.

Eye and Ear Infirmary
University of Illinois, Chicago

Each year brings innovations to procedures of oculoplastic surgery. Some of these I find helpful; others I modify or discard in preference to methods that have proved valuable through the years.

The Müller's muscle-conjunctiva resection procedure for ptosis continues to provide excellent, predictable results in ptotic lids that elevate to an almost normal level with application of phenylphrine drops into the upper fornix.[1] I now advocate an 8-mm resection if the lid elevates to normal with the phenylphrine test; the resection will vary from 6 to 9 mm if the level is slightly higher or lower, respectively, than normal.

The levator aponeurosis advancement-and-tuck procedure for ptosis is an alternative method to elevate eyelids with acquired ptosis.[2] Although a disinsertion of the levator aponeurosis seems to be the etiology in most cases of acquired ptosis, reattachment of the recessed levator to tarsus does not provide as high a success rate as does the Müller's muscle resection procedure. I therefore advocate the Müller's muscle procedure for lids with acquired ptosis that elevate to normal with phenylphrine and recommend the levator aponeurosis advancement-and-tuck procedure for those lids that do not elevate to normal with this test.

Epstein and I[3] recently have demonstrated that ptosis

secondary to levator aponeurosis disinsertion can also occur from the repeated insertion and removal of contact lenses.

The suture tarsorrhaphy system has decreased the incidence of exposure keratopathy after ptosis surgery.[4] The gradual opening of the eyelids, by the progressive removal of the lid sutures, permits the cornea to adapt slowly to its new unprotected state.

A graded excision of Müller's muscle, with or without stripping, and recession of the levator aponeurosis under sensory anesthesia without motor anesthesia brings thyroid-retracted lids to a normal level in about 95% of patients.[5,6] If the result is not acceptable, the simplified levator recession or internal vertical eyelid shortening procedure can bring the success rate to almost 100%.[7,8]

Basal cell cancer can be treated successfully almost 100% of the time by a full-thickness resection of the lid under frozen-section control.[9] It also seems to be the method of choice for cancer of the meibomian glands.[10]

The transmarginal rotation procedure for entropion has a greater than 90% success rate in the treatment of cicatricial entropion that is not associated with ocular pemphigoid.[11] By varying the distance of the incision from the lid margin and the position where the sutures exit in the margin, additional control of the procedure is obtained.[11] Pemphigoid is a more difficult problem, and the success rate of the transmarginal rotation procedure is only about 65%.

Hamako and Baylis[12] have described a new technique to treat lower lid retraction that may occur after cosmetic blepharoplasties. The authors release the internal lid adhesions from the inferior orbital rim and elevate the lid through a lateral canthal shortening, as described by Tenzel.[13] For severe cases, they advocate a graft of ear cartilage.[14] Ear cartilage is proving to be an excellent material to add vertical dimension to the retracted lower eyelid.

Conjunctivodacryocystorhinostomy with Silastic intubation of the canaliculi is a procedure advocated for those patients who have a partial obstruction of the upper and lower canaliculi, complete obstruction of the common canaliculus or a single canaliculus, or paresis of the orbicularis muscle.[15] It allows the surgeon to preserve the normal lacrimal apparatus and possibly to create patency of the obstructed pathways while simultaneously creating a new drainage channel if the reconstructed canaliculi again close.

Callahan's[16] method to reconstruct the temporally displaced medial canthus is ingenious. It avoids the time-consuming, complicated, and dangerous technique of transnasal wiring. A device similar to the piton used by mountain climbers is pounded into the nasal bone, and the medial canthal tendon is attached to it.

The contracted ocular socket continues to be relieved successfully by securing the midaspect of a full-thickness mucous membrane-lined custom-made conformer to the superior and inferior orbital rims.[17] All patients have had a spacious cul-de-sac formed by this procedure. The oral scar contracture has been reduced with the use of early exercises, in which the mouth is opened widely, while the cheek is pushed inward.

I now advocate that all pure isolated blowout fractures of the orbital floor be followed up until ocular motility and enophthalmos stabilize rather than wait the 4- to 6-month period of observation I originally recommended.[18,19] If persistence and stabilization of visually handicapping diplopia occur before 1 month after trauma, a standard orbital floor reconstruction is performed; if stabilization occurs after 1 month, extraocular muscle surgery is performed. If cosmetically unacceptable enophthalmos exists, it is treated with an orbital floor implant when it stabilizes, if associated with a downward sinking of the eye. A Müller's muscle conjunctival resection procedure is performed if the enophthalmos is associated with a narrow palpebral fissure that opens to normal with the phenylephrine test, and excision of skin and fat and elevation of the crease on the normal, contralateral upper lid is used if the enophthalmos is associated with a deep supratarsal sulcus.

I look forward to future advances in oculoplastic surgery.

References

1. Putterman A.M., Urist M.: Müller muscle-conjunctiva resection: Technique for treatment of blepharoptosis. *Arch. Ophthalmol.* 93:619, 1975.
2. Jones L.T., Quickert M.H., Wobig J.L.: The cure of ptosis

by aponeurotic repair. *Arch. Ophthalmol.* 92:629, 1975.
3. Epstein G., Putterman A.M.: Acquired blepharoptosis secondary to contact lens wear. *Am. J. Ophthalmol.* 91:634–639, 1981.
4. Putterman A.M.: Suture tarsorrhaphy system to control keratopathy after ptosis surgery. *Ophthalmic Surg.* 11:577–580, 1980.
5. Putterman A.M., Urist M.: Surgical treatment of upper eyelid retraction. *Arch. Ophthalmol.* 87:401, 1972.
6. Putterman A.M., Chalfin J.: Müller's muscle excision and levator recession in retracted upper lid. *Arch. Ophthalmol.* 97:1487–1491, 1979.
7. Putterman A.M., Urist M.J.: A simplified levator palpebrae superioris muscle recession to treat overcorrected blepharoptosis. *Am. J. Ophthalmol.* 77:358, 1974.
8. Putterman A.M.: Internal vertical eyelid shortening to treat surgically induced segmental blepharoptosis. *Am. J. Ophthalmol.* 82:122, 1976.
9. Putterman A.M., Chalfin J.: Frozen-section control in the surgery of basal cell carcinoma of the eyelid. *Am. J. Ophthalmol.* 876:802–809, 1979.
10. Epstein G., Putterman A.M.: Sebaceous adenocarcinoma of the eyelid. To be published.
11. Katzen L., Putterman A.M.: Transmarginal rotation entropion procedure. To be published.
12. Hamako C., Baylis H.: Lower eyelid retraction after blepharoplasty. *Am. J. Ophthalmol.* 89:517–521, 1980.
13. Tenzel R.R.: Treatment of lagophthalmos of the lower lid. *Arch. Ophthalmol.* 81:366, 1969.
14. Neuhaus H., Baylis H.: Complications of lower eyelid cosmetic surgery. In Putterman A.M. (ed.): *Cosmetic Oculoplastic Surgery.* New York, Grune & Stratton. In press.
15. Putterman A.M., Epstein G.: Combined Jones tube-canalicular intubation and conjunctivodacryocystorhinostomy. *Am. J. Ophthalmol.* 513–521, 1981.
16. Callahan M.A., Callahan A.: *Ophthalmic Plastic and Orbital Surgery.* Birmingham, Ala., Aesculapius Publishers, Inc., 1980, p. 164.
17. Putterman A.M., Scott R.: Deep ocular socket reconstruction. *Arch. Ophthalmol.* 95:1221, 1977.
18. Putterman A.M., Stevens T., Urist M.J.: Nonsurgical management of blowout fractures of the orbital floor. *Am. J. Ophthalmol.* 77:232, 1974.
19. Putterman A.M.: Late management of blowout fractures of the orbital floor, in Hornblass A. (ed.): *Third Symposium of Ophthalmic Plastic Surgery.* In press.

Chapter 1—LIDS, LACRIMAL APPARATUS AND ORBIT / 15

1–1 **Factors in Successful Surgical Management of Basal Cell Carcinoma of the Eyelids.** Basal cell carcinoma accounts for over 85% of all malignant epithelial tumors of the eyelids. Marcos T. Doxanas, W. Richard Green, and Charles E. Iliff (Johns Hopkins Med. Inst.) reviewed 126 cases of basal cell carcinoma of the lid managed by excision biopsy and 39 in which the margins of excision were monitored by frozen-section study. Excisions included 2 to 3 mm of surrounding, normal full-thickness skin and subepithelial tissue. Mean follow-up was 6½ years. About two thirds of the tumors were in the lower lid. Over half the patients were in their seventh and eighth decades.

Carcinomas had been inadequately excised in 21% of cases, in all of which frozen-section monitoring was omitted. Seven tumors recurred (4.2%), all in the group that had incomplete excision biopsy. In 8 other cases in the excision biopsy group the tumor margins were close to the surgical margins, but no recurrence was observed. Residual tumor was found in 5 of 7 cases in which reexcision was performed within 1 or 2 months after initial, incomplete excision. All recurrences were completely reexcised; 2 patients had exenterations. Basal cell carcinoma was not diagnosed preoperatively in about 40% of cases. Over half the lesions were nodular. Three recurrent tumors were of the morphea type, 3 were ulcerative lesions, and 1 was a nodular carcinoma.

Complete initial excision of basal cell carcinoma of the eyelid is important. Frozen-section monitoring of the surgical margins has an essential role in the management of these tumors. The ulcerative, multicentric, and morphea types of basal cell carcinoma frequently extend beyond the apparent area of clinical involvement because of dermal proliferation. When these types of tumor are incompletely excised, early reexcision is necessary, but the need for reexcision is reduced by frozen-section monitoring at initial operation. Close observation of incompletely excised nodular lesions appears to be acceptable.

1–2 **Incompletely Excised Basal Cell Carcinoma of the Ocular Adnexa.** Eugene O. Wiggs (Univ. of Colorado) asserts that adequate management of patients with incom-

---

(1–1) Am. J. Ophthalmol. 91:726–736, June 1981.
(1–2) Ophthalmic Surg. 12:891–896, December 1981.

pletely excised periocular basal cell carcinoma (BCC) requires evaluation of the relation between histologically carcinomatous surgical margins and recurrences. Close cooperation with a pathologist should minimize false positive results. Operation is generally considered to be the best approach to most BCCs, but this may not necessarily be true for patients with residual periocular disease. Radiotherapy is useful in patients who refuse further surgery and for palliation, but conjunctival keratinization may result, and multiple visits are necessary. Other options include cryotherapy and chemosurgery.

Nodular BCC is the least aggressive of the basal cell tumors. Operation with frozen-section control and chemosurgery are acceptable options. Cryotherapy spares tissue where a shortage exists, but it should not be used until the wound is reasonably strong. Cryotherapy may also be considered after major reconstruction where further surgery or chemosurgery might compromise a flap or skin graft, produce significant deformity, or result in corneal exposure. Careful observation has a role in the management of patients with incompletely excised BCCs of the eyelids after primary closure or lateral canthal lesions in certain circumstances.

Morpheaform, sclerosing, and ulcerative-invasive BCC are the most dangerous types. Residual lesions of these types require further careful and aggressive operation with frozen-section control or Mohs's chemosurgery. Repeat biopsy with frozen-section control is indicated at reconstruction after chemosurgery.

▶ [The authors of this article and the preceding one emphasize the generally accepted use of frozen-section monitoring of the tumor excision. Indeed, incomplete excisions only occurred when frozen-section technique was not used.] ◀

1-3 **Eyelid Tumors of Sweat Gland Origin** were described by M. Lahav, D. M. Albert, R. Bahr, and J. Craft. Tumors of sweat gland origin are not uncommon in the periocular region. These tumors may arise in two main types of sweat glands, eccrine and apocrine. The eccrine glands are also seen elsewhere in the skin. The apocrine glands are related to the pilosebaceous apparatus in the axilla, nipple, geni-

---

(1–3) Albrecht von Graefes Arch. Klin. Exp. Ophthalmol. 216:301–311, 1981.

tal, and anal regions. In the eyelid they appear as the specialized glands of Moll. Benign tumors of the sweat gland show a wide spectrum of differentiation, including syringoma, a benign hamartoma; porosyringoma, or clear cell myoepithelioma; and chondroid syringoma, or mixed tumors. The malignant counterparts of these tumors may be difficult to diagnose in view of the variability of the histopathologic patterns. Therefore, location, clinical behavior, and histochemical characteristics of the tumor should be considered. The authors recently examined 5 eyelid tumors that demonstrate the difficulties in the classification and diagnosis of such tumors.

The first 3 cases were diagnosed respectively as benign eccrine syringoma; mixed tumor of sweat gland origin, or chondroid syringoma; and benign mixed tumor, probably of sweat gland origin. The fourth case was diagnosed as benign sweat gland adenoma of ductal origin. However, because of its deeply infiltrative and scirrhous appearance and the clinical history, it was considered to be locally infiltrative. The fifth case is presented as follows:

Woman, 70, had a left lower lid lesion that had grown slowly for 3 years. The lesion was excised but recurred 3 years later. Surgical excision showed a brownish mass measuring $10 \times 5 \times 5$ mm. The chemical analysis of the mucinous substance suggested the presence of nonsulfated mucopolysaccharides or sialomucin. These findings and the results of the microscopic examination led to the diagnosis of mucus-secreting adenocarcinoma of sweat gland origin.

Because tumors of sweat gland origin may be infiltrative or may have metastatic potential despite their relatively benign appearance, great care should be taken to classify them correctly. The clinical history, biologic behavior, and morphologic and histochemical characteristics should all be considered in the diagnosis and management of these tumors.

1-4 **Lid Splitting and Posterior Lamella Cryosurgery for Congenital and Acquired Distichiasis.** Congenital distichiasis is a rare familial state in which an accessory row of lashes is present in or near the meibomian gland orifices.

(1-4) Arch. Ophthalmol. 99:631-634, April 1981.

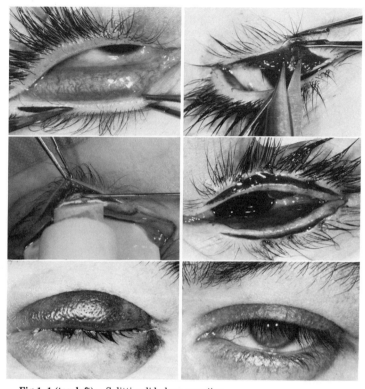

Fig 1–1 (top left).—Splitting lid along gray line.
Fig 1–2 (top right).—Sharp dissection of lid into anterior and posterior lamellae.
Fig 1–3 (center left).—Cryotherapy of posterior lamella with thermocouple in place.
Fig 1–4 (center right).—Anterior lamella recessed in posterior lamella.
Fig 1–5 (bottom left).—Lid edema evident 1 week after operation.
Fig 1–6 (bottom right).—Lid edema resolved 1 month after operation.
(Courtesy of Anderson, R. L., and Harvey, J. T.: Arch. Ophthalmol. 99:631–634, April 1981; copyright 1981, American Medical Association.)

Acquired distichiasis is seen in cases of Stevens-Johnson syndrome, ocular pemphigoid, and chemical and physical injury to the lids. Richard L. Anderson and John T. Harvey (Univ. of Iowa) devised a corrective operation and evaluated it in 13 lids with acquired distichiasis and, recently, in 4 lids with congenital distichiasis.

TECHNIQUE.—After injection of lidocaine with epinephrine and conjunctival instillation of phenylephrine, lid splitting is performed at the gray line (Fig 1–1), and dissection is carried out into the anterior and posterior lamellae (Fig 1–2), avoiding the normal anterior lash follicles. The posterior lamella is frozen to -20 to -25 C with the large, beveled tip of a nitrous oxide lid cryoprobe (Fig 1–3). A rapid freeze and slow thaw are followed by a second freeze and slow thaw. If the conjunctival surface of the lid is keratinized, curettage precedes cryosurgery. The anterior lamella then is recessed 2 to 3 mm from the lid margin with 6–0 chromic horizontal mattress sutures (Fig 1–4). The lashes are directed in a slightly everted position. Corticosteroid-neomycin ointment is used for at least a week postoperatively. If both lids are operated on, considerable swelling may be present, which resolves within a month of operation (Figs 1–5 and 1–6).

Seven of 13 lids with acquired distichiasis are symptom free after this operation. The other 6 lids have required minor cryosurgical touch-ups or occasional epilation of a trichiatic lash. A continuous margin of anterior lashes was obtained in 10 of the 13 lids. Conjunctival keratinization was substantially improved in most cases. Short-term follow-up of 4 patients treated for congenital distichiasis indicates good results.

Acquired distichiasis may represent reversion of the meibomian glands to complete pilosebaceous units. Congenital distichiasis probably represents failure of the primary epithelial germ to differentiate selectively into a sebaceous gland only. The authors' technique utilizes the advantages of cryosurgery and avoids many of its disadvantages.

1–5 **Complications of Cryosurgery.** John R. Wood and Richard L. Anderson (Univ. of Iowa) reviewed the complications occurring in 70 consecutive patients who had cryosurgery for trichiasis and lid lesions in a 2-year period, 58 of whom had adequate follow-up. The 30 male and 28 female patients had a mean age of 52 years. The average follow-up time was $9^1/_2$ months. A total of 133 lids were treated in this group. Fifty-three patients had trichiasis of varying causes. Four patients had benign lid lesions, and 1 had multiple basal cell carcinomas. Previous surgery for trichiasis had been done in 28% of affected patients. A nitrous oxide lid probe was used in all cases. In trichiasis, a freeze to -25 C was followed by thawing and then a refreeze to -20 C, epilation of lashes, and application of an antibiotic-steroid ointment.

Extensive lid edema followed cryosurgery, but patients generally had little or no pain postoperatively. A single treatment of double-freeze-thaw cryosurgery was adequate in 115 lids with trichiasis. There was some effect on symblepharon in patients with conjunctival shrinkage. Four of 6 patients with conjunctival keratinization showed loss of keratin and marked symptomatic improvement after treatment. Twelve lids showed evidence of misdirected, aberrant lashes in areas adjacent to the initial treatment site. Half of these patients had conjunctival shrinkage preoperatively. Fifteen patients had adverse reactions that were directly attributed to cryotherapy, including lid notch-necrosis, corneal ulcer formation, acceleration of symblepharon, xerosis, and severe cryotherapy reaction with pseudomembrane formation. One patient each had cellulitis and activation of herpes zoster, and 1 had visual loss. In all, 27% of the treated lids had complications. Complications occurred in 4 of 7 patients with reconstructed or irradiated lids who underwent cryotherapy.

About one fourth of eyelids subjected to cryotherapy had complications. Patients with conjunctival shrinkage preoperatively did poorly. No cases of epiphora or canalicular obstruction were observed. Cryosurgery probably remains the best means of managing trichiasis in difficult cases with a poor natural history, but it should be used cautiously in patients with conjunctival shrinkage and those with previously reconstructed or irradiated eyelids.

▶ [The success rate for the treatment of distichiasis is impressive for this difficult problem, but monitoring the temperature of the tissue with a thermocouple is essential and surgeons who do not have this equipment may not have such good results. The treatment of trichiasis without first splitting the lid is associated with some complications.] ◀

1-6 **Congenital Total Eversion of the Upper Eyelids.** In rare instances, infants may be born with total eversion of the upper eyelids and chemosis of the upper palpebral and conjunctival fornix. In severe cases, the conjunctival fornix may prolapse. K. O. Bentsi-Enchill (Univ. of Ghana) reviewed the findings in 8 cases of bilateral and 6 of unilateral congenital total eversion of the upper eyelids, seen in a 3-year period in Ghana. The infants were treated by lid suture only, by subconjunctival hyaluronidase injection and lid suture, or by hyaluronidase injection in one lid and lid suture after subconjunctival hyaluronidase injection in the other. Antibiotic eye ointment also was used. The dose of hyaluronidase injected was 750–1,500 units. Only topical anesthesia was used.

The typical appearance of unilateral total eversion is shown in Figure 1–7. None of the infants had Down's syndrome or any other abnormality. The longest time needed for the upper lid to revert to normal position after lid suture only was 4 days. With combined treatment, the lids were reverted with little or no edema on the first postoperative day, and the suture could be removed after 1–2 days without recurrence of lid eversion. Lid suture appeared to be necessary for early reversion of the eyelid position.

The lids of 150 consecutive newborn infants were also examined; 22 had upper lids that overlapped the lower lid margins to some degree.

Uterine contractions might cause eversion of the upper

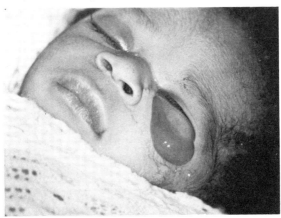

Fig 1–7.—Unilateral congenital total eversion of left upper eyelid. (Courtesy of Bentsi-Enchill, K. O.: Br. J. Ophthalmol. 65:209–213, March 1981.)

lid, and irritation of the exposed conjunctiva might produce acute blepharospasm, preventing spontaneous reversion. Conjunctival trauma then could lead to chemosis, further inhibiting reversion of the lid. The best treatment appears to be lid suture and subconjunctival hyaluronidase injection. Early correction reduces the risks of desiccation and infection of the exposed conjunctiva and decreases the hospital stay.

▶ [This rare disease seems easily treated and, in fact, lid suture alone solved the problem in 4 or less days. This seems safer than adding injections, and the short time should not cause sensory problems.] ◀

1–7 **Lid Surgery** is discussed by M. Hatt (Univ. of Zurich). The goal of plastic surgery is to reconstruct a normal functioning lid as accurately as possible. From the anatomic and physiologic point of view, the eyelid may be divided into three layers: a deep layer, comprising the tarsi and the canthal tendons with the levator aponeurosis and the lower lid retractors, the orbicularis muscle layer, and the skin. The function of the deep layer is to give form and stability to the lids. In treatment of lid injuries, minute reconstruction of this layer is of chief importance. The orbicularis muscle lies over the deep layer. In the upper lid it acts as antagonist to the levators and closes the lids. In the lower lid it has a dynamic part in retraction against gravity. Behind the orbital septum and between the deep and muscle layers lies the orbital adipose tissue. If exposed through injury, serious consequences are possible. Adipose tissue should not be removed but repaired. Frequently, it is enough to hold the septum and adipose tissue in their proper place by means of a faultless closure of the muscle layer. A drain is used in case of infection. The skin layer is thin and has a characteristic linear course. Because it has no subcutaneous fatty tissue, the skin is nourished through the muscle layer. Because of the danger of lagophthalmus of the upper lid and ectropion of the lower lid, vertical tension of the skin is prohibited.

From the beginning of surgery, special attention should be given to facial symmetry; therefore, both eyes should be kept open under sterile covering. In the management of

---

(1–7) Klin. Monatsbl. Augenheilkd. 178:244–247, April 1981.

Chapter 1—LIDS, LACRIMAL APPARATUS AND ORBIT / 23

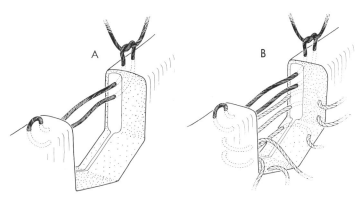

Fig 1–8.—Technique for lid closure. **A,** pattern of everted intermarginal 6–0 silk suture. **B,** pattern of 6–0 Dexon S or Vicryl sutures for adaptation of deep and muscle layers. (Courtesy of Hatt, M.: Klin. Monatsbl. Augenheilkd. 178:244–247, April 1981.)

Fig 1–9.—Technique for lid closure. **A,** closure of deep sutures and setting of additional sutures on lid edge. **B,** skin closure with inclusion of lid edge sutures in first knot. (Courtesy of Hatt, M.: Klin. Monatsbl. Augenheilkd. 178:244–247, April 1981.)

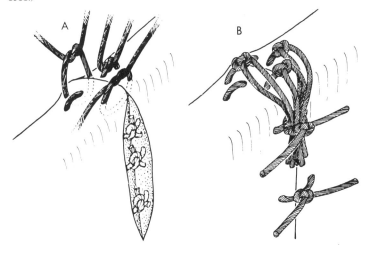

eyelid injuries, the meticulous reconstruction of the medial canthal tendon and canthus is extremely important. Only after reconstruction are the lids closed from medially to laterally and from deep to superficial tissues. The lid margin may be used as a guide in reconstruction (Figs 1–8 and 1–9). If the primary procedure is delayed, the injury should be covered with moist antibiotic compresses. The main sutures are removed after 5–7 days and the intermarginal sutures after 12 days.

1–8 **Use and Fate of Fascia Lata and Sclera in Ophthalmic Plastic and Reconstructive Surgery** are discussed by Charles K. Beyer and Daniel M. Albert (Harvard Med. School). Fascia lata is the best material to use in frontalis suspensions for ptosis (Fig 1–10). Nearly uni-

Fig 1–10.—Methods of frontalis suspension depicting different configurations of fascia in final position. (Courtesy of Beyer, C. K., and Albert, D. M.: Ophthalmology (Rochester) 88:869–886, September 1981.)

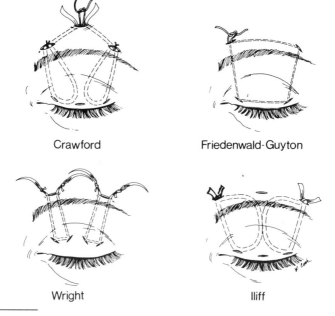

Chapter 1–LIDS, LACRIMAL APPARATUS AND ORBIT / 25

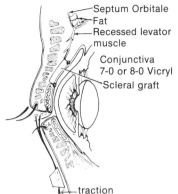

Fig 1–11.—Application of sclera in upper lid retraction. In this cross section, position of scleral graft is demonstrated. (Courtesy of Beyer, C. K., and Albert, D. M.: Ophthalmology (Rochester) 88:869–886, September 1981.)

versal success has been reported. Preserved fascia lata may be useful in reconstructing large excisions of the lid sector for tumor. A fascia lata sling may be helpful in lid malposition. Sclera has been proposed for use in place of fascia lata in ptosis surgery. Sclera also has been used in enucleation operations and in management of exposed and extruding implants. Other possible applications of sclera are in cicatricial upper lid entropion, lid reconstruction, and after overcorrection in ptosis surgery. The use of sclera in upper lid retraction is illustrated in Figure 1–11.

Examination of recovered homografts of preserved fascia lata showed mild fibroblastic infiltration for up to several years after implantation. Absorption was not apparent, and associated cellular reactions were not observed. In contrast to the histologically well-preserved fascia lata, scleral grafts exhibited significant degeneration with associated vascularization. Cellular and fibrotic reactions were not seen. Adverse tissue reactions and rejection have not occurred in the clinical use of scleral grafts.

Much remains to be learned of the fate of transplanted human tissues in ophthalmic surgery. Histologic evaluation of recovered implant materials will be most revealing. Neither animal studies nor clinical impressions are fully satisfactory means of determining the results of implantation of these tissues.

1–9 **Correction of Facial Contour Deformities With Prefabricated Sculptured Implants** is described by Richard K. Dortzbach, Sue C. Alexander, Francis C. Sutula, and Michael J. Hawes (Univ. of Wisconsin). Close cooperation between ophthalmologist and ocularist is necessary for optimal cosmetic results to be obtained with ocular prostheses.

Woman, 29, was seen 15 years after having sustained multiple facial fractures and trauma to the left eye in an automobile accident, resulting in enucleation. There was a deep left superior sulcus and a deformed right upper lid fold and crease. The left prosthesis was refitted by the modified impression technique, with silicone applied to a stone model rather than to the patient. The silicone mold was duplicated in methyl methacrylate, and implants of different volumes were fabricated. The implant that appeared to fit best in the subperiosteal space on the orbital floor was wired to the inferior orbital rim, beneath the periosteum (Figs 1–12 and 1–13). A blepharoplasty was done to revise the deformed right upper lid fold and crease. The appearances of both orbits improved.

Prefabricated sculptured implants are useful in correcting facial contour deformities. The implants are individu-

Fig 1–12 (left).—Deep superior sulcus. Orbital tissues sagging posteriorly and inferiorly.

Fig 1–13 (right).—Prefabricated implant placed on orbital floor beneath periosteum. Implant wired to inferior orbital rim, displacing orbital tissues anteriorly and superiorly to fill deep superior sulcus.

(Courtesy of Dortzbach, R. K., et al.: Ophthalmology (Rochester) 88:908–916, September 1981.)

(1–9) Ophthalmology (Rochester) 88:908–916, September 1981.

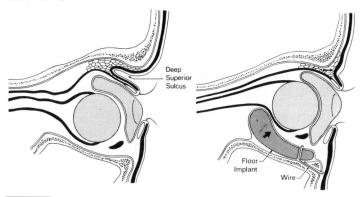

alized to correct the specific soft tissue or bony deformities, or both, in each case. Both bony and soft tissue defects can be corrected at the same time with the same implant. An implant can be placed beneath the periosteum or on top of the periosteum and wired to the underlying bone or fixed to the periosteum with Supramid Extra sutures. Correction of a superior sulcus deformity with a prefabricated orbital floor implant provides a measurable volume replacement and a stable structure, and it will not absorb. However, the implant should not be used where a seeing eye is present.

▶ [The authors of this article and the preceding one have described five implant techniques to solve problems otherwise impossible to repair. Nonetheless, there is still much to be learned about the long-term fate of implanted sclera, fascia lata, silicone and methyl methacrylate, as shown in the following article.] ◀

1–10 **Retraction of the Eyelids Secondary to Thyroid Ophthalmopathy: Its Surgical Correction With Sclera and the Fate of the Graft.** Joseph C. Flanagan examined the fate of grafted scleral material in the rabbit with regard to the use of this material in correcting eyelid retraction secondary to thyroid ophthalmopathy. Rabbit sclera was grafted into rabbit eyelids, and immunoperoxidase testing was carried out in 15 animals with bilateral scleral grafts by using absorbed guinea pig antirabbit sclera serum. A strong immunoperoxidase reaction was present in scleral grafts 1 to 2 weeks after surgery, when inflammation from the suture reaction was present. Peroxidase-positive inflammatory cells were present in the central part of the grafts in the second week. Scar tissue was not stained significantly. Scleral antigen remained 1 month after grafting, when suture material was no longer identifiable. Antigens persisted up to 8 months, long after evidence of inflammation had disappeared. Antigen remained present at 1 year but in reduced amounts.

Scleral grafts can be used to correct moderate to severe thyroidal lid retraction by using 2 mm of sclera for each millimeter of desired correction. Allogeneic scleral grafts in the rabbit eyelid survive for up to a year. Little histologic change is observed after the initial inflammatory reaction. Scleral antigen is detected in the grafts up to a year after surgery, although the amount declines over the postoperative period.

1-11 **The Natural History of Congenital Epiphora** due to an incompletely developed tear duct has been difficult to elucidate because of the availability of cure through probing. R. D. Suckling (Christchurch, New Zealand) reviewed the findings in 117 consecutive infants with congenital nonpatency of one or both tear ducts. In the first 31 infants, probing was delayed to age 10 months, when 17 eyes were still watering. In the next 43 children, probing of 13 eyes was delayed to age 14 months. In the last 43 children, probing of 11 eyes was delayed to age 21 months. Reprobing was necessary in 3 children in the first group, seen at an average age of 7.5 months, and in 4 in the second group, with an average age of 8.8 months when first seen. None in the third group, seen at an average age of 11.9 months, required reprobing.

There appears to be no risk in waiting for spontaneous opening of the congenitally blocked tear duct, apart from mild lid dermatitis due to tears and sensitivity to antibiotic drops if used. On the other hand, use of a general anesthetic carries a small risk to life as well as a small risk of morbidity and psychological upset. Probing can damage the lacrimal structures when not properly carried out. Epiphora is rarely observed in adults who were, for some reason, not treated in infancy.

▶ [In this series, a remarkable 94% of those infants left untreated until 21 months cured themselves.] ◀

1-12 **The Questionably Dry Eye.** The clinical picture can be confusing in patients with moderately depleted tear production. The differential diagnosis of the questionably dry eye includes chronic blepharoconjunctivitis, rosacea keratoconjunctivitis, allergic conjunctivitis, and other external eye diseases in early or atypical form. Ian A. Mackie (Moorfields Eye Hosp., London) and David V. Seal (Southampton, England) performed the Schirmer strip test in 41 subjects with normal eyes. False positive results were obviated by moving the strip to another site within the sac if no tear fluid appeared within 2 minutes. Tear lysozyme was

---

(1–11) N. Z. Med. J. 93:74–75, Feb. 11, 1981.

(1–12) Br. J. Ophthalmol. 65:2–9, January 1981.

measured in 255 eyes of 128 subjects. Studies were done in 20 patients with autoimmune disease, 23 with various external eye disorders not usually associated with dryness, 38 patients with questionably dry eyes; 30 with definite keratoconjunctivitis sicca; and 3 with a dry mouth and sore eyes.

The mean tear lysozyme ratio (TLR) in normal eyes was 2.25 units/µl, with a normal range of 1.05–4.75. Particulate matter in the tear film, which was seen in 23 of 75 questionably dry eyes, was associated with low lysozyme secretion. The mean TLR was reduced significantly in patients with questionably dry eyes even when particulate matter was not present, and also in patients with keratoconjunctivitis sicca. The mean Schirmer test value was not significantly reduced in patients with questionably dry eyes except when particulate matter was present. The mean value was significantly low in patients with keratoconjunctivitis sicca. The results of the two tests correlated well in this group, but not in patients with normal eyes. The lowest normal limit of the Schirmer test was set at 6 mm. The 3 patients with xerostomia had normal tear lysozyme levels with no evidence of keratoconjunctivitis sicca.

The Schirmer test is helpful in detecting eyes with severely depleted lysozyme secretion, but is unreliable in detecting eyes with moderately depleted lysozyme secretion. Xerostomia may occur in the absence of dry eyes. The questionably dry eye is best evaluated by the tear lysozyme test. A severely dry eye has a TLR below 0.5 units/µl and a Schirmer test value less than 6 mm.

▶ [The poor reliability of the Schirmer test is well known, but until now we had little else to help us with the frequent dry eye complaint. Measurement of the tear lysozyme concentration appears more reliable and sensitive than Schirmer testing. Further research is necessary to determine if there are other substances in tears that may change with decreased tear production.] ◀

1–13 **Meibomian Glands and Contact Lens Wear.** Antonio S. Henriquez and Donald R. Korb examined the meibomian glands of 38 consecutive patients with a primary complaint of contact lens intolerance, for which all conventional tests had failed to show a definite cause. Twelve subjects matched for age and sex who exhibited optimal contact lens toler-

(1–13) Br. J. Ophthalmol. 65:108–111, February 1981.

ance served as controls for bacteriologic and cytologic studies. The meibomian glands of the lower lid were studied by collecting samples of secretion at the lid margin after gentle or forceful expression.

The superficial oily layer of the tear film is chiefly a product of meibomian gland secretion. The glands are holocrine structures located within the tarsal plate of the lid. Duct obstruction presumably is more likely to occur where there is increased epithelial cell turnover, because of the accumulation of desquamated cells, especially near the lid margin (Fig 1–14). With stagnation, the duct dilates, sometimes without pouting of the orifices or inflammatory changes at the lid margin. Dead, desquamated epithelial cells in the stagnated secretions can provide a good culture medium for bacteria, but the presence of bacteria in smears was not always associated with clinical signs of inflammation or the presence of inflammatory cells in the secretions. Only 4 patients had specimens with large amounts of bacteria, and they had no inflammatory changes.

Contact lens intolerance associated with meibomian gland dysfunction may be due to mechanical obstruction of the glands by keratotic plugs, which can cause a change in the oily secretion, or to the release of bacteria or their toxic products, or both, into the precorneal tear film. Symptoms usually are absent unless the integrity of the tear film is impaired, possibly by either a contact lens or a significant change in environmental humidity or temperature. The most

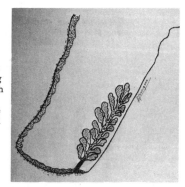

Fig 1–14.—Drawing illustrates mechanism of meibomian gland obstruction; desquamated epithelial cells from skin surface and inner ductal lining accumulate at exit of excretory duct, with formation of keratotic plug and subsequent stagnation of secretion inside gland. (Courtesy of Henriquez, A. S., and Korb, D. R.: Br. J. Ophthalmol. 65:108–111, February 1981.)

Chapter 1—LIDS, LACRIMAL APPARATUS AND ORBIT / 31

effective treatment relieves the obstruction by expressing the glands at appropriate intervals. Hot compresses and scrubs of the lid margins should be used at home on a daily basis.

▶ [The authors' implication is that meibomian gland orifices should be examined for epithelial plugs before contact lenses are prescribed.] ◀

1–14 **Endocrine Ophthalmopathy** is discussed by A. G. Bouzas (Athens). Endocrine ophthalmopathy usually is associated with hyperthyroidism, but it can also occur in euthyroid and even hypothyroid persons as well. The extraocular muscles may become swollen and markedly enlarged, and there also is an excess of orbital connective tissue and enlargement of the lacrimal gland. Mucopolysaccharides accumulate in the ground substance. Mast cells probably are responsible for protrusion of the eye. Retrobulbar connective tissue is increased and may prolapse forward through dehiscence into the orbital septum. The extraocular muscle changes include interstitial inflammatory edema with lymphocytes, macrophages, plasma cells, mast cells, and fatty infiltration.

Clinical changes progress from upper lid retraction and exophthalmos through soft tissue involvement and proptosis to extraocular muscle involvement. Finally the cornea is involved and vision is lost through optic nerve disease.

Ocular changes usually begin subacutely. Their course and duration vary widely in individual cases. Most often the ocular manifestations follow the treatment of hyperthyroidism. An association of open angle glaucoma with Graves' disease has been described. The pathogenesis of Graves' disease and endocrine ophthalmopathy remains unclear. Kriss demonstrated connections between the lymph drainage channels of the thyroid gland and the orbit. Extraocular muscle membrane has a particular affinity for thyroglobulin, and the binding of thyroglobulin-antithyroglobulin complexes to ocular muscle membranes may be pathogenically significant. High levels of circulating thyroglobulin antibody are found after treatment of hyperthyroidism.

Local treatment of endocrine ophthalmopathy includes the instillation of an antibiotic-decongestant preparation and

---

(1–14) Trans. Ophthalmol. Soc. U.K. 100:511–520, 1980.

the use of local adrenergic blocking agents, particularly guanethidine eye drops. When other measures including high-dose steroids have failed, orbital decompression is carried out. Careful control of associated thyroid dysfunction is important. Plastic surgery techniques are available to correct lid retraction, and extraocular muscle surgery may be indicated to correct secondary strabismus, diplopia, or disfigurement.

Orbital Graves' Disease: A Modification of the "NO SPECS" Classification. Henry J. L. Van Dyk (Louisiana State Univ., New Orleans) has reviewed both the original American Thyroid Association (ATA) classification of orbital changes in Graves' disease and the subsequent modification made by the ATA and has proposed some further changes. The modified classification of the ATA is outlined in Table 1. The mnemonic "NO SPECS" was retained in the modified classification. The criteria for grading of class II were dropped, and the designators of activity of the orbital process were omitted.

A further modification now is proposed that includes restoration of the listing of soft tissue signs; symptoms need not be included. The signs to be added, which may be subsumed under the mnemonic "RELIEF," are resistance to retrodisplacement of the eye, edema of the conjunctiva and caruncle, lacrimal gland enlargement, injection of the con-

TABLE 1.—ABRIDGED CLASSIFICATION OF EYE CHANGES OF GRAVES' DISEASE AS MODIFIED IN 1977

Class*	Definition
0	No physical signs or symptoms
I	Only signs, no symptoms (signs limited to upper eyelid retraction, stare, and eyelid lag)
II	Soft-tissue involvement (symptoms and signs)
III	Proptosis
IV	Extraocular muscle involvement
V	Corneal involvement
VI	Sight loss (optic nerve involvement)

*Each class usually, but not necessarily, includes the involvement indicated in preceding class.

TABLE 2.—PROPOSED SECOND MODIFICATION OF DETAILED
CLASSIFICATION OF ORBITAL CHANGES OF GRAVES' DISEASE*

Class	Grades	Orbital Signs
II		Resistance to retrodisplacement of eye
		Edema of conjunctiva/caruncle
		Lacrimal gland enlargement
		Injection of conjunctiva, focal or diffuse
		Edema of lids
		Fullness of lids
	0	Absent
	a	Minimal
	b	Moderate
	c	Marked

*First letter of each sign forms the mnemonic "RELIEF."

junctiva, edema of the lids, and fullness of the lids Table 2. The grades remain as before.

With the new classification, activity of the disease process is implied by specifying the grade within class II. An entirely satisfactory classification must await more knowledge of the pathogenesis and immunology of the process. It is hoped that restoration of specific soft tissue signs to class II of the ATA classification of orbital Graves' disease will provide greater clinical specificity in describing affected patients.

1–16 **Surgical Treatment of Thyroid-Related Upper Eyelid Retraction: Graded Müller's Muscle Excision and Levator Recession** is described by Allen M. Putterman (Univ. of Illinois). A method of excising Müller's muscle, with or without recession of the levator aponeurosis, yielded excellent cosmetic results in 47 of 53 consecutive upper lids in patients with thyroid ophthalmopathy. The other 6 patients had minor complications remedied by further surgery. Another 49 upper lids now have been managed, with equally good results on follow-up for up to 3 years. Only 1 of these patients required further surgery for residual lid retraction. The procedure is illustrated in Figure 1–15.

(1–16) Ophthalmology (Rochester) 88:507–512, June 1981.

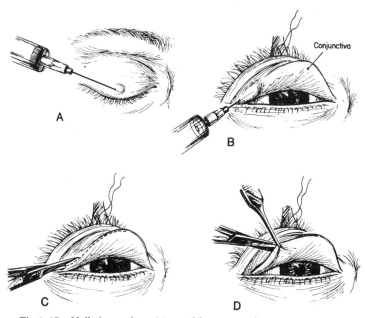

Fig 1–15.—Müller's muscle excision and levator muscle recession. **A,** subcutaneous administration of anesthetic for retraction suture. **B,** subconjunctival administration of anesthetic. **C,** conjunctival incision along temporal two thirds of superior tarsal border. **D,** dissection of conjunctiva from Müller's muscle. *(Continued.)*

TECHNIQUE.—Local anesthesia is used after premedication with promethazine and meperidine. The conjunctiva is entered just over the superior tarsal border at the temporal aspect of the lid and cut from the superior tarsal border with iris scissors to separate it from Müller's muscle. Müller's muscle then is cut from the tarsus temporally and undermined from the levator aponeurosis at the level of the superior tarsal border over the temporal two thirds of the lid. If the lid remains retracted with the patient sitting, the levator muscle must be released. The aponeurosis is lengthened stepwise, after which the detached part of Müller's muscle is excised. The conjunctiva then is sutured to the superior tarsal border, and a traction suture is inserted and left for a variable period.

This is the preferred treatment of thyroid-related retraction of the upper eyelid. It is a relatively simple procedure that is based on the physiologic and anatomical nature of

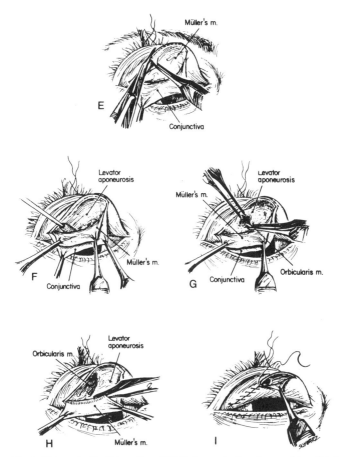

Fig 1–15 *(cont.).*—**E**, disinsertion of Müller's muscle from temporal two thirds of superior tarsal border. **F**, dissection of Müller's muscle from levator aponeurosis. **G**, stripping of levator aponeurosis. **H**, excision of Müller's muscle, also showing recessed levator aponeurosis. **I**, suture of conjunctiva to superior tarsal border. (Courtesy of Putterman, A. M.: Ophthalmology (Rochester) 88:507–512, June 1981.)

the disorder. When the second upper lid is treated, several weeks after the initial operation, the lid should be placed at the same level as that to which the first was placed at operation.

▶ [Surgery for upper eyelid retraction is sometimes necessary, although basic to the disease are its remissions and exacerbations. Guanethidine eye drops are sometimes effective, but are not routinely used in the United States.] ◄

1–17 **Diagnosis and Treatment of Thyroid Myopathy.** William E. Scott and Jill A. Thalacker (Univ. of Iowa, Iowa City) reviewed the results of treatment in 25 patients with thyroid myopathy, 23 of whom had a laboratory diagnosis of hyperthyroidism. Medical treatment of thyroid disease was given to 21 patients. All were hypothyroid and on supplemental treatment or were euthyroid for at least 6 months before ocular surgery. Twelve patients had a trial of prisms, and 6 temporarily wore a patch over 1 eye to eliminate diplopia. Prisms eliminated the need for surgery in only 3 cases. Five other patients had undergone orbital decompression before muscle surgery. The extraocular muscles involved are shown in the table. Adjustable sutures have been used in recessing the extraocular muscles. The inferior rectus was recessed 3–7 mm; the medial recti, 3.5–8.5 mm; and the superior recti, 4–5 mm.

All but 2 of the 22 patients who had surgery were followed for 6 months or longer. Full versions and normal motility were restored in only 4 cases. Four patients required a second procedure for postoperative hypertropia. All but 4 patients were able to fuse without prisms in the primary position. Ten patients were left with limited abduction, whereas 2 showed limited adduction postoperatively. Seven patients had mildly limited depression, and 10 had limited upgaze postoperatively.

Adjustable sutures are important in extraocular muscle surgery in patients with thyroid myopathy because the ex-

MUSCLE INVOLVEMENT IN 25 PATIENTS*

Muscles	No.	Percent
Inferior rectus	20/25	80%
Medial rectus	11/25	44%
Superior rectus	6/25	24%
Lateral rectus	0/25	0%

*Involvement may have occurred alone or in combination with other muscles.

act amount of recession needed often is difficult to determine in restrictive problems. Postoperative hypertropia in a few of the present patients is attributed to progression of the disease or masked involvement of the superior rectus, or both. A large majority of patients were left with some area of limitation postoperatively. An upgaze limitation is preferable to a downgaze problem because a reading position is more frequently required by adults.

1-18 **Graves' Ophthalmopathy: Immunologic Parameters Related to Corticosteroid Therapy.** Steroids have been used empirically in patients with Graves' ophthalmopathy. A decrease in thymus-derived rosette-forming lymphocytes has been described in most patients with active progressive Graves' ophthalmopathy. Robert C. Sergott, Norman T. Felberg, Peter J. Savino, John J. Blizzard, and Norman J. Schatz (Philadelphia) related the response to steroid therapy to T lymphocyte status in 17 steroid-responsive patients with progressive Graves' ophthalmopathy; the 10 women and 7 men had a mean age of 45.5 years. All patients had painful, restrictive ophthalmoplegia and proptosis exceeding 23 mm; 8 also had decreased visual acuity from dysthyroid optic neuropathy. All patients were euthyroid when steroid therapy was begun. Findings in 5 steroid-resistant patients, 3 women and 2 men with a mean age of 49.6 years, also were evaluated. Two had decreased visual acuity.

Both numbers and percentages of active and total rosette-forming cells increased after the institution of oral prednisone therapy in the steroid-responsive patients, but a significant decrease in active rosette-forming cells occurred in the steroid-resistant patients. The responsive patients had no significant changes in percentages of B cells and complement receptor rosettes. Steroid therapy increased the lymphoblast transformation response to phytohemagglutinin in a steroid-responsive patient, but decreased the response in a steroid-resistant patient.

Possible mechanisms for an increase in T lymphocytes with steroid therapy in steroid-responsive patients having Graves' ophthalmopathy include a change in the lympho-

---

(1–18) Invest. Ophthalmol. Vis. Sci. 20:173–182, February 1981.

cyte membrane; release of T cells from storage sites; prevention of the egress of circulating cells to sites of tissue damage; and maturation of T cells from T cell precursors. Elucidation of the mechanism should permit more precise treatment of Graves' ophthalmopathy. The goal is to determine which patients will improve with steroid treatment and which should receive other therapy.

▶ ["Therapeutic trials" of corticosteroids are common clinical practice but there are risks, so knowing which patients will respond ahead of time seems very desirable.] ◀

1–19 **Optic Nerve Involvement in Dysthyroidism.** The estimated prevalence of optic neuropathy in dysthyroidism is less than 5%, but it is a preventable cause of serious visual loss. Jonathan D. Trobe (Univ. of Florida, Gainesville) reviewed the findings in 21 patients, 14 of whom had at least a 3-month history and 7 of whom had noted visual loss for more than 6 months before initial evaluation. All 21 patients with visual loss reported congestive symptoms, which had preceded visual loss by at least 1 month and by an average of 4 months. Only 2 patients had exposure keratopathy sufficient to reduce visual acuity. Twelve patients had proptosis of more than 25 mm. All patients had lid retraction or edema, conjunctival injection or chemosis, and ductional defects. Ductions were comparably reduced in all directions in both eyes. The optic nerve head appeared normal in most cases. Where disk swelling is present, it is not distinctive.

Patients with Graves' optic neuropathy tend to be older than those with Graves' disease in general. Other clinical features are similar. The lack of marked proptosis in patients with optic neuropathy and the symmetrical restriction of motility suggest an orbital panmyositis.

Some untreated patients will recover spontaneously, but permanent deficits can be disabling. Dramatic improvement in vision has been described with oral corticosteroids as well as supervoltage irradiation. Surgical decompression of the orbit may be effective; recently, removal of the orbital floor and parts of the nasal orbital wall, as described by Ogura, has been recommended. Patients with chronic

---

(1–19) Ophthalmology (Rochester) 88:488–492, June 1981.

sclerosing disease have a poorer prognosis than those with acute congestive features. Early diagnosis is of critical importance. Where patients are refractory to one type of treatment, another may prove to be effective.

▶ [It is obvious that thyroid ophthalmopathy continues to present the ophthalmologist with extraordinarily difficult problems. Upper eyelid retraction may be a serious problem, although many cases seem to resolve spontaneously if the patient is willing to wait a relatively long time. Myopathy, however, is more serious because resulting diplopia may be incapacitating. The use of adjustable sutures is important in these difficult surgical cases (see the introductory article, "The Adjustable Suture," in Chapter 2). Optic nerve involvement, although rare, results in loss of vision and must be treated early if there is to be recovery.] ◀

1–20 **Periorbital and Orbital Cellulitis in Childhood.** L. P. Noel, W. N. Clarke, and T. A. Peacocke (Children's Hosp. of Eastern Ontario, Ottawa) reviewed the findings in 47 children seen from 1977 to 1979 with a diagnosis of orbital or periorbital cellulitis. The 25 children with orbital cellulitis had a mean age of 6 years. All had marked lid swelling, 10 had chemosis, and 7 had restricted extraocular muscle movements. Four children had proptosis. Papilledema was seen in the 1 patient who developed a brain abscess. Sinusitis was observed roentgenographically in 22 cases. The most common organisms isolated from blood, eye, nose, and throat specimens were *Hemophilus influenzae,* hemolytic streptococci and *Staphylococcus aureus*. Most patients received combined intravenous ampicillin and cloxacillin therapy, and all but 1 responded well to antibiotic treatment. The patient who developed a brain abscess from spread of frontal sinusitis required neurosurgical drainage.

The 22 patients with periorbital cellulitis had a mean age of 5 years. An external site of infection was seen in all cases. Five patients had primary bacterial conjunctivitis. Mild sinusitis was seen in 2 of the 8 patients examined. The most common causative organisms were *S. aureus, H. influenzae,* and hemolytic streptococci. About half the patients received combined intravenous cloxacillin and ampicillin therapy, but antibiotic treatment was quite varied in this group.

Blood and conjunctival cultures had the highest yield in

(1–20) Can. J. Ophthalmol. 16:178–180, October 1981.

these cases and should be obtained in all cases of orbital cellulitis. Many cases of periorbital cellulitis due to bacterial conjunctivitis or a hordeolum could have been treated more efficiently with topical antibiotic administration on an outpatient basis, but they were not distinguished from more serious preseptal infections. All cases of presumed orbital or periorbital cellulitis should be assessed as soon as possible by an ophthalmologist.

1–21 **Infraorbital Fold in Atopic Dermatitis.** It has been suggested that a linear wrinkle beneath the margin of the lower eyelid is an indication of atopy. Masami Uehara (Shiga Univ. of Med. Science, Seta, Japan) sought evidence of the infraorbital fold in 300 consecutive patients with atopic dermatitis and in 11 patients with allergic contact dermatitis of the lower lids. A linear wrinkle of the lower lid was seen in 74 (25%) of the 300 patients and an eczematous or lichenified lesion of the lower lids in 69 (23%). Of the latter patients, 57 (83%) showed an infraorbital fold. Eight of 17 patients with an infraorbital fold but no lower lid dermatitis had a history of recalcitrant dermatitis of the lower lids. Fifty (85%) of 59 patients with bilateral infraorbital

Fig 1–16.—Girl, aged 14, with atopic dermatitis with infraorbital fold and lower eyelid dermatitis bilaterally. (Courtesy of Uehara, M.: Arch. Dermatol. 117:627–629, October 1981; copyright 1981, American Medical Association.)

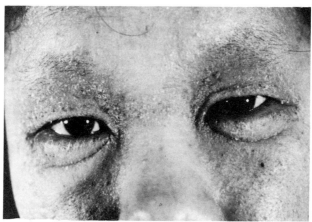

folds also had lower lid dermatitis bilaterally (Fig 1–16). All but 1 of 15 patients with a unilateral infraorbital fold exhibited the fold in the lower lid where dermatitis was present. The incidence of an infraorbital fold in 300 age- and sex-matched control subjects was 2.3%. A fold was present in 8 of the 11 patients with allergic contact dermatitis of the lower lids.

This study failed to show that a linear wrinkle of the lower eyelid is a phenotypic marker of atopy. An infraorbital fold was present only rarely in normal subjects but occurred frequently in patients with allergic contact dermatitis who had chronic eczematous changes in the lower eyelids. It seems likely that an infraorbital fold develops when the lower lid is involved by a chronic eczematous dermatitis of any cause. Its frequent occurrence in patients with atopic dermatitis may simply reflect the fact that the eyelid is a site of predilection for this condition.

2. Motility

The Adjustable Suture

EUGENE R. FOLK, M.D.
MARILYN T. MILLER, M.D.

Eye and Ear Infirmary
University of Illinois, Chicago

The adjustable suture procedure is the "hot" item at strabismus meetings in much the same manner that discussions on implants draw crowds at cataract meetings. Adjustable sutures are not a novel idea, as noted by Helveston,[1] along with Ellis,[2] and Scott et al.[3] One of us happened to be sitting next to one of the senior ophthalmologists (renowned for his work in intraocular tumors) during the 1965 Academy meeting when he remarked, with reference to the presentation of Thorsen, Jampolsky, and Scott[4] on the use of the adjustable sutures, that he had heard that same lecture at the same Academy in Chicago 30 years previously.—Oh well, nothing is really new.

The principle of a second chance is appealing to all strabismologists (which perhaps indicates the current status of strabismus therapy). The essence of the adjustable suture is to place the muscle in such a manner that the muscle can be advanced or loosened postoperatively when the patient is fully alert (this is very important, as adjustment in a sedated patient does not work well). The best known description of this technique is presented by Jampolsky.[5] Scott et al.[3] report a slight modification of the method. The adjustable suture usually is placed on the recessed muscle, but may be done on a resected muscle.

Initially, the classic indications for the adjustable suture were thyroid myopathy, superior oblique palsies and reoperations—especially reoperations for overcorrection. However, as the strabismus surgeons have become more comfortable with the technique, it has become the procedure of choice in most adults.[5-7] It is truly amazing the degree of shift and manipulation that most patients tolerate with little or no discomfort. As one becomes more experienced with the technique, more confidence is developed and the adjustment is easier.

There are divergent opinions concerning several aspects of this operation. Jampolsky[5] and Rosenbaum[7] deliberately overrecess so that adjustment is almost always necessary; the rationale is that it is easier to bring the muscle forward than to attempt to have it slip back or push it back. However, Scott et al.[3] advocate placing the muscle where the surgeon feels it should be and adjusting when the eyes are not straight at the first postoperative visit. With this technique, fewer adjustments are necessary, but undercorrections are more frequent. Nevertheless, we prefer this system because the adjustment is not free from problems, and it is better not to have to do any manipulation if you can avoid it.

There is also a question about timing the adjustment. Some propose it should be done the afternoon of surgery, while others perform the adjustment the following morning. It probably makes little difference as long as the patient is fully awake. Adjustments in the patient who is sedated or drowsy may cause you to make decisions that are not justified.

The major problem is deciding on the optimum position of the eyes at the time of the postoperative adjustment. In a study by Rosenbaum et al.,[8] relatively little change was found to occur in the postoperative period after the adjustment had been made. However, some patients do show differences in the ocular alignment during the next few weeks or months after surgery. The correlation of the eye position on the first postoperative day with the final result is not clearly known and may vary with a number of factors, as the patients are a very heterogeneous group with regard to etiology of the disorder, age, previous surgery, and other factors. The diplopia patient is usually adjusted for single binocular vision in the primary position, but this optimum position may not exist in all fields of gaze, especially the crucial down position. At times, one has to give preference to one of these positions during the adjustment. There has not been sufficient discussion in the literature about this exceedingly important aspect of the adjustable suture technique. The most pertinent comment about this subject is the observation of Scott et al.: "One usually knows where you do not want the eye to be." Eliminating this undesirable postoperative position is the attraction to the strabismologist.

Another infrequently mentioned problem is the increased pain and prolonged recovery time for the patient with this technique. There are a few patients with whom "just a slight adjustment" becomes a formidable experience for both patient and ophthalmologist. Also, the adjustable suture technique frequently requires a modification in the ophthalmologist's schedule. It is useful to have the option of making the adjustment either the day of operation or the next morning if there is no disadvantage to the desired outcome of the surgery.

In summary, the adjustable suture operation is an excellent addition to our surgical options. The importance of slight variations in technique should be established over the next few years as we gain more experience and have an opportunity to observe the natural history of patients who have had this procedure.

References

1. Helveston E.: *Atlas of Strabismus Surgery*. St. Louis, Mosby, 1977.
2. Helveston E., Ellis F.: Adjustable sutures for horizontal and vertical strabismus. *Am. J. Ophthalmol.* 28:18, 1975.
3. Scott W.E., Martin-Casals A., Jackson V.B.: Adjustable sutures in strabismus surgery. *J. Pediatr. Ophthalmol.* 14:71, 1977.
4. Thorsen J.C., Jampolsky A., Scott A.B.: Topical anesthesia for strabismus surgery. *Trans. Am. Acad. Ophthalmol. Otolaryngol.* 76:968, 1966.
5. Jampolsky A.: Current techniques of adjustable suture surgery. *Am. J. Ophthalmol.* 88:406, 1979.
6. Jampolsky A.: Strabismus re-operation techniques. *Trans. Am. Acad. Ophthalmol. Otolaryngol.* 79:704, 1975.

7. Rosenbaum A.L.: The use of adjustable suture procedures in strabismus surgery. *Am. J. Ophthalmol.* 28:88, 1978.
8. Rosenbaum A.K., Metz H.S., Carlson M., Jampolsky A.: Adjustable rectus muscle recession surgery: A follow-up study. *Arch. Ophthalmol.* 95:817, 1977.

2-1 **Photographic Screening for Strabismus and High Refractive Errors of Children Aged 1–4 Years.** The early detection of abnormal refractive errors is necessary to prevent squint or amblyopia, or both. Kari Kaakinen (Univ. of Helsinki) developed a simple photographic method of screening for squint and high refractive errors in children that involves simultaneous photographing of the corneal and fundus reflexes. The method was used on 182 children aged 1–4 years in the course of annual screening at a children's health care center. Mydriatic and cycloplegic drops were not used. Twenty randomly selected children with normal photographs were evaluated clinically.

All the normal photograph subjects had normal clinical examinations. Two cases of marked esodeviation were detected from photographs. Both these patients had an apparent squint on clinical examination. One of 5 patients with possible microstrabismus had about +2 degrees of microesotropia, whereas 4 patients had straight eyes. Two cases of hyperopia and 2 of anisocoria were detected. Four subjects were incorrectly thought to have possible microstrabismus and 2, asymmetrical fundus reflexes. The rate of technical failure was 2.7%.

This simple photographic method is useful in rapidly screening young children for strabismus and gross refractive errors. Paramedical personnel can apply the method after a short training period. A more complicated and sensitive photographic method for measuring refractive errors in children and for assessing astigmatism has also been developed.

2-2 **Development of Monofixation Syndrome in Congenital Esotropia.** Patients have been described who, in addition to a deviation of 8 PD or less on prism and cover testing, have a central scotoma, stereopsis, and good fusional vergences. The eyes of patients with this monofixa-

(2-1) Acta Ophthalmol. (Copenh.) 59:38–44, February 1981.
(2-2) J. Pediatr. Ophthalmol. Strabismus 18:42–44, Jan.–Feb. 1981.

DEVELOPMENT OF MONOFIXATION SYNDROME IN CONGENITAL ESOTROPIA*		
Months*	Patients	%
6-12	5 of 11	45%
13-24	7 of 17	41%
25-36	1 of 11	9%
37-66	0 of 11	0%
Totals:	13 of 50	26%

*Age at which surgically aligned to 8 PD or less of esotropia.

tion syndrome (MS) remain aligned for a long period. Rene Vazquez, Joseph H. Calhoun, and R. D. Harley (Philadelphia) attempted to determine whether the MS reduces the likelihood of horizontal strabismus or manifest vertical deviation developing. A study was made of 125 patients with constant esotropia before the age of 6 months and with 8 PD or less of esotropia by the cover-uncover test after the last operation. No amblyopia or organic visual deficit was present. Patients were more than 4½ years old at the time of study, and the average age was 9 years. The average time from the last surgical procedure was 5.3 years.

Development of the MS is shown in the table. The syndrome developed most frequently in patients who were operated on before age 2 years and was not observed in those operated on after age 3 years. The horizontal alignment remained stable an average of 8½ years after the last surgical procedure in the 13 patients with MS. Four patients had dissociated vertical deviation. Six patients had overaction of the inferior obliques, 3 of them after straightening to 8 PD or less of esotropia. No patient with dissociated vertical deviation had a manifest hypertropia in either eye. Of patients without MS, 30% had dissociated vertical deviation and 40.5% had overaction of the inferior obliques. Six of the 11 patients with dissociated vertical deviation had a manifest hypertropia of either or both eyes for more than half the day.

About half of patients with congenital esotropia had MS if aligned before age 2 years. Manifest hypertropia develops more frequently in patients with dissociated vertical deviation who do not have MS. Exotropia is more likely to develop in subsequent years in patients without MS. The overall need for further surgery is reduced by the development of MS.

▶ [The debate about early versus late surgery for congenital esotropia continues. These authors show that the monofixation syndrome develops more frequently in patients having early surgery. Moreover, in patients who have the monofixation syndrome, there is a decrease in the likelihood that further surgery will be necessary.] ◀

2–3 **Therapy of Anisometropic Amblyopia.** Jane D. Kivlin and John T. Flynn (Univ. of Miami) reviewed data on 67 patients with anisometropic amblyopia seen in the past 15 years, excluding patients with strabismus, congenital glaucoma, and other organic ocular problems. Nearly all patients were detected on routine screening, usually at school. Average age at presentation was 7 years. Refractive errors of the amblyopic eyes ranged from -18 to $+8$ D, with anisometropia of -19 to $+6$ D. Hyperopic and myopic differences each accounted for 40% of cases. The median initial corrected acuity in the amblyopic eye was 20/70; 7 patients had acuity of 20/40 or better. Treatment was with glasses only in 21 patients, glasses followed by patching in 17, and patching from the outset in 25. Two patients were not treated. Two thirds of patients completed recommended treatment and were followed for more than 1 year.

Both initial vision and best vision achieved correlated significantly with amount of anisometropia in both myopic and hyperopic patients. Best vision achieved also correlated with initial vision (Fig 2–1) in the overall group and in the myopic patients. Apart from the patients whose initial acuity was 20/40 or better, 28% of subjects achieved 20/20 vision, and another 42% achieved 20/40 or better. Patients with stereopsis had better initial and better final vision. Treatment with glasses only and with both glasses and patching gave comparable results. Median time to maximum vision was 8 months. Ten treatment failures were due to incorrect spectacle prescriptions. Three patients developed deviation of alignment with constant diplopia while being patched. Three of 35 patients who had vision of 20/40 or better after treatment relapsed on later follow-up.

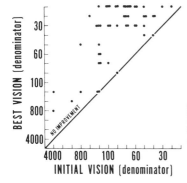

Fig 2–1.—Best vision achieved vs. initial vision (all patients). (Courtesy of Kivlin, J. D., and Flynn, J. T.: J. Pediatr. Ophthalmol. Strabismus 18:47–56, Sept.–Oct., 1981.)

Patients with lower amounts of anisometropia tend to do well with glasses alone. Although many patients in this study had extreme anisometropia or markedly poor vision, the group as a whole did well. Even highly myopic patients have been treated successfully. Several months may be necessary, and full astigmatic correction and continued use of glasses are important.

2–4 **New Clinical Aspects of Stimulus Deprivation Amblyopia.** Stimulus deprivation amblyopia is a reduction in visual acuity in patients in whom foveal visual stimulation was absent or inadequate early in life. The causes include complete congenital blepharoptosis, surgical tarsorrhaphy, prolonged bandaging of 1 eye, corneal opacities, cataracts, and severe uncorrected refractive errors. Gunter K. von Noorden (Baylor College of Medicine, Houston) reviewed findings in 11 patients with stimulus deprivation amblyopia.

Amblyopia was associated with unilateral visual deprivation starting before age 6 and lasting 1 month to 3 years. The cause of visual deprivation could not be related to the severity of amblyopia. The severity of amblyopia varied in patients having comparable periods of visual deprivation. Two patients had eccentric fixation in the amblyopic eye. With 1 exception, no patient with an onset of amblyopia before age 30 months responded to treatment, but treatment did not begin until they were aged 2½ years or older.

(2–4) Am. J. Ophthalmol. 92:416–421, September 1981.

Treatment was effective in 2 of 4 patients who became amblyopic at or after age 30 months.

Visual deprivation in infants may sometimes be unavoidable; however, early treatment offers a good chance of visual recovery, thus it must not be delayed until the child is aged 30 months or older. The risk of causing amblyopia in the patched eye must be considered during treatment. This may be avoided by switching the patch to the deprived eye at regular intervals. The findings in 1 patient treated successfully during infancy indicated that the deleterious effects of visual deprivation from birth may be preventable. Distinction between stimulus deprivation amblyopia and occlusion amblyopia no longer appears justified.

2–5 **Contact Lenses in Management of Myopic Anisometropic Amblyopia.** Amblyopia secondary to unilateral severe myopia has a poor prognosis with either pleoptic therapy or occlusion therapy. Marilyn Mets and Ronald L. Price (Cleveland Clinic) evaluated contact lens correction of the refractive error with occlusion in 16 patients seen during 3 years with anisometropic myopia with amblyopia. The amblyopic eye had a spherical equivalent of at least -5.00 diopters and there was a difference between the eyes of at least 5.00 diopters (D). All patients used contact lens correction of the refractive error in the more myopic eye. The 10 girls and 6 boys had a mean age at the outset of 5 years. The mean spherical equivalent of the more myopic eye was -10.00 D, and the mean difference between the eyes was 10.25 D. Eight patients had strabismus; 3 had esotropia and 5, exotropia.

Ten patients achieved final acuities of 6/12 or better. Three others improved by 2 or more Snellen lines, whereas 3 patients showed little if any improvement (Fig 2–2). The latter patients had myelinated retinal nerve fibers. None of the others had retinal abnormalities that could cause a significant reduction in visual acuity. The patients who improved but not to 6/12 or better had the greatest myopia in the amblyopic eye and began treatment with the poorest visual acuity. Presence of strabismus did not appear to influence the final visual outcome. Contact lens wear did not present a problem in these children. All patients achieved

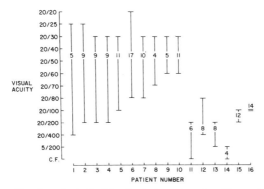

Fig 2–2.—Visual results in the 16 patients shown in order of decreasing response to occlusion. Lower bar indicates preocclusion visual acuity and upper bar, final visual acuity. (Courtesy of Mets, M., and Price, R. L.: Am. J. Ophthalmol. 91:484–489, April 1981.

6–8 hours of continuous lens wear within 10 days of receiving their lenses, and no significant complications occurred.

These results compare favorably to those achieved by spectacle correction in cases of amblyopia secondary to unilateral severe myopia. With contact lenses the correction is in place more of the time, and the wearer generally is unaware of their presence. Peripheral distortion is absent, leading to more comfortable vision. Most patients with strabismus responded well to occlusion. Contact lenses do not appear to prevent binocularity in anisometropic myopia.

2–6 **Extended-Wear Soft Contact Lenses in the Treatment of Strabismic Amblyopia.** Interest has been expressed in the use of extended-wear soft contact lenses, which can be used continuously for several months and are particularly suitable for children, in patients with strabismic amblyopia. J. Elmer, Y. A. Fahmy, M. Nyholm, and K. Nørskov (Copenhagen) evaluated an extended-wear, lathe-cut soft lens, the Duragel 75, Scanles 24 h, containing 76% water, in 18 amblyopic patients aged 4 to 9 years. Fourteen had a manifest convergent squint and 4 a divergent squint. Each had a central acuity of 6/60 or better in the amblyopic eye. Plaster occlusion was abandoned for various reasons

(2–6) Acta Ophthalmol. (Copenh.) 59:546–551, August 1981.

in these cases, including plaster allergy, cosmetic reasons, and refusal of the child to wear plaster.

Only 1 of the 18 children failed to reach an acuity of 6/9. Eleven achieved equal vision, and 7 reached alternation. Patients responded to treatment in 2 to 13 weeks. Occlusion amblyopia was not observed. Ten of the 17 patients who completed treatment had eccentric fixation at the outset, but only 2 remained parafoveally eccentric at the end of treatment. Ten patients lost lenses. Three had deposits and 2 exhibited irritation. Conjunctivitis developed in 5 children, a rate similar to that in other reports of use of extended-wear soft contact lenses. No corneal or intraocular infections occurred.

High-power plus extended-wear soft contact lenses are an alternative treatment for strabismic amblyopia. The stability of improved visual acuity is uncertain. Inadequately motivated children may consciously or unconsciously blink the lens out of the eye. In deep amblyopia, contact lens occlusion has been strengthened by applying oculoguttae atropine 0.5% once a day in the nonamblyopic eye.

2–7 **Evaluation of CAM Treatment for Amblyopia: A Controlled Study.** Campbell et al. recently described the CAM Vision Stimulator treatment for amblyopia. This technique consists of having the child view a series of slowly rotating square wave gratings of high contrast with the amblyopic eye while playing drawing games over the grating; however, control procedures were lacking. Milan E. Tytla and Louise S. Labow-Daily attempted to replicate the initial findings with several tests, including single and linear acuity and contrast sensitivity studies, in 9 test children, aged 5–12 years, with amblyopia and 6 controls. The latter children played games over a gray disk of the same mean luminance as the treatment gratings. Contrast sensitivity to vertical sinusoidal gratings was measured for the two eyes separately.

Slow, steady improvement in single-letter acuity was noted in most children as treatment progressed, but average linear acuity gains did not approach those of single-letter acuity; the study and control groups performed similarly. Amblyopic contrast sensitivity before treatment was progressively reduced as spatial frequency increased. Contrast sensitivity sometimes improved in both study and control children. There was no change in the size of deviation in strabismic patients. A change in fixation was noted in 2 study patients and 1 control; all changed from steady paramacular to steady macular fixation. Stereoacuity improved in 2 patients and 2 controls. These changes were not related to changes in acuity or contrast sensitivity. Intractable diplopia did not develop.

The "physiologic" nature of the CAM treatment of amblyopia is appealing, but the findings here indicate that the presence of gratings has no role in improvement of vision. It may be the minimal occlusion that is the effective part of the treatment in children whose vision improves. Sensitivity to contrast did improve in several children, and this could not be attributed to increased familiarity with the technique or to criterion shifts.

▶ [With the exception of CAM treatment, one should be enthusiastic about the therapy of amblyopia. An underlying theme that runs through these papers, however, is intense and careful patient care. High plus contact lenses are difficult to handle and wear and, indeed, 10 of 18 were lost. The physicians were persistent and the patients did well. The relapse rate is high, and long-term care is essential. Treatment for the amblyopia must be adapted to the patient, begun early, and continued for months, with careful follow-up for years.] ◀

2–8 **Surgical Results in Intermittent Exotropia.** Intermittent exotropia is generally considered to be a surgical problem, but undercorrection is a frequent result. William N. Clarke and Leon P. Noel (Ottawa) reviewed the results of operation for intermittent exotropia in 51 girls and 27 boys whose average age at operation was 7.9 years. The average time from initial assessment to operation was 15.7 months, and the average postoperative follow-up was 20.8 months. Thirty-three patients had acceptable results, with a residual deviation between 8 PD of esophoria and 8 PD of exophoria at all distances, with no tropia and with full stereopsis. Thirty-nine patients were undercorrected and 6 were overcorrected.

Acceptable results were obtained in 6 of 12 patients with

(2–8) Can. J. Ophthalmol. 16:66–69, April 1981.

pseudodivergence excess, 19 of 41 with basic exotropia, and 8 of 18 not assessed with +3.00 lenses. The 1 patient with true divergence excess was undercorrected. Nearly two thirds of children had either a real hypertropia or a dissociated vertical divergence besides the horizontal deviation. Forty-seven patients had lateral incomitance greater than 25%. In 11 patients there was a significant vertical incomitance requiring oblique muscle surgery, horizontal muscle shifts, or both. Ten patients had had previous operations. All but 13 patients underwent unilateral recession and resection.

The overall "cure" rate in this series was 42%. The frequency of surgical undercorrection was disappointingly high at 50%. It is reasonable to offer operation when good measurements of the quality and quantity of deviation have been obtained. As many muscles as required to achieve alignment in one procedure must be operated on. Purposeful overcorrection is necessary. A relatively advanced age at initial operation predisposes to undercorrection. Regular review of the results of operation for intermittent exotropia is important.

2-9 **Intermittent Exotropia: Is Surgery Necessary?** The proper management of intermittent exotropia is unclear. Judith Newman and Malcolm L. Mazow (Univ. of Texas, Houston) reviewed the outcome in 60 cases of intermittent exotropia seen in the past 7 years. The patients had acquired exotropia with no more than a 1-line difference in acuity between the eyes, no hyperdeviation more than 10 PD, no significant "A" or "V" pattern, and no gross adhesive syndrome. Four of the 12 patients operated on previously had surgical corrections. The average age at the start of medical therapy was 8 years and that at the time of surgery, 6 years. Most patients had a basic type of exodeviation. Nine patients in each group had hyperdeviation. An average exodeviation of 20 diopters (D) of exotropia in 30 patients was managed medically by alternate patching and convergence exercises where indicated. Thirty patients with an average exotropia of 32 D had operations. Basic exodeviations were treated by a recess-resect procedure, whereas divergence excess deviations were treated by bilateral lateral rectus recessions.

(2–9) Ophthalmic Surg. 12:199–202, March 1981.

Chapter 2–MOTILITY / 55

RESULTS OF MEDICAL AND SURGICAL TREATMENT RELATED TO AGE AND FUSION STATUS

Functional Status		Age		Fusion	
		Under 4	4 and over	Central	Peripheral or None
Medical 30 (pts)	Cure 21(pts)	4	17	6	13
	Failure 9(pts)	3	6	4	1 (24 measured)
Surgical 30 (pts)	Cure 23(pts)	6	17	8	8
	Failure 7(pts)	2	5	6	3 (25 measured)

Follow-up averaged 2 years for both groups. Two thirds of all patients with an exodeviation of less than 30 PD were functionally cured, as were two thirds of the surgically treated patients. More than half the medical cures and more than two thirds of surgical cures were associated with constant exophoria. The results are related to age at treatment and to fusion status in the table.

All medical methods were successful in the present series. Medical management is apparently acceptable when an intermittent exotropia of less than 30 PD occurs. The surgical cure rate may exceed the medical cure rate in patients younger than age 4 years, but results in more cases are needed before any conclusions may be made. Most patients have at least a peripheral fusion potential. Central fusion is apparently not necessary for clinical cure in patients with intermittent exotropia.

▶ [The surgical cure rate of intermittent exotropia is so poor that a real question is raised about whether to operate on any of the patients.] ◀

2–10 **Surgical Therapy For Convergence Insufficiency** is discussed by John S. Hermann (New York). Convergence insufficiency is characterized by an exodeviation greater at near than at distance, definite symptoms of asthenopia with near work, and decreased amplitudes of convergence. Typically, adolescents and young adults engaged in near work are affected. The symptoms often are out of proportion to

---

(2–10) J. Pediatr. Ophthalmol. Strabismus 18:28–31, Jan.–Feb. 1981.

the deviation. Suppression rarely occurs. A few patients fail to respond to orthoptics, glasses, prisms, drugs, or other medical measures. Fourteen such patients underwent resection of both medial recti for symptoms of intractable convergence insufficiency. These patients were seen in a 10-year period when about 1,200 patients were treated by orthoptic methods for convergence insufficiency. Fresnel prisms were used postoperatively if there was a consecutive esotropia with diplopia at distance.

The cases are summarized in the table. The average age was 23.5 years, and the average duration of symptoms of asthenopia was 3½ years. The average preoperative exodeviation was 10.3Δ at distance and 25.2Δ at near. The av-

SUMMARY OF PREOPERATIVE AND POSTOPERATIVE FINDINGS

Case No	Age Sex	Pre-Op Deviation	Bimedial Resection mm.	Post-Op Deviation 1 Week	Last Examination Deviation	Follow-Up (Months)
1	27 M	X-16 Δ X'-25 Δ	4.5	ET-10 Δ	No Follow-Up	—
2	16 F	X-12 Δ X'-40 Δ	4.5	ET-20 Δ ORTHO	E-4 Δ ORTHO	13
3	30 F	X-16 Δ X'-25 Δ	4.0	ET-16 Δ ET'-10 Δ	E-2 Δ ORTHO	13
4	26 F	X-14 Δ X'-25 Δ	4.0	ET-10 Δ E'-4 Δ	X-14 Δ X'-14 Δ	27
5	25 F	X-4 Δ X'-20 Δ	3.5	ET-20 Δ ET'-10 Δ	X-4 Δ X'-20 Δ	18
6	19 4	X-2 Δ X'20 Δ	4.0	ET-20 Δ X'2 Δ	ORTHO X'-8 Δ	13
7	41 M	X-25 Δ X'-35 Δ	4.5	X-10 Δ X'-14 Δ	X-6 Δ X'-6 Δ	6
8	16 F	ORTHO X'20 Δ	4.0	ET-16 Δ E(T)'-8 Δ	X-10 Δ X'-10 Δ	46
9	22 M	X-8 Δ X'-20 Δ	3.5	ET-14 Δ ET'-14 Δ	X-6 Δ X'-16 Δ	61
10	30 F	X-8 Δ X'-25 Δ	3.5	ET-16 Δ ET'-14 Δ	E-8 Δ E'-12 Δ	10
11	23 F	X-16 Δ X'-25 Δ	4.0	ET-25 Δ ET'14 Δ	X-2 Δ X'-4 Δ	106
12	30 F	X-8 Δ X'-18 Δ	3.5	ET-18 Δ E'-4 Δ	ORTHO X'-14 Δ	10
13	10 F	X-4 Δ X'-25 Δ	3.5	ET-25 Δ E'-4 Δ	X-2 Δ X'-16 Δ	3
14	14 F	X 12 Δ X'-30 Δ	4.0	ET-2 Δ X'-12 Δ	X-2 Δ X'-12 Δ	1

erage esodeviation at distance a week postoperatively was 15.1Δ. Asthenopic symptoms at near resolved within about a month after surgery, and esotropia and diplopia at distance resolved in about 3 months. On follow-up averaging 32 months, a 4.5-mm bimedial resection resolved an average of 16Δ at distance and 40Δ at near; a 4-mm resection resolved 4.4Δ at distance and 15.8Δ at near; and a 3.5-mm resection resolved 2Δ at distance and 10Δ at near. The longterm average exophoria at distance was 2.2Δ and at near, 7.4Δ. No patient has required further surgery, and all have had dramatic symptomatic relief.

Resection of both medial rectus muscles led to marked symptomatic relief in all these patients with intractable convergence insufficiency. Exophoria at near will return, but not the symptoms. Temporary diplopia due to consecutive esotropia is a necessary surgical result, and is relieved by fresnel prisms.

▶ [Is there a small, select group of patients with convergence insufficiency who do not respond to medical treatment and thus qualify for surgery? This article is certain to generate controversy.] ◀

2–11 **Anterior Transposition of the Inferior Oblique.** Occasionally overaction of the inferior oblique persists after surgery designed to weaken the muscle. Richard L. Elliott and Sheldon J. Nankin (Santa Ana, Calif.) have modified the standard inferior oblique recession by reattaching the muscle slightly anterior to the temporal border of the insertion of the inferior rectus.

TECHNIQUE.—An inferior temporal fornix incision is made, and a suture is passed beneath the insertion of the lateral rectus and fastened to the head drape with the eye in a fully elevated and adducted position. The inferior oblique then is placed on a tenotomy hook and dissected free from its fascial attachments, and a 6-0 Vicryl suture is placed through it near its point of insertion and locked at both borders. The muscle is disinserted from the sclera and the other suture released. The suture needles are passed through superficial sclera just anterior to the temporal insertion site of the inferior rectus and the sutures tied (Fig 2–3). The conjunctiva is closed with 6-0 plain gut.

Of 64 anterior transpositions done in 5 years, 28 were bilateral, and 21 were combined with a standard recession

---

(2–11) J. Pediatr. Ophthalmol. Strabismus 18:35–38, May–June, 1981.

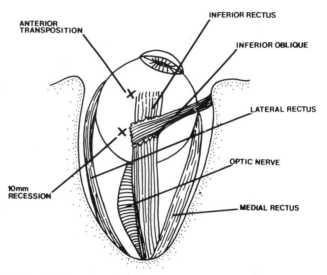

Fig 2–3.—Attachment site for anterior transposition of inferior oblique to sclera is depicted slightly anterior and immediately adjacent to temporal edge of insertion of inferior rectus. (Courtesy of Elliott, R. L., and Nankin, S. J.: J. Pediatr. Ophthalmol. Strabismus 18:35–38, May–June, 1981.)

procedure. Follow-up averaged 12 months. Previous oblique operations had been performed on seven eyes. About two thirds of the anterior transpositions were done for 3+ to 4+ overactions, as were 11% of 90 standard recession procedures performed in the same period. A −3.0 net change in the amount of overaction of the inferior oblique followed anterior transposition, compared with a −2.0 net change for standard recession procedures. Both procedures effectively reduced primary position hypertropia where present. A −1 to −2 primary position elevation deficiency followed 11 of 15 unilateral anterior transpositions but only 4 of 16 unilateral recession procedures. Anterior transposition produced further weakening in all eyes with previous inferior oblique recessions. No changes in palpebral fissure width have been observed. There have been no symptoms related to torsion.

The anterior transposition is a relatively easy procedure

for use in persistent and, possibly, marked cases of inferior oblique overaction.

▶ [Many techniques have been advocated for the weakening of overacting inferior oblique muscles. Some simply cut the muscle loose from its insertion and let it reattach on its own, while others carefully suture it in a recessed position. These authors recommend anterior transposition, which seems theoretically sound. They compared their results with standard recessions but they apparently did not use a randomized, prospective method of patient selection, so we can not be certain their method is actually better than recession. In favor of their technique, however, is the fact that it does appear to be easier to carry out.] ◀

2-12 **Benign Recurrent VI Nerve Palsy in Childhood.** Sixth nerve palsies acquired in childhood usually signify a serious posterior fossa disorder. Some acquired forms are benign and self-limited, but recurrent benign sixth nerve palsy is rare. Wayne W. Bixenman and Gunter K. von Noorden (Houston) describe a child who had six well-documented episodes of benign sixth nerve palsy in her first 3 years.

Girl, aged 2 months, had right-sided esotropia of sudden onset 3 days after a slight "cold." The right eye could not be abducted beyond the midline. Other ophthalmologic and neurologic findings were normal, and the esotropia resolved over the next 10 days. A similar episode occurred 8 months later, 3 weeks after onset of an upper respiratory tract infection and right-sided serous otitis media. The esotropia failed to respond to occlusion therapy, and right medial rectus recession and lateral rectus resection were carried out. Right-sided esotropia developed in association with upper respiratory infection at age 17 months. Left medial rectus recession and lateral rectus resection were performed. Right-sided esotropia recurred at age 2 years, a few days before an upper respiratory tract infection, and responded to alternate-day occlusion therapy of the left eye. There were two subsequent recurrences, both managed by alternate occlusion. The patient will be considered for bilateral superior oblique tenectomy and further horizontal rectus muscle surgery after the measurements have stabilized.

Only 2 previous cases of recurrent benign sixth nerve palsy have been reported. The condition may have the same immunologic basis as other parainfectious neuropathies. After recovery from an initial episode, the abducens nerve may be predisposed to recurrent inflammation and loss of function. Most often the recurrences are triggered by febrile ill-

---

(2–12) J. Pediatr. Ophthalmol. Strabismus 18:29–34, May–June, 1981.

nesses of childhood. An incomitant esotropia due to sixth nerve palsy may evolve into a comitant esotropia that may or may not improve. Vigorous occlusion therapy is indicated. Strabismus surgery should be done once the esotropia becomes comitant and the angle of deviation is stable for 4 to 6 weeks. Maintenance occlusion is necessary so long as improvement progresses.

2–13 **Masked Bilateral Superior Oblique Paresis.** John S. Hermann (New York) observed superior oblique paresis in the contralateral eye in 9 of 57 patients treated surgically for unilateral superior oblique paresis. Masked bilateral superior oblique paresis has been described by several workers. Bilaterality should be presumed in all cases of superior oblique paresis until ruled out, and attempts should be made on multiple occasions to elicit contralateral inferior oblique overaction.

Boy, 15, was seen because of the left eye shooting up in right gaze and diplopia in superior and right gaze. He had been unconscious after a head injury at age 6. Prismatic therapy combined with orthoptic treatment to improve the horizontal vergences did not lead to symptomatic improvement over several months. Marked overaction of the left inferior oblique and right inferior rectus was observed. There was no overaction of the right inferior oblique on extreme left gaze. An 8-mm recession of the left inferior oblique was done, combined with a 2.5-mm recession of the right inferior rectus. Vertical diplopia had recurred 2 months after operation, and the right-sided hyperdeviation was increasing. Right superior oblique paresis with overaction of the right inferior oblique was confirmed the next month. A 9-mm recession of the right inferior oblique was then performed, and the symptoms resolved. No hyperdeviation was observed on head tilt testing 3 years later.

Souza-Dias suggested that there is an inhibitional palsy of the contralateral inferior oblique because of a secondary ipsilateral superior rectus overaction in these cases. A large excyclotorsion and a large V pattern may be clues to bilateral superior oblique paresis. Even an insignificant V pattern should suggest the possibility of a masked paresis.

2–14 **Double Elevator Palsy** is diagnosed in patients with a monocular limitation of elevation. The limitation is the same in primary gaze, adduction, and abduction. Some patients may have a true elevator weakness, and others an inferior restriction, or both may be present. Henry S. Metz (Univ. of Rochester) recently encountered 2 patients with orbital cellulitis and a unilateral limitation of elevation as the only motility defect. The diagnosis was confirmed by computed tomography and by the lid swelling. In 11 patients with monocular limitation of upgaze and no deviation in the primary position, excluding cases of blowout fracture, thyroid ophthalmopathy, third-nerve palsy, and orbital inflammation or tumor, the average limitation of upgaze was between -2 and -3. Vertical saccadic velocity studies showed average upward and downward saccadic velocities of 255 and 230 degrees per second, respectively. Eight other patients with an average upgaze limitation of -3 had an average deviation in primary position of 20 PD. Four patients with an average limitation of elevation of -4 had an average deviation in the primary position of 30 PD. Only 4 of the 23 patients had evidence of true elevator palsy.

Most patients with monocular limitation of elevation probably have an inferior restriction. The mechanism of "double elevator palsy" rarely is applicable to these cases. Where inferior restriction is the major cause, the tight inferior rectus muscle should be recessed and a conjunctival recession performed. Recession of up to 8 mm may be necessary. Inferior rectus recession may be unwise if there is no deviation in the primary position. Patients with evidence of superior rectus palsy may benefit from transposition surgery, with complete transposition of the medial and lateral recti to the insertion of the palsied superior rectus muscle. As much as 35 PD of hypotropia can be corrected in this manner. Only a modest increase in elevation may result in cases of complete superior rectus paralysis. An inferior restriction, if present, must be released before transposition surgery can be effective.

▶ [The author points out that most cases of monocular limitation of elevation are due to inferior restrictions. Indeed, when the elevation limitation is due to elevator palsy, it is rarely double but usually only involves the superior rectus.] ◀

2-15 **Dynamic Vergence Eye Movements in Strabismus and Amblyopia: Asymmetric Vergence.** Vergence and saccadic movements occur in the eyes of normal persons, but dynamic aspects of vergence in patients with strabismus and/or amblyopia have received little attention. Robert V. Kenyon, Kenneth J. Ciuffreda, and Lawrence Stark (Univ. of California School of Optometry, Berkeley) investigated line-of-sight asymmetric disparity vergence in 7 patients with intermittent strabismus, constant strabismus with amblyopia, or amblyopia without strabismus. The mean age was 23 years. Two adult control subjects also were studied. Binocular horizontal eye position was assessed using an infrared reflection technique. Targets were placed along the line of sight at 25 or 50 cm from the estimated center of rotation of the eye, producing a disparity of about 6.8 degrees.

Patients with strabismus exhibited markedly unequal vergence amplitudes. Relative vergence amplitude equaled 20%, with the smaller movement in the "on-axis" eye. The saccades corrected only positional errors induced by small vergence movements in the dominant eye. Not all amblyopic patients exhibited the absence of disparity vergence. Accommodative vergence responses in patients were similar to those in control subjects with the nondominant eye covered. The asymmetric vergence responses of patients could not be attributed to dominant eye stimulation. With the dominant "off-axis" eye covered, the accommodative vergence response appeared to be absent or grossly abnormal in deep amblyopia and unrelated to the presence of strabismus.

Patients with strabismus and amblyopia use accommodative vergence rather than disparity vergence to track asymmetric vergence stimuli. In the 4-prism diopter base-out test, if both disparity and blur are produced, the esotrope would be expected to exhibit a saccade plus accommodative vergence, both driven by the dominant eye. A goal of fusion training in strabismic and amblyopic patients would be normal static and dynamic fusional responses in both instrument and free space for both symmetric and asymmetric disparity vergence stimulus conditions.

▶ [When a prism is placed in front of the normal eye in a patient with amblyopia, the amblyopic eye moves to a new position. According to this study, the amblyopic eye may also move with an accommodative vergence which would confound the assessment of the strabismus.] ◀

2-16 Ocular Torsion and the Primary Retinal Meridians.

Ocular torsion is considered to be a partial compensatory mechanism for retinal tilt. Dynamic torsion is thought to have a larger amplitude than static torsion. Robert S. Jampel (Wayne State Univ., Detroit) measured ocular torsion during and after head and body tilt, ocular convergence, and conjugate gaze in 15 normal subjects and 400 patients without extraocular motor defects. A biomicroscope was used.

No static torsion was measured in normal subjects for head or body tilts for any fixation point that maintained the eye in a stable orbital position. No static torsion was observed on head tilting with the subjects prone, supine, or lying on their sides. No true ocular torsion was observed in 200 patients aged 7–87 years at head tilts of about 30–60 degrees (Fig 2–4). Cine studies of 8 normal subjects with the corneal eggshell membrane technique showed that head tilts of more than 3 degrees per second were associated with

Fig 2–4.—Experimental results for one subject; angle is formed by lower edge of illuminated slit on iris, and dashed line is drawn through distinct iris markings *(arrowheads)*. Acute angle measures 49 degrees and is same in all frames; if intorsion took place, acute angle would become larger. **A,** head is rotated 11 degrees; **B,** 19 degrees; **C,** 30 degrees; **D,** 43 degrees; **E,** 77 degrees; **F,** 89 degrees. (Courtesy of Jampel, R. S.: Am. J. Ophthalmol. 91:14–24, January 1981.)

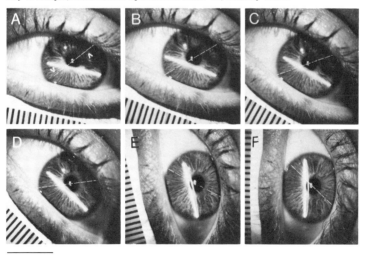

saccadic, small-amplitude torsional movements that preceded the head movements. No persistent torsion was observed. The torsional eye movements did not lag behind the head movements. Torsion was not observed in symmetric or asymmetric convergence in normal subjects or in 200 consecutive patients, aged 2–74 years, with clinically normal eye movements. In no case was cyclophoria observed with the routine cover-uncover and alternating-cover tests.

Several factors may produce experimental artifacts of pseudotorsion. Ocular torsion occurs during head tilt and under conditions in which integrative brain mechanisms are disordered, as well as under special experimental conditions that elicit ocular adjustments to factors not usually present in the visual environment. The absence of static ocular torsion is a factor in the normal oculomotor physiology of man. The primary retinal meridians are aligned with one another during binocular fixation, regardless of the position of the head or the point of ocular fixation. The vestibular and oculomotor systems work together to inhibit ocular torsion. The eyes are oriented to a plane in the brain rather than to the horizon.

▶ [Doctor Jampel has questioned the existence of ocular torsion in human beings and subhuman primates. As he points out, this is a critical issue in oculomotor physiology, and his fine work is sure to generate interest and further studies of ocular torsion.] ◀

2–17 **Etiology, Treatment, and Prevention of the "Slipped Muscle."** A "lost" muscle is a well-described entity in strabismus surgery, resulting from detachment of a newly sutured muscle from the sclera and its retraction into the orbit. Jeffrey N. Bloom and Marshall M. Parks (Children's Hosp. Natl. Med. Center, Washington, D.C.) recently encountered 9 patients with consecutive exotropia in whom the medial rectus muscle slipped posteriorly within its capsule while the capsule remained attached at the site of recession. In a tenth patient, a consecutive hypotropia due to posterior slippage of the superior rectus muscle within its capsule developed after recession of the muscle.

If a suture is passed only through the capsule before disinserting the tendon (Fig 2–5), the free end will retract posteriorly within the capsule after the capsule is resu-

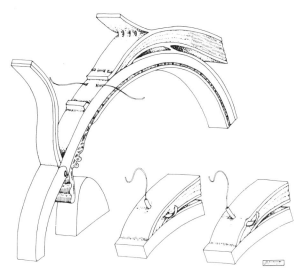

Fig 2–5.—Far right diagram illustrates tangential passage of needle through only superficial capsule. Middle diagram demonstrates proper placement of needle through body of tendon. (Courtesy of Bloom, J. N., and Parks, M. M.: J. Pediatr. Ophthalmol. Strabismus 18:6–11, Jan.–Feb. 1981.)

tured to the sclera. Muscle power is decreased as a result, although some contractile force may remain. The force decreases as the slipped muscle remains in a chronically contracted state.

Both slipped and lost muscles present with exotropia, reduced adduction, and proptosis with widening of the palpebral fissure on attempted adduction. If the muscle capsule is traced posteriorly the slipped muscle often will be found at the point where it penetrates Tenon's capsule. Care is needed to avoid dissection of the friable muscle capsule away from its scleral attachment. Unsuccessful, repeated surgery for a consecutive deviation should lead to suspicion of a slipped muscle. Either synthetic or nonsynthetic sutures may be associated with a slipped muscle. The needle should be placed within the full substance of the tendon at initial surgery. When locking bites at the edges of the tendon are taken, the needle should be directed perpendicularly rather than tangentially. Proper suture placement should be checked routinely after disinsertion.

3. Vision, Refraction, and Contact Lenses

3–1 **How Good Is Normal Visual Acuity? Study of Letter Acuity Thresholds as a Function of Age.** Most contemporary visual acuity charts are based on Snellen's value for normal acuity of 6/6, but acuity levels better than 6/6 have been found to be common in normal persons. L. Frisén and M. Frisén (Univ. of Göteborg) determined acuity in 100 normal subjects, using a finely graduated letter chart under optimized test conditions. Each line contained 10 letters of similar difficulty, arranged in random order; letter heights were 10% less than the norm throughout. The chart was placed 5.3 m from the subject. Acuity was tested bilaterally in 70 subjects.

Acuity levels are related to age at various correct response thresholds in Figure 3–1. The same trend with age was seen in all sets of observations, although there was considerable variation between subjects. In double determinations on 10 subjects, reproducibility appeared to be fairly good for the 50% and 90% thresholds, but was much worse for the 100% threshold. The most marked fall in acuity occurred after the age of 60 years. The average difference between the two eyes was 0.04.

An acuity level of only 1.0 is quite unusual in clinically normal eyes examined under optimal conditions, and it appears quite reasonable to complain if acuity falls to the level of 1.0. Age must be taken into account when evaluating a given acuity result. Acuity charts containing 1.0 as the most difficult test line are not appropriate for the early detection of visual abnormalities. A useful chart would contain several lines of letters more difficult than 1.0. The use of a

(3–1) Albrecht Von Graefes Arch. Klin. Exp. Ophthalmol. 215:149–157, January 1981.

68 / OPHTHALMOLOGY

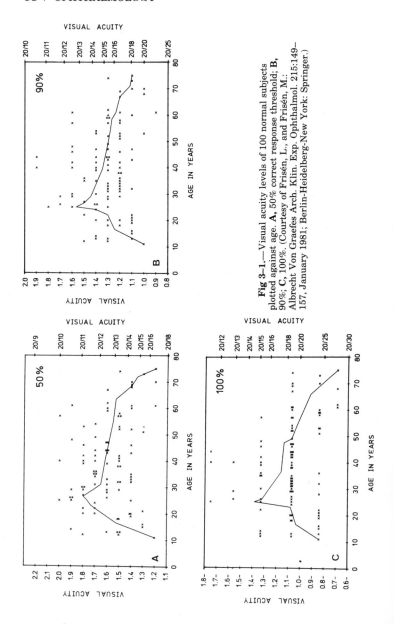

Fig 3-1.—Visual acuity levels of 100 normal subjects plotted against age. **A**, 50% correct response threshold; **B**, 90%; **C**, 100%. (Courtesy of Frisén, L., and Frisén, M.: Albrecht Von Graefes Arch. Klin. Exp. Ophthalmol. 215:149–157, January 1981; Berlin-Heidelberg-New York: Springer.)

fractional response criterion, such as the 50% threshold, is necessary in critical work.

▶ [Acuity measurements would be much improved if 50% correct in a given line was used as the end point. Moreover, patients, especially the young, should all be pressed beyond the 6/6 line.] ◀

3–2 **A Comparison of the Frisby, Random-Dot E, TNO, and Randot Circles Stereotests in Screening and Office Use.** The best commercial random-dot stereogram (RDS) test for use in detecting clinically significant strabismus, amblyopia, and anisometropia in children remains unclear. Kurt Simons (Albany Med. College) evaluated the Frisby, Random-Dot E (RDE), and TNO tests and also the Randot circles test, which is designed to avoid the monocular clue artifact of the Titmus circles, in three populations. Studies were done in 110 children aged 3–5 years at three day-care centers and nursery schools; 79 children of similar age in a community vision screening program; and 72 patients with strabismus or amblyopia, or both, aged 4–36 years.

Four of 110 children in the day-care center and nursery school sample had binocular dysfunction. The Frisby and RDE tests were both failed by 1 subject who passed the TNO test, for an over referral rate of 0.9% in both instances. In the community screening program, 1 subject with intermittent esotropia missed detection by the Frisby test at both screening and rescreening. Another probably was an overreferral for the Frisby test, and the Frisby also overreferred 2 other subjects. The RDE overreferred 1 subject, as did the visual acuity test. The Frisby and RDE tests both "underreferred" at least 1 subject, and probably 2, with refractive errors. Nine subjects in the patient sample seemed to pass the Frisby test through the use of cruder stereoscopic cues than are available with the other tests or through the use of monocular cues. Three patients failed the RDE while passing the TNO or the Frisby and TNO tests. The TNO test produced anomalous findings in 5 cases. Finer stereoacuities usually were achieved on the circles test where there was a difference from the three RDS tests.

The RDE appears to be the test of choice for vision screening. The TNO seems most useful for retesting chil-

---

(3–2) Arch. Ophthalmol. 99:446–452, March 1981.

dren who have failed or given equivocal responses to the RDE test in a screening setting. In an office setting, the TNO is the best choice for obtaining initial RDS stereoacuity thresholds. The Randot circles test seems particularly useful in clinical settings because it provides a reliable grade measure of binocular function when this is too poor to be tested by RDS methods.

▶ [Population screening may be the only way to detect the large numbers of persons (1 in 20) who have strabismus, amblyopia, and anisometropia. Stereotesting may be a reasonable method of large-scale screening.] ◀

3–3 **Near Work and Familial Resemblances in Ocular Refraction: Population Study in Newfoundland.** J. C. Bear, A. Richler, and G. Burke (Univ. of Newfoundland) investigated the influences of near work and educational level on familial patterns of ocular refraction in a rural Newfoundland population, because of epidemiologic evidence that the near work associated with formal education can cause myopia. Study was made of 971 persons aged 5 years and older in three adjoining communities on the west coast of the Great Northern Peninsula of Newfoundland, a geographically isolated area. About 80% of the population aged 5 and older were refracted. Fourteen subjects with myopia greater than -6 D or right eye amblyopia were excluded.

When the effects of near work and education were evaluated by adjusting refraction for age and sex and comparing correlations among relatives before and after further linear regression adjustments of refraction, reductions in sib-sib correlations and offspring-parent regressions were observed, suggesting that the environmental factors inflated intrafamilial resemblances in refraction. Offspring-parent similarities were consistently greatest for the 15 to 29-year age interval, perhaps because these subjects were at an age at which refraction is relatively stable. Resemblances for children aged 5 to 14 years may have been relatively low because refractions in these children are changing relatively rapidly.

Near work, as a feature of common familial environ-

(3–3) Clin. Genet. 19:462–472, June 1981.

ment, can inflate estimates of the genetic contribution to variation in refraction if not taken into account. The contribution of genetic dominance to sib-sib correlations is unclear. Longitudinal data on changes in refraction from childhood to adulthood are needed for appropriate comparison of the refractions of persons of different ages. The particular features of near work that influence refraction must be better specified.

▶ [It is persuasive that near work contributes to myopia, but the many specifics have not been worked out. This is a fine report that helps us understand the many difficulties of these kinds of studies.] ◀

3-4 **Subjective Visual Disturbances Based on Glasses or Contact Lenses in Cataract Patients With Lens Extraction** were discussed by D. Rähle (Univ. of Zurich). The conventional correction given to patients after lens extraction consists of cataract glasses or contact lenses. However, patients fitted with either of these devices are known to have difficulty with some everyday activities and to experience visual disturbances. The newer operative possibility is the implantation of an artificial plastic lens. Such a lens causes neither magnification nor restriction of the visual field. However, this type of surgery is associated with somewhat high short- and long-term risks and should not be performed unless the disadvantages of the classic cataract operation are perceived to be disturbing to a particular patient.

Using a questionnaire with 43 patients, the frequency of disturbances reported by patients fitted with glasses or contact lenses was investigated and a definition of the specific problems was attempted. The conditions required of participating patients were as follows: at the time of the investigation, the last cataract surgery was less than 4 years ago; fairly good vision existed (the limit of corrected farsightedness and nearsightedness within 0.6); the aphakic eye was used in everyday life and did not show additional rough ophthalmologic changes. The author depended on case histories for data on the latter. Finally, he considered the tendency of the visual impairment to improve with time. Walking downstairs was the activity most frequently af-

(3-4) Schweiz. Med. Wochenschr. 111:260–265, February 1981. (Ger.)

fected, followed by sewing (threading a needle impossible), walking upstairs (uncertainty, stumbling), shopping (colliding with others), reaching (easy tiring), writing, eating (frequent spilling), and walking straight. Problems with walking downstairs, shopping, traveling, and eating were frequently reported by patients using glasses, while problems with seeing in the distance, reading, and writing were complaints of patients using contact lenses. With the exception of reading and writing, there was little possibility of adaptation. The "Jack-in-the-box" phenomenon and restriction of the visual field were the most common disturbances, and they did not tend to improve. Magnification of the retinal image and the other visual disturbances studied did, however, improve markedly with time.

When questioned about the difference in vision before and after cataract surgery, 37 patients gave a positive answer. Judging in retrospect, only 15 of the 43 patients would have decided in favor of an intraocular lens transplant. Virtually all the patients were satisfied with their aphakia correction.

3–5 **Empirical Fitting of Hard Contact Lenses in Infants and Young Children.** Contact lenses may be indicated for infants and young children with a variety of disorders. In unilateral aphakia the visual prognosis is poor, unless proper optical correction is provided. Previously, fitting of hard lenses has involved general anesthesia. Hydrophilic lenses may be unsuitable for many aphakic patients, and frequent replacement may be necessary. Richard A. Saunders (Med. Univ. of South Carolina) and F. Daryel Ellis (Indiana Univ.) describe a method of empirically fitting hard contact lenses without use of "K" readings and without general anesthesia for children younger than age 18 months.

TECHNIQUE.—A trial lens of approximate dioptric power is first inserted, and fluorescein is instilled into the cul-de-sac. The pattern is evaluated with a Burton magnifier. A proper fit shows a "double-ring" sign with a central fluorescein pool about three-fourths the diameter of the contact lens and a peripheral ring. Generally a lens ½ to 1 D flatter in radius than that generating a small central bubble is appropriate. Proper tightness is confirmed by moving the lens around the cornea with the patient's

(3–5) Ophthalmology (Rochester) 88:127–130, February 1981.

Chapter 3–VISION, REFRACTION, AND CONTACT LENSES / 73

lids or an index finger. A refraction should be done with and without the trial lens in place. A steep fit is preferred. A good aphakic fit generally results in 2 D or more of positive tear meniscus. It is usual to over-plus aphakic infants by 1 to 3 D to provide best vision at their usual working range.

About 20 patients have been fitted in this way in the past 2½ years. Only 1 could not be fitted successfully. The rest retained their contact lenses without undue ocular irritation or frequent loss, although some eventually came to represent contact lens failures for other reasons. Given the questionable safety of intraocular lens implantation, hard corneal contact lenses are the method of choice for optical correction in infants and young children with unilateral aphakia.

3–6 **Extended-Wear Contact Lenses for Myopic Correction.** Walter J. Stark and Neil F. Marin (Johns Hopkins Hosp.) investigated the use of extended-wear soft contact lenses in correcting myopia in 106 patients who wore the Permalens (perfilcon A) successfully for 4 to 8 years. The median period of lens use was 4.9 years. The patients were generally from a working-class background in Great Britain. The 72 women and 34 men had a mean age of 34.3 years. With 1 exception, all patients wore the lens for periods of at least 2 months without removing it, and most removed the lens for cleaning less often than every 4 months.

Acuity with the contact lens alone was 20/30 or better in 82% of the 207 eyes fitted in the 106 patients. It was 20/40 or better in 95% of eyes. The average length of radial corneal vascularization was 1.02 mm superiorly and 0.39 mm inferiorly, significantly more than in control myopic patients who had not worn contact lenses. In 8.7% of the 207 eyes the vessels extended more than 1.5 mm in from the limbus. The degree of vascularization could not be correlated with the duration of contact lens wear. Punctate corneal staining was seen in 3% of eyes and conjunctival injection in 1%. Review of data on 153 other patients who successfully wore the lens but were not examined revealed six episodes of corneal abrasion in 5 patients, but no corneal scarring or visual loss. Conjunctivitis was the reason for discontinuing use of the extended-wear lens in 25 of 30 other cases. Four patients had corneal abrasion and 1 had a sterile punctate keratitis. Twenty of these 30 patients were wearing another type of daily wear or extended-wear contact lens at follow-up.

These results are encouraging. No complications resulting in reduced acuity or corneal scarring have been observed. Extended-wear soft contact lenses may provide a valuable alternative for patients seeking surgical correction of myopia. Caution is needed, however, to avoid indiscriminate use of extended-wear contact lenses to correct myopia.

3–7 **Extended-Wear Contact Lenses for Aphakic Correction—Experiences With the Cooper Permalens: A Preliminary Report.** P. Thomas Manchester, Jr., has carried out a study of extended-wear contact lenses to determine whether they are practical and helpful for aphakic patients older than age 45 years. A total of 116 eyes in 86 patients were fitted with the Cooper Permalens Perfilcon A contact lens in the past year. The success rate was 71%, based on use of the lens for a month or longer. Causes of failure are listed in the table. At least 9 patients were poorly motivated and never should have been encouraged to try the lenses; when these 14 eyes were eliminated from the study, a success rate of 80% was obtained. Dry eyes appear not to contraindicate the use of this lens in a patient who is followed closely and can be expected to use artificial tears regularly. In eyes with corneal edema, the lenses appeared to fit loosely. Seven patients had the "tight lens syndrome," despite fitting of the loosest available lens. Refraction over the Cooper lenses gave unpredictable results. Vision with Cooper lenses plus glasses often was somewhat worse than with cataract glasses or hard contact lenses, but near vision usually was better.

No failures were due to infection or loss of lens in this series. Several patients who discontinued wearing the lenses because of corneal edema or unsatisfactory fit have obtained satisfactory results with other types of extended-wear lenses such as the Sauflon or the CSI lens. Follow-up to

Causes of Failure With Cooper Permalens	
Poor motivation	14
Dry eyes	2
Corneal edema	10
Unsatisfactory fit	8
Total	34

date is short, and future failures may occur because of frequent lens loss, deposits on lenses, papillary hypertrophy, or corneal vascularization. Nevertheless, patients can be advised that the chance of successful use of Cooper lenses is about 80% in well-motivated subjects. The extended-wear lens is a good alternative to secondary lens implantation in patients who are already aphakic.

▶ [This article and the three preceding ones all emphasize the use of contact lenses instead of surgery. The Rähle study was not a prospective randomized clinical trial, but the conclusion that only approximately one fourth of cataract patients would choose an intraocular lens must certainly shock implant surgeons. A simple method of hard contact lens fitting for infants is recommended primarily to avoid implants. Extended-wear contact lenses are recommended as an alternative to both radial keratotomy in myopic patients and secondary implants in aphakic patients. It certainly seems appropriate to be as conservative as we can be at present when corneal surgery and, to some extent, implant surgery are relatively new. Which procedures will dominate our practices in the future, however, is not yet clear, and we can only hope for a continuation of careful research to assess the various methods for the benefit of our patients.] ◀

4. Conjunctiva

Acute Hemorrhagic Conjunctivitis

JOEL SUGAR, M.D.

Eye and Ear Infirmary,
University of Illinois, Chicago

At times, there are reports of entities of little apparent clinical importance to western ophthalmology. Such seemed the report that appeared in the 1976 issue of the YEAR BOOK, when reference was last made to articles over the preceding few years of hemorrhagic conjunctivitis of pandemic proportions occurring in the Far East.[1, 2] This problem remained distant only until 1981, when the first significant outbreak of acute hemorrhagic conjunctivitis caused by enterovirus 70 was reported in the western hemisphere.[3-7]

The first epidemic was reported in Ghana in 1969.[8] Subsequently, large outbreaks occurred in Japan, Taiwan, Hong Kong, India, Morocco, Singapore, Thailand, and Indonesia. Smaller outbreaks followed in England, France, and Yugoslavia. Involvement in the western hemisphere was limited to occasional cases in refugees until the summer of 1981, when outbreaks were reported in South America, Central America, and the Caribbean. Subsequently, an epidemic occurred in Key West and then Miami, Florida, with more than 3,500 cases reported in Miami between September 8, and October 9, 1981. A smaller secondary outbreak followed in North Carolina.[7] While these outbreaks subsequently have declined, recognition of the entity remains essential for control of future outbreaks.

The clinical picture of acute hemorrhagic conjunctivitis consists of a sudden onset of mixed papillary and follicular conjunctival injection and irritation with conjunctival and subconjunctival hemorrhages, profuse tearing, and often preauricular adenopathy (77%) and lid edema (66%).[5] The hemorrhages start and are often most dense superiorly. Punctate keratopathy, which is most marked superiorly, occurs as well.[8] Although symptoms may begin in one eye, the other eye usually is involved within hours. Symptoms and signs last 3 to 5 days. Strikingly, the patients usually do not have fever or upper respiratory symptoms. The incubation period is less than 24 hours, and secondary involvement of family members and contacts is high. Transmission appears to be by hand-to-eye contact. The short incubation period and high secondary attack rate promote explosive epidemics. Permanent ocular sequelae are not seen except with rare secondary bacterial infection.[9] Occasional neurologic sequelae with a "poliomyelitis-like" radiculomyelitis occurred in the outbreaks in the Far East,[10] but with the exception of a single case of Bell's palsy,[7] no neurologic sequelae have been reported in the western hemisphere as of the time of this writing.

Laboratory evaluation includes conjunctival scrapings, which show multiple lymphocytes and some polymorphonuclear leukocytes. Culture requires special techniques and is unrewarding in routine clinical laboratories. Differential diagnosis includes adenovirus conjunctivitis, which may occasionally be associated with subconjunctival hemorrhages and lid ecchymoses but is more likely to be unilateral or asymmetric, or both. In addition, the time course between contact and onset of disease is usually significantly more prolonged, being 1 to 2 weeks. Herpes and inclusion conjunctivitis must be included in the differential diagnosis but are unlikely to be confused. Bacterial conjunctivitis due to *Streptococcus pneumoniae, Hemophilus influenzae,* or *Neisseria* organisms can be differentiated by conjunctival scrapings.

The virus involved has been identified as a picornavirus of the enterovirus type.[11] It has been called "enterovirus 70" and also called "Apollo" virus because the first outbreak in 1969 occurred at the time of the Apollo moon landing. Although most outbreaks have been from the same virus, the episode that occurred in Singapore in 1970 was caused by a virus antigenically different from the outbreak in Singapore in 1971 and from most outbreaks that have occurred subsequently.

No specific treatment is available for this viral conjunctivitis. It is important, however, aggressively to attempt to limit outbreaks by restricting infected patients from going to their place of employment or to school during the active phase, which appears to be less than 1 week in duration. Likewise, eye clinics and other facilities where these patients are seen should be set up in such a way that ophthalmologists and ophthalmic equipment do not serve as vectors for further spread of the disease.

It is difficult to know whether further outbreaks will occur in the United States. Most outbreaks have taken place in tropical climates during warm weather, and that factor may restrict outbreaks to the southern United States. Awareness of this entity, however, is essential so that appropriate patient management can limit the spread of this disease should further outbreak occur.

References
1. Dawson C. R.: Introduction to chapter "The Conjunctiva," in Hughes W. F. (ed.): 1973 YEAR BOOK OF OPHTHALMOLOGY. Chicago, Year Book Medical Publishers, Inc., 1973. pp. 61–64.
2. Yang F. Y., et al.: Epidemic Hemorrhagic Keratoconjunctivitis, in Hughes W. F. (ed.): 1976 YEAR BOOK OF OPHTHALMOLOGY. Chicago, Year Book Medical Publishers, Inc., 1976. pp. 54–55.
3. Center for Disease Control: Acute hemorrhagic conjunctivitis: Latin America. *Morbid Mortal Weekly Rep.* 30:450–451, 1981.
4. Center for Disease Control: Acute hemorrhagic conjunctivitis: Key West, Florida. *Morbid Mortal Weekly Rep.* 30:463–464, 1981.
5. Center for Disease Control: Acute hemorrhagic conjunctivitis: Florida. *Morbid Mortal Weekly Rep.* 30:465–466, 1981.
6. Center for Disease Control: Acute hemorrhagic conjunctivitis: Panama and Belize, 1981. *Morbid Mortal Weekly Rep.* 30:497–500, 1981.
7. Center for Disease Control: Acute hemorrhagic conjunctivitis: Florida, North Carolina. *Morbid Mortal Weekly Rep.* 30:501–502, 1981.
8. Chatterjee S., Quarcoopome C. O., and Apenteng A.: Unusual

type of epidemic conjunctivitis in Ghana. *Br. J. Ophthalmol.* 54:628–630, 1970.
9. Wolken S. H.: Acute hemorrhagic conjunctivitis. *Surv. Ophthalmol.* 19:71–84, 1974.
10. Green I. J., Huns T. P., and Sung S. M.: Neurologic complications with elevated antibody titer after acute hemorrhagic conjunctivitis. *Am. J. Ophthalmol.* 80:832–834, 1975.
11. Hatch M. H., Malison M. D., and Palmer E. L.: Isolation of enterovirus 70 from patients with acute hemorrhagic conjunctivitis in Key West, Florida. *N. Engl. J. Med.* 305:1647–1648, 1981.

4–1 **Adult Inclusion Conjunctivitis: Clinical Characteristics and Corneal Changes.** Susan Stenson (New York Univ. Med. Center) reviewed 25 consecutive cases of inclusion conjunctivitis in adults. All patients with acute or chronic follicular conjunctivitis were included. There were 18 acute and 7 chronic cases. The average age of the 16 men and 9 women was 26 years. Infection was bilateral in 16 cases. In 4 cases the sexual partner had had concomitant conjunctivitis. Systemic symptoms were infrequent, but 12 patients had some genitourinary complaints on careful questioning. Upper tarsal involvement predominated in several cases. Hemorrhages were not observed. Twenty patients had corneal changes, particularly in the upper half of the cornea; epithelial keratitis was the usual finding. Treatment was with topical erythromycin ointment and oral tetracycline for 3 weeks. All patients except 1 recovered completely. Scarring occurred in only 1 patient with severe membranous follicular conjunctivitis and epithelial keratitis.

The clinical features of viral and chlamydial follicular conjunctivitis are compared in the table. Although the clinical features of inclusion conjunctivitis and trachoma differ, overlap does exist. Several types of superficial corneal involvement have been described in adult inclusion conjunctivitis, and all but 5 of 25 patients in the present series had significant corneal changes. Superficial epithelial keratitis was the most common finding. In contrast to viral conjunctivitis, upper corneal involvement predominates, and keratitis often is observed early in the course of disease. A

(4–1) Arch. Ophthalmol. 99:605–608, April 1981.

Chapter 4–THE CONJUNCTIVA / 81

COMPARISON OF VIRAL AND CHLAMYDIAL FOLLICULAR CONJUNCTIVITIS

	Inclusion	Viral
incubation	4-19 Days	3-7 Days
Unilateral, bilateral	Usually bilateral	Usually unilateral
Ages	Young adults; neonates	All ages
Systemic findings	Genitourinary	Respiratory
Discharge	Mucopurulent	Watery
Course	Chronic	Self-limited
Adenopathy	+ +	+ + +
Follicles	+ + +	+ + +
Scarring	Rare	Rare
Keratitis	Common; epithelial and subepithelial; frequent limbal involvement; upper half of the cornea	Common; early epithelial; late subepithelial; diffuse involvement
Cytologic findings	Inclusion bodies; polymorphic	Mononuclear response
Response to tetracycline	+	—
Response to steroid	—	+

lack of response to topical steroids helps distinguish the keratitis of adult inclusion conjunctivitis from that associated with viral conjunctivitis.

4–2 **Clinical Features and Diagnosis of Adult Atopic Keratoconjunctivitis and the Effect of Treatment With Sodium Cromoglycate.** Uncertainty persists as to the relation between vernal disease and adult atopic keratoconjunctivitis. Jeffrey L. Jay (Univ. of Glasgow) report the findings in 17 atopic adults with various types of keratitis and conjunctivitis, most of whom were treated with topical sodium cromoglycate, which is useful in the control of vernal catarrh in children. The diagnosis was confirmed by determining the serum IgE level by the radioimmunosorbent technique. Patients were treated with 2% sodium cromoglycate drops 4 times daily for 3 months or longer. Nine patients underwent a double-masked crossover trial with cromoglycate and a matching placebo preparation, each used for 6 weeks.

All but 3 patients were male; the mean age was 35 years. Ocular symptoms had been present for a mean of 7 years. Fourteen patients had a history of eczema, and 11 reported

---

(4–2) Br. J. Ophthalmol. 65:335–340, May 1981.

asthma or wheezing. Seven patients had hay fever, and 16 described perennial symptoms. Nine patients had findings resembling those of the tarsal or limbal forms of vernal keratoconjunctivitis in children, including thickening or ptosis of the lids with edema during exacerbations, and giant or cobblestone papillae of the upper tarsal conjunctiva. Three of these patients had indolent ovoid corneal ulcers with subsequent plaque formation. The usual findings in the other 8 patients were a fine papillary conjunctival reaction and punctate epithelial keratitis. Three patients had predominantly unilateral involvement. Many patients had normal peripheral eosinophil counts. Ten of 15 patients reported symptomatic improvement while using cromoglycate, but complete resolution of the signs was not observed. In the double-blind trial, 4 of 9 patients had less ocular inflammation by clinical examination while using the active preparation. Patients with typical and atypical findings responded similarly.

A substantial number of adults with atopic keratoconjunctivitis have relatively nonspecific ocular findings, but many respond to treatment with sodium cromoglycate. Many patients have had a complete remission of symptoms for several months and have been able to discontinue treatment. Other medications may be useful in refractory cases or during severe exacerbations, and the surgical removal of corneal plaques may be necessary.

4–3 **A Clinical Comparison of Topical Clobetasone Butyrate and Sodium Cromoglycate in Allergic Conjunctivitis.** Clobetasone butyrate is apparently as effective an anti-inflammatory agent as betamethasone, while, at the same time, Clobetasone has less effect on the intraocular pressure. Sodium cromoglycate has been under study for use in the treatment of allergic conjunctivitis. A. W. Frankland and S. R. Walker (St. Mary's Hosp., London) compared these agents in 21 male and 18 female patients (mean age, 24.6 years) who had had allergic conjunctivitis in association with nasal symptoms during the hay fever season and who had positive skin prick tests to grass pollen extracts. Ocular symptoms had been present for 3 to 27 years and lasted an average of 12 weeks each year. Irritation and lacrimation were the most common symptoms, occurring with sneezing and nasal discharge. The double-blind study lasted 4–8 weeks. A betamethasone inhaler was used to prevent nasal symptoms. The two eyes were treated 4 times daily with 0.1% clobetasone butyrate and 2% sodium cromoglycate.

Both cromoglycate and clobetasone provided relief of ocular symptoms. Clobetasone butyrate produced a better response in 20 patients and cromoglycate in 5 cases, whereas in 10 cases the responses were comparable. Nasal symptoms were controlled successfully by the betamethasone valerate nasal aerosol in 29 patients. At the end of the study, 27 patients preferred clobetasone butyrate to sodium cromoglycate; 12 patients had no preference for either drug. The favorable response to clobetasone was related not only to its efficacy, but also to the absence of the local stinging sensation caused by the cromoglycate eye drops.

Clobetasone butyrate was advantageous in the management of allergic conjunctivitis in hay fever patients in this study, in comparison with sodium cromoglycate. Clobetasone produces little or no rise in intraocular pressure in patients who may have an increase when using other steroids. Little risk of steroid-induced glaucoma develops when clobetasone is used for 4–6 weeks during the hay fever season.

▶ [Sodium cromoglycate is a nonsteroid antiallergic compound efficacious in the treatment of allergic conjunctivitis. It is probably not as effective as even weak corticosteroids, but there are, thus far, no known serious complications and it appears far safer to use than corticosteroids.] ◀

4–4 **Orally Administered Tetracycline for Phlyctenular Keratoconjunctivitis.** Phlyctenular keratoconjunctivitis is a nodular conjunctival or corneal condition seen mainly in children, which is associated with the proteins of various bacteria other than tubercle bacilli and is considered to be a nonspecific delayed hypersensitivity reaction to foreign protein. Prolonged corticosteroid therapy does not always eliminate disease and may cause ocular complications. Gerald W. Zaidman and Stuart I. Brown (Univ. of Pittsburgh)

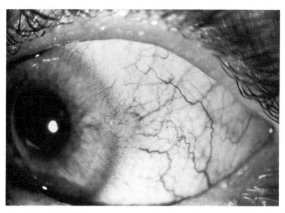

Fig 4–1.—Left eye showing corneoscleral limbic phlyctenule surrounded by conjunctival hyperemia. (Courtesy of Zaidman, G. W., and Brown, S. I.: Am. J. Ophthalmol. 92:178–182, August 1981.)

used oral tetracycline treatment in 6 patients with phlyctenular keratoconjunctivitis, 3 of whom had failed to respond to prolonged topical corticosteroid and antibiotic therapy. The 5 girls and 1 boy had an average age of 10 years. Three patients had had symptoms for 2 years or longer. All patients had neovascularization of the inferior part of the cornea, associated with thinning in 4, and 3 patients had acute limbic phlyctenulae. The appearances in 1 case are shown in Figure 4–1.

The patients received 250 mg of tetracycline two to four times daily. Symptoms resolved completely, and the facial pustules present in 4 patients disappeared. Three patients presently are receiving 250 mg of tetracycline daily, and 2 are taking 250 mg twice daily; 1 is not receiving treatment. One patient had a brief, mild recurrence of conjunctival hyperemia, but no other recurrences have been seen during follow-up. There were no side effects from tetracycline therapy. Corneal neovascularization and opacifications have regressed in all patients.

Oral tetracycline therapy is effective in recalcitrant cases of nontuberculous phlyctenular keratoconjunctivitis. Tetracycline can be used in place of corticosteroid therapy in patients with corticosteroid-induced side effects. Tetracycline was tried in this disorder because of its similarity to ocular rosacea. Presently treatment with 250 mg of tetracycline two or three times daily is recommended until the patient has been asymptomatic for 3 weeks. The dosage then is reduced by 250 mg a day every 3 or 4 weeks to 250 mg daily.

▶ [It seems unusual that an antibiotic is effective in a presumably immune disease, but the finding is of considerable value. The authors state that there were no complications although an 8-year-old child might have tooth coloration problems because the antibiotic is administered for a long time. This is certainly minor in comparison to the disease or effects of the use of long-term corticosteroids.] ◀

4–5 **Conjunctival Melanomas: Prognostic Factors: Review and Analysis of a Series** of 19 cases of primary conjunctival melanoma seen in 1955 to 1974 and followed up for at least 5 years is presented by J. Brooks Crawford. Eight patients developed metastases and died of their disease. Younger patients had a poorer prognosis. Five patients who died had initial resection before age 37 years; all 11 survivors had initial treatment of lesions after age 37. No relation could be found between sex or the duration of symptoms and the course of disease. All surviving patients but 1 had recurrences, and only 3 patients died of metastases before having a local recurrence.

Tumors arising in the caruncle, fornix, or palpebral conjunctiva had a worse prognosis than those arising on the bulbar conjunctiva. Depth of invasion did not correlate significantly with the prognosis, but the number of mitoses was a factor. No influence of the extension of tumor to the surgical margin was apparent. The degree of inflammatory response was inversely related to the risk of developing distant disease. Three of 4 patients having exenteration died of metastatic disease.

Tumor thickness and type of melanoma were not significant prognostic factors in these cases of conjunctival melanoma. An attempt at classifying the lesions by the Clark-McGovern scheme was unsuccessful and did not predict the outcome. Unfavorable prognostic factors in this series included age less than 37 years; tumor in the caruncle, fornix, or palpebral conjunctiva; 4 or more mitoses in 40 high,

4-6 **Benign Pigmented Lesion of the Eyelid Associated With Acquired Ocular Melanosis.** Primary acquired ocular melanosis is a rare condition that may affect the bulbar or palpebral conjunctiva, or both. The potential for malignant transformation makes its recognition important. Roberta F. Palestine, Alan G. Palestine, Charles H. Dicken, and Thomas J. Liesegang (Mayo Clinic and Found.) encountered a patient with both acquired melanosis of the upper eyelid and a pigmented lesion of the lid margin.

Woman, 44, had had a small, pigmented lesion removed from the inferior border of the left upper eyelid 16 months before. Examination showed a flat, 10 × 6-mm, deeply pigmented area of palpebral conjunctiva extending to the lid margin (Figs 4–2 and 4–3). The area was nearly contiguous with the site of the previously removed lesion. Biopsy specimens of the pigmented area showed hyperpigmented epithelial cells, occasional nevus cells, and slight pigment incontinence. Review of sections of the lesion removed 16 motnhs earlier showed clumped and scattered pigmented cells in the dermis and an occasional nevus cell at the dermoepidermal junction. The pigment was identified as melanin.

Fig 4–2 (left).—Acquired ocular melanosis, shown by eversion of left upper eyelid.
Fig 4–3 (right).—Lesion cannot be seen without eyelid eversion. Mild erythema is present because of preceding eyelid eversion and manipulation.
(Courtesy of Palestine, R. F., et al.: Arch. Dermatol. 117:579–581, September 1981; copyright 1981, American Medical Association.)

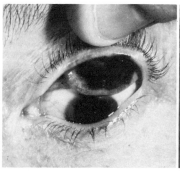
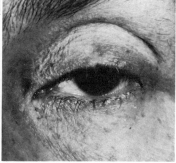

Little change in the conjunctival melanosis was observed on reexamination nearly 4 years later.

Malignant change has been reported in 17% of cases of primary acquired ocular melanosis, usually occurring 5 to 10 years after the onset in patients aged 40 to 50 years. Acquired ocular melanosis may involve the skin of the lid margin directly. It is not certain that the pigmented skin lesion in this patient was directly related to the acquired ocular melanosis, but it is a possibility. When pigmented lesions of the eyelid are examined or excised, the conjunctival surfaces should also be examined to identify concomitant acquired ocular melanosis.

4–7 **Cryotherapy for Precancerous Melanosis (Atypical Melanocytic Hyperplasia) of the Conjunctiva.** Seymour Brownstein, Frederick A. Jakobiec, Ralph D. Wilkinson, John Lombardo, and W. Bruce Jackson utilized cryotherapy in 2 patients with progressive, diffuse precancerous melanosis of the conjunctiva. One patient had two sessions of treatment for involvement of the contigous cutaneous parts of both eyelids. Both patients showed a good response of the melanocytic process to cryotherapy, with slough of the superficial conjunctiva and reepithelialization from adjacent areas. One patient had incomplete regression in the perilimbal region, which was later excised. Neither patient has had a recurrence in more than 7 months of follow-up. Both patients had serious complications, and 1 with severe and extensive disease had corneal and lenticular opacities. Other complications included trichiasis, corneal abrasions, iritis, and mild ptosis.

Cryotherapy led to control of diffuse precancerous melanosis of the conjunctiva in these 2 patients, but complications were more serious than in 2 previous patients with invasive melanoma who required more extensive surgery and multiple applications of cryotherapy. The present patients were elderly, in contrast to the previous patients, and impaired healing may have been responsible for persistent corneal epithelial defects in 1 case. The possibility of obtaining effective control and possible cure of disease in these cases must be weighed against the risk of serious side effects from cryotherapy. Side effects may be minimized by careful patient selection and variations in technique, including the possible concomitant use of other treatment measures.

▶ [This article and the two preceding ones demonstrate the seriousness of conjunctival melanomas. Perhaps most important, they must be recognized, and this may require eversion of both eyelids.] ◀

4–8 **Erythroplasia (Queyart) of Conjunctiva.** Erythroplasia of Queyrat (EQ) is a squamous cell carcinoma in situ that resembles Bowen's disease of the skin histologically, but it more often progresses to invasive squamous carcinoma and metastasizes early. In contrast to Bowen's disease, there is no internal malignancy and no association with arsenic ingestion. Ray S. Dixon and George R. Mikhail (Henry Ford Hosp.) encountered two cases of EQ of the conjunctiva in patients with a long history of basal cell carcinoma of the eyelid.

Man, 55, with hypothyroidism, had had basal cell carcinoma of the right upper eyelid, which was excised and irradiated 6 years earlier. Chronic radiation dermatitis was present, and basal cell

Fig 4–4.—Nodule on right lower eyelid *(arrow)* proved to be invasive squamous cell carcinoma. (Courtesy of Dixon, R. S., and Mikhail, G. R.: J. Am. Acad. Dermatol. 4:160–165, February 1981.)

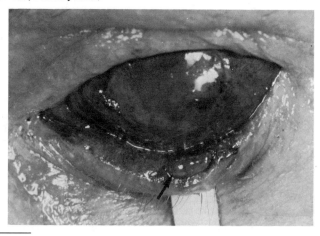

cancer was excised from the right outer canthus a few months before referral with inflammation of the right palpebral and bulbar conjunctivas. The globe exhibited radiation keratoconjunctivitis, and the lens was opaque. The palpebral conjunctiva was erythematous, velvety, and chemotic. Biopsy showed an irregularly acanthotic epidermis with numerous intraepidermal dysplastic cells and atypical mitoses. The dermis contained a marked infiltrate of lymphocytes and plasma cells. Residual basal cell cancer was found during serial excisions of the lesion. Two nodules of invasive squamous cancer later developed on the medial part of the limbus and on the conjunctiva of the right lower lid (Fig 4–4) and were also excised by the microscopic control method. The patient was tumor free for the next 2 years.

The cause of EQ is unknown. The authors' cases show the importance of obtaining biopsy material from patients with refractory conjunctivitis, particularly if there is a history of irradiation of the eyelid region. Microscopically controlled surgical excision with serial examination of layers of tissue by the Mohs technique is ideal in these cases, assuring complete removal of growths with maximum conservation of normal tissues.

▶ [The authors suggest biopsy of chronic conjunctivitis. This is easily carried out by using a chalazion clamp and pinning the tissue to a tongue blade for fixation. Most would probably not agree with routine conjunctival biopsy, but it may be essential if there is a history of irradiation.] ◀

4–9 **Ocular Cicatricial Pemphigoid** is reviewed by Bartly J. Mondino and Stuart I. Brown (Univ. of Pittsburgh). Ocular cicatricial pemphigoid (OCP) is a chronic progressive disease characterized by conjunctival shrinkage, entropion, trichiasis, xerosis, and, finally, reduced vision from corneal opacification. It is a relatively rare disease that generally occurs late in life. The skin appears to be affected less often than the mucous membranes. Mucosal involvement is seen in the nose, oral cavity, pharynx, larynx, esophagus, anus, and vagina, as well as in the conjunctiva. The eyes may be affected simultaneously or separately. Initially, there are irritation, burning, and tearing, and corneal involvement later leads to photophobia and reduced vision. The essential process is fibrosis beneath the conjunctival epithelium. The tear film is reduced and unstable. About half of patients with OCP have elevated IgA levels.

(4–9) Ophthalmology (Rochester) 88:95–100, February 1981.

Surgery may involve a risk of inciting acute disease activity in OCP. Most cases progress when followed up over the long term, but the course of the disease is variable. Progression may be more rapid in the later stages. Artificial tears may be helpful in early and moderately advanced cases of OCP. Antibiotics should be used on the basis of specific sensitivity testing. Staphylococcal blepharitis can be managed by lid scrubs and antibiotic ointment. Entropion with trichiasis can be corrected early in the course using oculoplastic surgical techniques. When the fornices are adequately deep, therapeutic soft contact lenses may be used to protect the cornea from trichiasis and drying. Systemic steroid therapy is of definite value in the treatment of acute manifestations of OCP. The value of long-term systemic immunosuppressive therapy is currently being evaluated. In the final stages, with ankyloblepharon and a keratinized ocular surface, a keratoprosthesis may be useful in restoring sight.

4–10 **Cytologic Changes of the Conjunctiva in Immunoglobulin-Producing Dyscrasias.** Giant cells with intracytoplasmic periodic acid-Schiff (PAS)-positive material were found in conjunctival scrapings from a patient with scleritis and macroglobulinemia. Whether the conjunctival changes were related to the immunoglobulin-producing dyscrasia or whether the conditions were independent of one another was unclear. Maria Spinak (Montefiore Hosp., New York) reviewed the ocular findings in 15 patients with documented immunoglobulin-producing dyscrasias to resolve this problem. The findings are presented in the table. Thirteen patients had clinically normal conjunctivae, but one had abnormal epithelial cells in cytologic preparations that included rouleaux-like formations, islands of rosette-like cells, and giant multinucleated cells. Giant cells with PAS-positive particles were present in a patient with recurrent episcleritis. Smears from a patient with conjunctival lymphomatous involvement showed lymphocytes and cells intermediate between lymphocytes and plasma cells; some cells showed intranuclear eosinophilic PAS-positive

CONJUNCTIVAL FINDINGS IN PATIENTS WITH IMMUNOGLOBULIN-
PRODUCING DYSCRASIAS

Patient	Age	Sex	Gross Ocular Symptoms	Diagnosis	Conjunctival Cytological Findings
PR	67	F	—	Macroglobulinemia	Negative
AB	55	M	—	Hypergammaglobulinemia	Multinucleation or rosette-like formation cells
BD	65	F	—	Hypergammaglobulinemia	Multinucleation or rosette-like formation cells
JW	69	M	—	Hypergammaglobulinemia	Multinucleation or rosette-like formation cells
MA	51	M	—	Multiple myeloma	Multinucleation or rosette-like formation cells and rouleaux-like formation
BT	74	M	—	Multiple myeloma	Dutcher bodies. Some epithelial cell hypertrophy
RP	67	M	—	Multiple myeloma	Multinuclear or rosette-like formation and numerous lymphocytes
BN	65	M	—	Multiple myeloma	Multinuclear or rosette-like formation, lymphocytes and hypertrophic epithelial cells; giant pale cells with granular PAS-positive granules, numerous lymphocytes
GR	78	M	—	Multiple myeloma	Multinuclear or rosette-like formation
HF	73	F	—	Multiple myeloma	Giant cells; folding of nuclei
RP	63	F	—	Lymphoma	Negative
JH	70	F	—	Macroglobulinemia	Negative
CA	72	F	Recurrent episcleritis	Macroglobulinemia	See text
PG	65	F	Conjunctival lymphocytic infiltration	Macroglobulinemia	See text

inclusions (Dutcher bodies). Dutcher bodies also were present in a patient with clinically normal findings.

Three fourths of clinically normal patients without ocular symptoms in this study had conjunctival epithelial-cell changes on cytologic study, in association with an immunoglobulin-producing dyscrasia. The rosette and rouleaux-like formations may be related to the hyperviscosity associated with macroglobulinemia. The giant PAS-positive cells may be large macrophages filled with PAS-positive immunoglobulin derived from the extracellular spaces of the conjunctival connective tissue. Lymphocytoid plasma cells also have been described in patients with immunoglobulin-producing dyscrasias. The conjunctiva is well-endowed with lymphoid tissue, and cytologic preparations may be a sensitive indicator of systemic immunoglobulin-producing dyscrasias. When positive findings are obtained, serum electrophoresis should be performed.

▶ [It is interesting to note that 10 of 13 patients with completely normal-appearing conjunctiva had abnormal cytology.] ◀

5. Cornea and Sclera

Refractive Surgery

STEVEN G. KRAMER, M.D., PH. D.

University of California, San Francisco

The statement has been made so often that it is now trite to suggest that just as the 1970s were the decade of vitreous surgery, the 1980s will be the decade of corneal surgery. Technologic advancements in ophthalmology have been so rapid in recent years that a bandwagon psychology seems to have developed within the profession.

Few ophthalmologists wish to remain standing in the cold as their colleagues surge ahead with new techniques demanded by a public ever seeking the very best that medical technology has to offer. Thus, it is an understatement to say that there is intense interest among ophthalmologists in refractive surgery.

The refractive surgery procedures divide themselves broadly into two groups. First is that group of procedures known as *refractive keratoplasties,* originated by Jose Barraquer, in which corneal tissue is frozen, lathed to a new shape, thus altering its refractive characteristics, and replaced on or added to the patient's eye. Second is *refractive keratotomy,* in which cuts are made in the cornea that are designed to alter its refractive characteristics.

Refractive keratoplasty can be subdivided further into three groups: (1) *keratomileusis,* a procedure in which a lamellar segment of the patient's cornea is removed, frozen, and lathed to either a hyperopic or a myopic configuration and then replaced on the patient's eye; (2) *keratophakia,* in which a piece of donor cornea is frozen, lathed, and implanted into a lamellar bed within the patient's cornea; and (3) *epikeratophakia,* a procedure developed by Werblin and Kaufman, in which a piece of donor cornea is frozen, lathed, and then sutured to the surface of the recipient cornea after only the epithelium has been removed. In this last procedure, Bowman's membrane is left essentially intact, and only a peripheral wedge of stroma is removed to allow suturing of the donor button that then is said to act essentially as a "living contact lens."

It should be noted that in all three approaches to refractive keratoplasty, living keratocytes are destroyed during the freezing process, and the patient's own reshaped cornea (in the case of keratomileusis) or the donor button (in the case of keratophakia and epikeratophakia) must be repopulated by keratocytes from the recipient and must be covered by epithelium from the recipient postoperatively. In addition, healing and remolding of the cornea with visual recovery are relatively slow, more in the nature of the postoperative recovery from keratoplasty than from cataract extraction with lens implantation, for example.

Nevertheless, patients with preexisting aphakia, contraindications to lens implantation, keratoconus, high myopia, and other relatively nontreatable refractive abnormalities may be offered some renewed hope by the continuing development of these procedures. It must be said that epikeratophakia probably has the greatest potential from the standpoint of surgical practicality, inasmuch as buttons may be prepared in advance and there is little invasion of the main corneal substance during the course of the procedure. From the standpoint of corneal biology, however, it remains to be confirmed that epikeratophakia buttons are repopulated adequately with keratocytes and can be recovered with epithelium successfully in all cases over the long term. Clearly, these new procedures are highly complex and bear continued, careful study in controlled clinical and laboratory research environments.

Refractive keratotomy is most well known as *radial keratotomy,* first tried by Sato as an internal and external operation and more recently developed and popularized by Fyodorov as an external procedure. This operation has made an unprecedented appearance on the American ophthalmic scene. It challenges our traditional view of indications for invasive surgery of the globe, offering more cosmetic and psychologic than functional benefit for the majority of patients for whom it is intended. The rapid rise of both professional and public interest in radial keratotomy, in my opinion, has been based in significant measure on economics and public demand stimulated by manipulation of the media.

Some ophthalmic surgeons, experiencing increasing crowding in their chosen field of specialty or subspecialty, are intrigued with the availability of a new, highly remunerative operation that can be done on an entirely new population of patients. It has been estimated that if all eligible patients in the United States were to have the operation, each and every ophthalmologist could anticipate a substantial increase in surgical revenue. To induce payment by third parties for refractive "services" such as radial keratotomy, some enterprising individuals have suggested the term "corneal dysplasia" as an alternative for "myopia."

Notwithstanding these motives for the development of radial keratotomy, it must be acknowledged that Americans seem to detest their glasses to a degree that has been astonishing to ophthalmologists. We should face the disquieting fact that radial keratotomy operations are being performed in the United States at a geometrically increasing rate, and numerous 2-day courses in keratotomy technique are being held throughout the United States at tuitions of up to $1,000.

As more people subject themselves to radial keratotomy, complications are appearing. Anterior chamber perforation probably occurs in at least 10% of eyes, although it usually is considered "inconsequential." Isolated unfortunate cases of lens capsule rupture, anterior synechia formation, significant central endothelial cell loss, and persistent epithelialization of incisions with excessive scarring have occurred. Many patients experience variable visual acuity, glare, inadequate correction, and regression toward the original refractive error. Glasses or contact lenses are often necessary to attain 20/20 vision postoperatively, while occasional patients may not return to 20/20 vision because of persistent corneal instability. In addition, long-term complications have yet to be evaluated adequately. For example, a decrease in central endothelial cell counts that is progressive with time after radial keratotomy in monkey eyes has recently been reported.

Before ophthalmologists become candidates for a windfall profits tax, it would seem wise for the profession as a whole to assess the current status and development of radial keratotomy in the most critical terms. In those terms at the moment, I believe that radial keratotomy is an unsatisfactory operation. It is not at all clear that this type of surgery is safe, predictable, or effective. No controlled clinical trial of the procedure has been published. Degree of correction and incidence of complications are uncertain, and the most significant variable of all—the surgical technique itself—is highly inconsistent. The length, spacing, and particularly the depth of the incisions have been very difficult to control. One study has shown that incision depth varied from 20% of corneal thickness to frank perforation into the anterior chamber.

I believe every effort should be made to develop technology (using animal models) that will produce a significantly more consistent surgical technique and outcome than are possible with present methods. Only if the surgical technique is truly standardized does it seem possible to me to do a meaningful evaluation of this type of procedure. That such an evaluation must be sought seems undeniable in the face of the large number of young, healthy, human eyes that are likely to have this type of surgery.

Even if the incisions can be made with absolute precision, it remains to be shown whether the biologic response of the cornea is predictable, whether the operation is effective in the long run, and whether it can be done safely without significant complications. Finally, we should consider that almost any incidence of complications is unacceptable for an invasive operation on a 20/20 eye.

5–1 **UCLA Clinical Trial of Radial Keratotomy: Preliminary Report.** Fyodorov's radial keratotomy for myopia has generated great interest in both ophthalmologists and the

---

(5–1) Ophthalmology (Rochester) 88:729–736, August 1981.

COMPARISON OF EYES WITH 20/40 OR BETTER UNCORRECTED VISUAL
ACUITY, CHANGES IN MYOPIA, AND DEGREE OF CORNEAL FLATTENING
FOR EACH DIOPTRIC CATEGORY OF PREOPERATIVE MYOPIA

Preoperative Myopia (Diopters)	No.* Eyes	Visual Acuity 20/40 or Better (%)	Mean Decrease in Myopia (Diopters)	Mean Corneal Flattening (Diopters)
2–3*	4*	100*	2.9 ± 0.4*	2.6 ± 0.4*
3–4	16	63	3.3 ± 1.4	3.0 ± 1.5
4–5	12	58	3.1 ± 1.2	3.4 ± 1.2
5–6*	4*	50*	4.5 ± 1.5*	3.5 ± 0.9*
6–7	6	17	3.1 ± 2.5	3.1 ± 2.5
7–8	7	14	4.1 ± 2.1	3.6 ± 0.8
8–14*	3*	0*	6.2 ± 3.3*	4.0 ± 2.0*
Total	52	52	3.4 ± 2.2	3.3 ± 1.5

*Not statistically comparable due to small number of eyes in group.

public. Kenneth J. Hoffer, John J. Darin, Thomas H. Pettit, John D. Hofbauer, Richard Elander, and Jeremy E. Levenson (Univ. of California, Los Angeles) report the preliminary results in a clinical trial of radial keratotomy, begun in late 1979. Excluded were patients younger than age 18 years, those with myopia of less than 2 diopters (D), those with progressive myopia or astigmatism greater than 4 D, and those with a history of any ocular disease other than mild amblyopia. Sixteen corneal incisions were made in a radial manner, attempting to incise 90% of the corneal thickness.

Data were available from 52 eyes of the first 43 patients with follow-up after operation. Mean age of the patients was 31 years. All patients had an uncorrected preoperative acuity worse than 20/200, and 59% were limited to counting fingers. At 3 months after operation, acuity was 20/20 or better in 25% and 20/40 or better in 52%; 21% of the eyes retained or returned to their preoperative uncorrected acuity range of worse than 20/200. Two eyes had good results but regressed. The mean central keratometry reading was 44 D before operation and 41 D afterward. The mean postoperative corneal flattening was 3.3 D. Myopia decreased 2–5 D in 70% of the eyes. In 25% of the eyes, N overcorrection hyperopic refraction was obtained. The results are summarized in the table. Overall endothelial cell loss was 10%. About one third of the patients had an annoying glare. Over one third of the eyes experienced transient variable vision.

Radial keratotomy offers hope to persons encumbered by myopic correction, but it is unpredictable at present, causes occasional visual complications, and has a potential for endothelial cell loss. It should continue to be considered an experimental procedure clinically until more long-term data are available.

5-2 **Radial Keratotomy: An Analysis of the American Experience.** In 1979, Fyodorov and Durnev reported a significant reduction in myopia and excellent unaided visual acuity after a radial keratotomy procedure. Leo D. Bores, William Myers, and John Cowder have reviewed the findings of the National Radial Keratotomy Study Group on 400 eyes of 223 patients, all of whom were followed up at least 12 months. All patients had bilateral nonprogressive myopia of -2 to -11 diopters (D) and underwent partial-thickness radial keratotomy bilaterally. Ninety-seven eyes were treated in a 7-month period in 1979 (group 1), and 303 were treated in the subsequent 14 months (group 2). Sixteen radial incisions were made in each eye from a preset central optical zone. Topical anesthesia was used.

Major discomfort rarely lasted more than 24 hours after

TABLE 1.—Postoperative Sequelae

Sequela	Group 1 (%)	Group 2 (%)
Subconjunctival hemorrhage	39(41.2)	22(7)
Upper lid edema	16(16.4)	48(15.8)
Epithelial defects	11(11.3)	18(5.9)
Stromal edema (14d)	90(92.8)	91(30)
Stromal edema (30d)	29(28.9)	26(8.8)
Stromal edema (45d)	0	0
Cells/flare (trace)	5(5.4)	15(4.9)
Cells/flare (significant)	0	0
Foreign body sensation (>7d)	2(2.1)	6(1.9)
Photophobia (<14d)	14(14.4)	297(98)
Photophobia (>14d)	4(4.2)	15(5.2)

(5–2) Ann. Ophthalmol. 13:941–948, August 1981.

TABLE 2.—ADDITIONAL POSTOPERATIVE SEQUELAE

Sequela	Group 1 (%)	Group 2 (%)
Keratitis (mild)	1(1)	6(1.9)
Fibrous proliferation	1(1)	0
Night glare (<3 months)	87(89.7)	273(90.3)
Night glare (>3 months)	3(4)	12(4)
Vision fluctuation (<3 months)	90(92.8)	271(89.4)
Vision fluctuation (>3 months)	6(1.9)	30(10)
Induced astigmatism (>6 months)	3(3.2)	2(0.6)
Endothelial cell count	↓4%	↓6.3%
Neovascularization	3(3.2)	0

operation. Limbal subconjunctival hemorrhage was much less frequent in group 2 patients, in whom the incision did not cross the limbus (Table 1). Corneal epithelial defects also were less frequent in group 2 patients. Iritis was observed in 5% of both groups. Fewer than 2% of patients in both groups had mild keratitis (Table 2). All patients had fluctuating vision. Keratometric changes were marked in the first 1–2 weeks after surgery. Most patients in both groups had corneal astigmatism in the first 2 months after operation. Hyperopia developed in 3 eyes in group 1. Residual refraction was 3.1 D in group 1 patients and 1.2 D in group 2 patients. Neovascularization of incisions, attributed to use of extended-wear soft contact lenses, occurred in 3 patients in group 1.

Radial keratotomy appears to be safe when properly performed and to be effective in reducing moderate degrees of myopia. Postoperative morbidity is reduced by avoiding cutting across the limbus. Refraction nearly always stabilizes 3–6 months after surgery and appears to be maintained thereafter. Keratotomy is not intended to replace glasses or contact lenses, but may be suitable for patients who cannot wear contact lenses; thus, the benefits of a partial reduction in myopia should not be underestimated. Persons who do work requiring a certain visual acuity without correction may also be candidates for radial keratotomy. The authors have been using this procedure for 30 months.

▶ [These two reports on radial keratotomy emphasize that the procedure is experimental and requires careful study. At this time, the indications have not been spelled out clearly, and this seems the central issue.] ◀

5-3 **Keratophakia Update.** Richard C. Troutman, Casimir Swinger, and Michael Goldstein have since 1977 attempted 32 keratophakias, 29 of them primary and 3 secondary, on aphakic eyes and have completed 29 cases at the first attempt. Another case was completed later. Two eyes had a wound dehiscence and had to be resutured. The patients, aged 35–84 years, were followed up for 3–23 months.

In earlier cases, the dioptic correction was about 28.5% less than that calculated to correct the aphakic error, whereas in later cases it was within 6.5% of the calculated dioptic power. The spherical equivalent refraction improved from $+2.07$ hyperopia to -0.86 myopia in the later cases. The keratometer results were comparably improved. With an improved computer program and instrumentation, the range of error in both refraction and keratometry was reduced. Significantly more of the later patients had acuity of 20/40 or better without correction. All 3 secondarily treated patients achieved good vision. In all, 85% of patients obtained at least 20/40 vision. Sixty percent of all patients were fully rehabilitated within 3 months of the procedure and 75%, within 6 months. Specular microscopy has shown less than 7% cell loss. Optical clarity of the tissues is excellent, despite a slight increase in corneal thickness. Only 1 patient had a retinal detachment, which was readily repaired.

Patients now are advised to have a standard cataract extraction and try the Permalens or a silicone continuous-wear contact lens before attempting keratophakia. Younger patients or any patients with good potential vision who do not undergo intraocular lens implantation and are unable to wear a contact lens now may undergo keratophakia.

5-4 **Keratophakia: Clinical Evaluation.** Daniel M. Taylor, Alan L. Stern, Kenneth G. Romanchuk, and Louis R. Keil-

---

(5-3) Ophthalmology (Rochester) 88:36–38, January 1981.
(5-4) Ibid., pp. 1141–1150, November 1981.

son examined the practicality and efficacy of the keratophakia and keratomileusis procedures of Barraquer in 13 cases of secondary keratophakia procedures in 1980–1981. All patients were unilaterally aphakic or pseudophakic in the fellow eye and were unable to wear a contact lens. They were poor candidates for intraocular lens implantation. Eight patients had secondary exotropia of the aphakic eye. All had good vision in the fellow eye. After removal of a 0.3-mm-thick lamellar cap from the recipient, a lenticule, which was processed by computerized specifications, was placed under the cap and tied under a surgical keratometer. The eye was patched for 48 hours postoperatively and was treated with 5% homatropine and antibiotic-steroid drops.

Excellent anatomical results were obtained in all cases. No immediate surgical complications or serious early postoperative complications occurred. In the 10 patients followed up for 6 months or longer, dramatic visual improvement was obtained, with a high level of patient satisfaction. Visual recovery occurred slowly, however. Seven of 10 patients had an acuity of 20/30 to 20/40 after 6–12 months. All patients have considerable peripheral and some paracentral irregular astigmatism. Average postoperative keratometric readings were reasonably close to the predicted final radius of curvature. Specular microscopy showed little or no endothelial cell loss from the procedure.

Although general conclusions cannot be drawn from this limited sample, the early visual results are somewhat disappointing when compared with results obtained with intraocular lenses and continuous-wear contact lenses. There are many opportunities for technical complications during grinding and insertion of the lenticule. The procedure is specifically indicated for young patients with contact lens intolerance and for older aphakic patients with endothelial damage in whom secondary intraocular lens insertion is contraindicated. The keratophakia procedure is not a viable alternative, however, for routine cataract patients and should not be used as a primary procedure. Further studies may show that the prolonged time of visual recovery is justified if most patients are free of complications and regain stable 20/20 vision.

▶ [Visual recovery is extremely slow after keratophakia and keratomileusis. This factor must be considered in the decision to carry out the procedures.] ◄

5-5 Keratophakia and Keratomileusis: Comparison of Pathologic Features in Penetrating Keratoplasty Specimens.

Frederick A. Jakobiec, Paul Koch, Takeo Iwamoto, Winston Harrison, and Richard Troutman (New York) examined keratoplasty specimens from a patient having two keratophakia procedures and another patient having keratophakia followed by a keratomileusis procedure.

The lenticle-bearing keratoplasty specimen exhibited preservation of the lamellar architecture of the surrounding corneal stroma with intact keratocytes and a thin interface scar surrounding the lenticle. The central part of the lenticle showed excellent preservation of the donor stromal lamellae. In the keratomileusis-penetrating keratoplasty specimen there was bullous separation of the corneal epithelium as well as basal cell swelling and a degenerative subepithelial fibrous pannus. Viable keratocytes were abundant in the donor stroma, but only a few degenerated keratocytes were present in the keratomileusis stroma.

In keratophakia, the anterior stroma is dissected in a la-

Fig 5–1.—Operative sequence in a keratophakia procedure. **A,** host's superficial corneal lamellae are dissected away from the deep stroma. **B,** lenticle *(crosshatched area)* is fashioned on the cryolathe out of a donor corneal button. **C,** donor lenticle is sandwiched between superficial and deep portions of host's stroma. **D,** lenticle is shown in situ between the sutured superficial and deep portions of the host's corneal stroma. (Courtesy of Jakobiec, F. A., et al.: Ophthalmology (Rochester) 88:1251–1259, December 1981.)

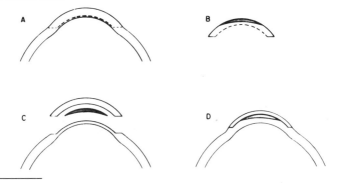

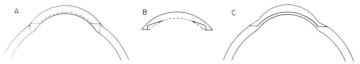

Fig 5–2.—Operative sequence in a keratomileusis procedure. **A,** host's superficial stroma is dissected from the deep stroma. **B,** host's anterior stroma is shaped on a cryolathe so as to correct for the refractive error. In the present report, a donor cornea was used to shape an anterior stromal keratomileusis button instead of the patient's own stroma. **C,** reshaped anterior corneal stroma is resutured onto host's deep corneal stroma. (Courtesy of Jakobiec, F. A., et al.: Ophthalmology (Rochester) 88:1251–1259, December 1981.)

mellar manner free from the deep corneal stroma (Fig 5–1) and replaced over a lenticle of stromal collagen from a donor cornea, fashioned on a cryolathe to correct the refractive error. In keratomileusis (Fig 5–2), the anterior stroma is dissected away in a lamellar manner, frozen and cryolathed, and resutured to the deep stroma. Active fibroblasts were observed in interface wounds in the present cases. The keratomileusis specimen showed complete repopulation of the anterior donor stroma by host keratocytes at 7 months. Keratomileusis is technically a more difficult procedure, but when satisfactorily performed, it permits a rapid return of visual acuity to preoperative levels. Slower recovery of acuity after keratophakia may be related to slow repopulation of the lenticle stroma by host keratocytes and distortion of acuity by the two interface scars. There is only one interface scar in keratomileusis. Remodeling of these scars probably takes well over a year after either procedure.

▶ [The Greek word for molding is spelled "smileusis," so that "keratomileusis" should actually have another "s": "keratosmileusis."] ◀

5–6 **Epikeratophakia—Surgical Correction of Aphakia: III. Preliminary Results of a Prospective Clinical Trial.** Theodore P. Werblin, Herbert E. Kaufman, Miles H. Friedlander, and Nicole Granet (Louisiana State Univ.) report the results in 14 patients randomized to keratomileusis or epikeratophakia and in 12 others who underwent the epikeratophakia procedure and had follow-up for at least 1 month. Aphakic patients older than age 10 years with sta-

PATIENTS UNDERGOING REFRACTIVE SURGERY

Patient No./ Age, yr/Sex	Visual Acuity			Length of Follow-up, mo
	Preoperative (Best)*	Postoperative (Spectacle)	Postoperative (Best)*	
		Epikeratophakia†		
1/81/F	20/50	20/50	20/50	8
2/85/M	20/40	20/300	20/40	4
3/59/F	20/20	20/80	20/30	4
4/50/M	20/20	20/40	20/20	3
5/62/F	20/20	20/300	20/50	3
6/42/F	20/30	20/50	20/80	3
7/68/M	20/25	20/40	20/40	3
8/15/M	20/20	20/20	20/20	3
9/70/F	20/25	20/80	20/50	2
10/61/F	20/20	20/50	20/50	2
11/66/M	20/25	20/400	20/400	2
12/28/M	20/20	20/300	20/100	2
13/80/F	...	20/400	20/100	2
14/34/M	20/25	20/40	20/25	2
15/59/M	20/20	20/200	20/200	2
16/77/M	20/20	20/60	20/40	1
17/70/M	20/20	20/60	20/60	1
18/74/M	20/20	20/200	20/200	1
19/77/F	20/20	Not done	20/400	1
		Keratomileusis		
1/60/M	20/20	20/200	20/100	3
2/62/F	20/20	20/40	20/25	3
3/63/M	20/20	< 20/400	20/200	3
4/25/M	20/60	20/200	20/200	3
5/38/F	20/20	20/60	20/30	3
6/23/M	20/25	20/200	20/50	2
7/70/F	20/25	20/50	20/50	2

*Best corrected visual acuity with a contact lens.
†One patient whose graft was removed has been excluded. Patient 8 received two grafts. First graft was lost as result of trauma; data herein are derived from postoperative course of second, successful graft.

ble acuities were candidates for the study. They were either not candidates for or not satisfied with other means of correction. Each had acuity of 20/40 or better in the fellow eye. Epikeratophakia involves removal of the corneal epithelium with alcohol and suturing in place of a prelathed lamellar corneal graft with 10–0 nylon sutures. The lenticules were obtained from donor corneal tissue unsuitable for penetrating keratoplasty.

Twenty patients received 21 epikeratophakia grafts (table). One graft was lost from a persistent epithelial defect and necrosis and 1 from trauma. The other grafts eventually appeared to be normal in clarity. Problems with graft epithelialization and recurrent epithelial defects have been nearly eliminated with use of a bandage soft lens for 3 or 4 weeks after operation. Several patients in both treatment groups reported photophobia in the early postoperative period. Many patients described a form of diplopia that developed as uncorrected acuity improved in the eye that was operated on. Acuity with spectacles was significantly better and was achieved more rapidly after epikeratophakia than after keratomileusis. A small but significant increase in corneal astigmatism was observed. The chief problem with the final refractive results was undercorrection, which averaged 4.6 D in the patients who had epikeratophakia. The oldest surviving epikeratophakia graft has been stable for about 7 months.

Epikeratophakia has been at least as successful as keratomileusis in terms of visual potential and visual recovery. A tendency to undercorrection is a major problem with this procedure. Because no lamellar dissection of the central visual axis is necessary, the procedure is reversible.

▶ [This article and the 5 that precede it have been carefully selected to furnish conservative, careful clinical information on what can only be described as experimental corneal surgery. Nonetheless, it is not clear what the criteria for surgery are and, indeed, they seem to be rapidly changing. Steven G. Kramer has written a fine introduction to this chapter, and the reader is referred to his thoughtful discussion.] ◀

5-7 **Factors Affecting the Outcome of Corneal Transplantation** are discussed by D. J. Coster (Flinders Univ. of South Australia, Bedford Park). The prognosis of corneal grafts has improved with the development of antimicrobial and anti-inflammatory therapy, and a high degree of success now is obtained with keratoplasty. Ninety-one patients having 132 penetrating corneal grafts for sequelae of herpetic keratitis in 1967–1978 were observed for up to 10 years after surgery. Forty-seven grafts eventually failed, including all 14 lamellar grafts. The outcome also was related to the degree of corneal vascularization at the time of surgery and to the presence of anterior segment inflammation. Donor age, but not the number of previous grafts, was a factor. Allograft rejection occurred in two thirds of failures. In only 20% of cases was developing graft rejection reversed by topical steroid therapy. Recurrent epithelial disease accounted for 11% of failures. Rejection frequently was associated with epithelial herpetic recurrence and bacterial infection.

Allograft rejection now is the chief obstacle to successful corneal grafting. Patients with extensive vascularization are at an increased risk of rejection. The role of cytotoxic antibodies to donor material remains unclear. Apart from progress in serologic screening and matching, the need for immunosuppression will continue. Cyclosporin A has been found to be effective in organ allografting in a wide range of animals, but any potential immunosuppressive agent must be evaluated in the setting in which it is to be used. Studies in rabbits have shown marked prolongation of graft survival with systemic cyclosporin A therapy, but not with topical treatment. Most persons in the world who are blind from corneal opacification have extensive outer eye disease that precludes corneal replacement. Their need is for better means of improving the environment of the outer eye so that they will become candidates for corneal transplantation.

5–8 **Selecting Patients for Penetrating Keratoplasty** is reviewed by George O. Waring III (Emory Univ.). Corneal transplantation is as much a psychologic and social event as an exercise in medical transplantation. The patient must understand the importance of careful attention to the graft for 1 to 2 years after operation and that there is a lifelong potential for opacification. Provision should be made for postoperative supervision, adequate economic resources, and reliable transportation. The risks and rewards of keratoplasty both are increased in a monocular patient with corneal opacification. Patient and physician must agree on the goal of keratoplasty. Good communication between the referring ophthalmologist and the corneal surgeon is important.

Noncorneal problems that may jeopardize graft clarity, including systemic disease, must be taken into account. An

Corneal Disease	Probability of Graft Clarity
Corneal Diseases Arranged in Order of Probability for Prolonged Graft Clarity	
Keratoconus	90%
Familial stromal dystrophy (eg, macular, granular, lattice)	
Central quiet avascular opacity (eg, traumatic, microbial ulceration, diskiform keratitis, minor chemical burn)	
Central Fuchs' endothelial dystrophy	
Aphakic or pseudophakic corneal edema	80%
Interstitial keratitis	
Failed corneal graft <8.0 mm	
Phlyctenular keratitis	
Scar with iridocorneal adhesion	70%
Stromal herpes simplex keratitis	
Blast injuries	
Trachomatous scarring with pannus	
Advanced Fuchs' endothelial dystrophy	
Total aphakic or pseudophakic corneal edema	50%
Central descemetocele	
Heavily vascularized, scarred, edematous corneas	30%
Congenital corneal opacities (eg, Peters' anomaly, sclerocornea)	
Severe chemical, thermal, or radiation injury	
Cicatricial pemphigoid; erythema multiforme	<10%

adequate tear film is important in the outcome. Too often, a clear corneal graft fails to improve acuity because of preexistent vitreoretinal disease. The most important recurrent condition after keratoplasty is herpes simplex keratitis. Evaluation of the thickness and vascularization of the host cornea helps predict the chance of long-term graft clarity after keratoplasty. The quality of the host corneal stroma and epithelium is also important. The chance of prolonged graft clarity associated with various corneal diseases is shown in the table.

Both the operator's judgment in preoperative and postoperative matters and his operative skills influence long-term graft clarity. Most well-trained ocular microsurgeons who have the services of a reliable eye bank and are facile in modern methods of intraocular surgery can perform a technically successful penetrating keratoplasty, but proper patient selection and postoperative management are important.

▶ [There are still obvious immunologic problems to be solved, but both this article and the preceding one rightly empahsize external eye disease, such as inadequate tears and infection.] ◀

5–9 **Current Techniques for Improved Visual Results After Penetrating Keratoplasty** are discussed by William M. Bourne (Mayo Clinic). The proportion of corneal transplants remaining clear for a year or longer now approaches 90% or more, but a truly successful procedure allows the eye to see with the best acuity of which its retina is capable. Ideally, this vision should be obtained relatively soon after surgery and should last a lifetime. A double running suture technique is preferable to use of a single running suture. In the double running suture method, the first 10–0 nylon suture is placed with 12 deep loops near Descemet's membrane perpendicular to the wound and tied tightly. After the four interrupted fixation sutures are removed, the second 11–0 nylon suture is placed in the same direction but less deeply and is tied less tightly than the first. It is inserted parallel to the first suture without torque to eliminate the tendency for the graft to rotate when the first suture is removed 2 months after keratoplasty. The second suture is removed 1 year after the procedure. When

Fig 5–3.—Mean endothelial cell density at five serial postoperative examinations in 24 penetrating corneal transplants without rejection or vitreocorneal contact. (Courtesy of Bourne, W. M.: Ophthalmic Surg. 12:321–327, May 1981.)

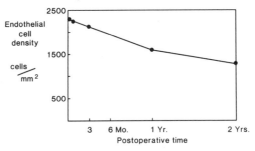

high astigmatism occurs, it can be reduced substantially by surgical relaxing incisions or wedge resections, but the results to date have been unpredictable with respect to the degree of astigmatic correction obtained.

Increased longevity of corneal grafts occurs when more endothelial cells are successfully transplanted by improving the quality of donor tissue and by reducing operative cell loss. It is useful to screen donor tissue by specular microscopy. Preoperative digital ocular massage and use of a scleral ring have significantly reduced cell loss in phakic grafts. Postoperative inflammation should be treated early with steroids. An anterior vitrectomy through the pars plana may be indicated if increased cell loss results from vitreocorneal contact. Chronic endothelial cell loss can be monitored in transplants (Fig 5–3), and attempts can be made to prevent cell death with antiinflammatory or other therapy where excessive loss is observed. Specular microscopy is the basis for all these measures, which should improve the long-term results of penetrating keratoplasty.

Visual Prognosis in Aphakic Bullous Keratopathy Treated by Penetrating Keratoplasty: A Retrospective Study of 73 Cases. Although clear corneal grafts have been reported in up to 95% of cases of aphakic bullous keratopathy, only about 50% of patients have had vision of 20/100 or better after 1–2 years. W. Stanley Muenzler and Willard K. Harms (Univ. of Oklahoma, Oklahoma City) reviewed the results obtained by corneal transplantation in 73 consecutive patients with aphakic bullous keratopathy who had follow-up for at least 2 years. All eyes had limbus-to-limbus edema, and none had preoperative vision better than 20/200. Oversized donor corneas were used in 44% of cases. Topical steroids were administered until the eyes were white and quiet. Four patients had correction with contact lenses postoperatively; the rest had spectacles.

Fifty-seven eyes (78%) had clear grafts at 2 years, and 67% achieved an acuity of 20/100 or better. Eight eyes with clear grafts had less than 20/100 vision at 2 years. Four of these had senile macular degeneration, and 2 had glaucoma. Another eye had a retinal detachment. Of all 24 eyes without at least 20/100 vision at 2 years, half had glaucoma, and one-fourth had macular dysfunction. Fewer than half of the grafts in glaucomatous eyes were clear at 2 years, and only one-third had an acuity of 20/100 or better. Seven of 10 eyes with poor visual results had glaucoma. Better results were associated with the use of oversized donor corneas.

Sixty-seven percent of eyes in this series with aphakic bullous keratopathy achieved 20/100 or better vision 2 years after corneal transplantation. Damage from glaucoma was the most common cause of failure. The long-term visual prognosis may be improved by using oversized donor corneas and manual vitrectomy techniques. Manual vitrectomy with cellulose sponges and scissors gives results at least as good as those obtained by mechanical vitrectomy.

▶ [Final visual acuity should not be assessed until at least 2 years after corneal transplantation. Special suturing techniques and partial anterior vitrectomy in aphakic transplants have been helpful. Methods to protect the endothelium during the surgical procedure are also of importance. Sodium hyaluronate has been extraordinarily helpful in maintaining the anterior chamber and appears to protect the endothelium during suturing. Sodium hyaluronate does have a tendency to increase the intraocular pressure for a few days postoperatively, however.] ◀

5–11 **Prolonged Donor Cornea Preservation in Organ Culture: Long-Term Clinical Evaluation.** Donald J. Doughman has examined the factors that are possibly involved in the contamination of organ-cultured corneal tissue by studying the type and frequency of donor eye contamination when it arrives at the eye bank, by comparing the effectiveness of immersing the globe in neosporin or gentamicin, and by determining the effectiveness of gentamicin, penicillin, and amphotericin B in preventing contamination during organ culture. In addition, the usefulness of a new terminal sterility check procedure was investigated. A total of 230 eyes were included in the study. Organ culture was performed using sterile technique in a vertical laminar flow hood. Clinical study included 124 penetrating keratoplasties in 116 patients, using corneas stored by the 37 C organ culture method. A total of 114 keratoplasties in 104 patients were evaluable.

(5–11) Trans. Am. Ophthalmol. Soc. 78:567–628, 1980.

Of the 230 eyes in the microbiologic study, 152 were contaminated by a total of 176 organisms. Neosporin sterilized only 36% of eyes, and gentamicin sterilized 78%. Gentamicin immersion did not combat *Pseudomonas aeruginosa* or *Proteus mirabilis* effectively. The overall rate of contamination during organ culture storage for 20 months was 4.7%, or 0.55% per month. In the clinical series, donor corneas were stored by organ culture incubation at 37 C for an average of 16.5 days. Twenty-two of 114 transplants have failed, but there were no primary graft failures. Forty-six of 61 successful transplants provided 20/40 or better vision. Some donor corneas were placed in M-K medium 16 hours before operation to improve visualization of the anterior chamber during surgery, but a delay in deturgescence still was noted in aphakic grafts.

The leading cause of graft failure was immune rejection, followed by uncontrolled glaucoma. Two failures were due to wound dehiscence, 1 in a patient with radiation keratitis and secondary fungal infection and 1 in a patient who had had herpes simplex keratouveitis and had a *Staphylococcus aureus* infection in a stitch after operation. The rate of recurrent herpes simplex was 40% (4 of 10 cases). Two stitch abscesses occurred, and there was 1 case of *Torulopsis glabrata* endophthalmitis.

Contamination of donor corneal tissue is a constant risk during organ culture. A terminal sterility check must be done by well-trained microbiologists experienced in such procedures. The 37 C organ culture technique does permit long-term storage of donor material for penetrating keratoplasty.

Time Series Analysis of Allograft Reactions After Penetrating Keratoplasties. Problems in preservation of donor endothelium and treatment of graft reactions continue to limit the success rate of penetrating keratoplasty. Zenro Inaba, Shigetoshi Nagataki, and Teruo Tanishima (Univ. of Tokyo) carried out a time series analysis of allograft reactions in 283 penetrating keratoplasties done from 1971 to 1979. The 184 male and 99 female patients were aged 4 months to 78 years. Donor eyes were removed within

---

(5–12) Jpn. J. Ophthalmol. 25:47–59, 1981.

12 hours after death, and the keratoplasties were performed within 12 hours after enucleation. All operations were done with the operating microscope. Patients received 0.1% dexamethasone and antibiotics topically three times a day and 1% atropine or homatropine once a day for as long as necessary.

Seventy-seven patients had allograft reactions, and 28 grafts eventually became opaque, despite massive topical and systemic corticosteroid therapy. Patients with leukoma did less well than patients with keratoconus. Reactions were more frequent in the group of 35 regraft cases, in 30% of which final opacification developed. Among primary grafts, final opacification was more frequent in patients with preoperative corneal vascularization. The cumulative probability of allograft reaction increased with the duration of postoperative follow-up, reaching a plateau after 2,000 to 3,000 days. The interval before failure was shorter in cases with a donor age over 60 years.

These observations suggest the second-set reaction that occurs in the graft transplanted to a previously sensitized host. Aged donor tissues may be likelier to undergo rejection. Allograft reactions occurred earlier in preoperatively vascularized corneas, but this series included no heavily vascularized corneas.

5–13 **Transplantation Immunology of Penetrating Keratoplasty.** Allograft rejection now appears to be the most important cause of delayed corneal graft failure in man. Walter J. Stark (Johns Hopkins Med. Inst., Baltimore) obtained serums before and after corneal transplantation and examined them for lymphocytotoxic antibodies, using a modified microcytotoxicity test. Human leukocyte antigen (HLA) typing also was performed. Studies were done in 78 patients without detectable lymphocytotoxic antibodies before keratoplasty. A total of 59 patients had no antibodies postoperatively; however, 8 of these patients (14%) had an immune graft response, as did 68% of patients with anti-HLA antibodies after keratoplasty (Fig 5–4). No cell killing of appropriate targets was observed through use of the antibody-dependent cell-mediated cytotoxicity assay in pa-

(5–13) Trans. Am. Ophthalmol. Soc. 78:1079–1117, 1980.

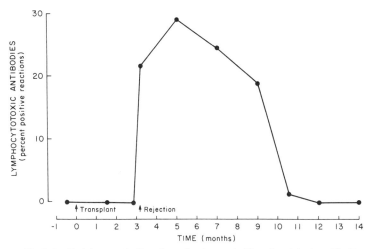

Fig 5–4.—Serial serum testing shows development of lymphocytotoxic antibodies at time of corneal allograft rejection. (Courtesy of Stark, W. J.: Trans. Am. Ophthalmol. Soc. 78:1079–1117, 1980.)

tients rejecting corneal transplants. Direct cell-mediated cytolysis could not be related to the clinical state of patients. Evidence of cell-mediated immunity was obtained by the leukocyte migration inhibition assay with pooled human corneal antigens.

In 1973–1978, 86 penetrating keratoplasties were done in patients with significant stromal vascularization in at least three quadrants, which extended into the visual axis. Three fourths of patients had had at least 1 transplant failure in the same eye, and the rest had been exposed to foreign HLA antigens by contralateral keratoplasty, blood transfusion, or pregnancy. The mean patient age was 60 years. Serums were cross-matched individually against potential corneal donor lymphocytes. A total of 78% of the grafts were clear at an average follow-up of 16.6 months, while 15% have failed from immune rejection. All but 1 of the graft failures due to rejection occurred within 6 months of surgery; the average interval was 3½ months. One fourth of all patients had evidence of immunity. Reversibility of allograft reactions was related to the HLA match (table). No significant correlation was apparent.

Donor-Recipient HLA Match and Reversibility of Allograft Reaction

Number of HLA antigens matched	Number of patients	Total number of immune events (reaction or rejection)	Allograft reaction (graft clear)	Percent reversed
0	51	14 (27%)	7	50
1	35	9 (26%)	3	33
2	11	1 (9%)	1	100
3	5	2 (40%)	0	0
4	1	0	0	—
Total	103	26 (25%)	11	42

Cultured corneal cells contain HLA antigens, and humoral and cellular immunity can develop at the time of corneal graft rejection. Usual cross-match testing does not require matching of individual HLA antigens. A trial is currently under way to determine the value of such matching in high-risk cases.

▶ [The allograft reaction incidence varies greatly, but allograft rejection is the most frequent cause of late graft failure. It is not yet certain if cross-match testing is of value, but a double-masked clinical trial is under way.] ◀

5–14 **Transplantation of Lacerated Corneas.** Satisfactory vision may not be obtained after repair of a corneal laceration because of severe central scarring and irregular astigmatism. Thomas G. Sharkey and Stuart I. Brown (Univ. of Pittsburgh) reviewed the results of penetrating keratoplasty in 8 patients aged 5 to 43 years with healed corneal lacerations extending through the corneoscleral limbus. In 7 eyes the laceration extended 2 to 3 mm beyond the limbus into the sclera. Three eyes had previously undergone cataract extraction. The host cornea was trephined to a depth of two thirds of the corneal thickness. Iris remnants and retrocorneal connective tissue were removed as was feasible, and anterior vitrectomy was done where necessary. Flattening of the cornea was compensated for in 5 instances.

The results are summarized in the table. Intraocular

CLINICAL SUMMARY OF EIGHT PATIENTS

Case, Sex, Age (yr)	Surgical Procedure	Intraocular Pressure Preoperative	Intraocular Pressure Postoperative	Postoperative Retinal Detachment	Graft Status
1, M, 26	Laceration repaired; cataract extracted	Normal	Controlled with cyclocryotherapy	No	Transparent centrally; 3 yr after surgery, visual acuity was 6/15 (20/50)
2, F, 42	Laceration repaired; cataract extracted	Normal	Controlled medically	Yes	Transparent
3, F, 12	Laceration repaired; cataract extracted	Normal	Controlled medically	Yes (reattached)	Transparent; 3 yr after surgery, visual acuity was 6/30 (20/100)
4 F, 8	Laceration repaired; cataract extracted	Normal	< 5 mm Hg	Yes	Transparent
5, M, 4	Laceration repaired	< 5 mm Hg	Controlled medically	Yes	Transparent
6, M, 15	Laceration repaired	Normal	Controlled with cyclocryotherapy	No	Transparent; 5 yr after surgery, visual acuity was 6/60 (20/200)
7, M, 42	Laceration repaired	Normal	Controlled medically	No	Transparent; 20 mo after surgery, visual acuity was 6/12 (20/40)
8, F, 4	Laceration repaired; lens expulsed at time of trauma	< 5 mm Hg	Controlled medically	Yes	Transparent

pressures above 35 mm Hg developed in 7 of 8 eyes within 3 weeks after operation. Two patients required cyclocryotherapy. Retinal detachment was present before or after operation in 4 eyes. Reattachment operations were successful in 1 of 2 eyes. Another patient was found preoperatively to have an inoperable traction detachment of the inferior portion of the retina that progressed to total detachment.

Retinal detachment may occur in eyes with corneal lacerations involving the corneoscleral limbus, where thick fibrous tissue ingrowth occurs in the anterior segment. Late rises in intraocular pressure frequently develop in such eyes. Despite these complications, corneal transplantation can be worthwhile, even in the presence of retinal detachment. Transparent grafts resulted in all cases in this series, and the intraocular pressure was controlled in all patients. Four patients gained functional to good vision.

▶ [There is a tendency to carry out more extensive surgery at the time of the injury, using the microscope for lenectomy and vitrectomy as needed. It may be that the incidence of late fibrous bands and retinal detachment will be decreased and corneal transplantation still more reasonable.] ◀

5–15 **Corneal Endothelial Replacement: I. In Vitro Formation of an Endothelial Monolayer.** Replacement of damaged corneal endothelium with cultured endothelial cells at keratoplasty may provide a new approach to surgical management of endothelial decompensation. Jorge A. Alvarado, Denis Gospodarowicz, and Gary Greenburg (Univ. of California Med. Center, San Francisco) have developed a

Fig 5–5.—Reconstruction of the corneal endothelium at 5 (A), 10 (B), 30 (C), and 60 minutes (D), and at 72 hours (E). The field shown in B was selected to demonstrate that the cells have become flattened by this time, and it is not representative of the number of cells present by this incubation time. Light microscopy; ×1,100. (Courtesy of Alvarado, J. A., et al.: Invest. Ophthalmol. Vis. Sci. 21:300–316, August 1981.)

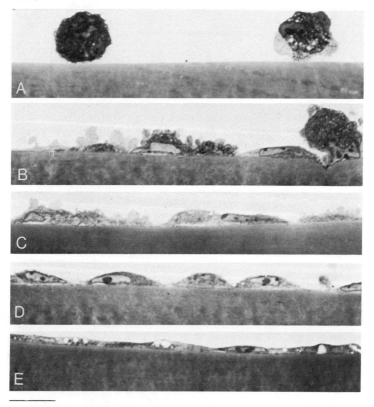

technique that allows the use of cultured corneal endothelial cells, passaged for prolonged periods, in animals at keratoplasty.

METHOD.—Bovine corneal endothelial cells were maintained in Dulbecco's modified Eagle's medium containing 10% calf serum and fibroblast growth factor and were passaged weekly. The cultured cells then were seeded onto a corneal button denuded of its own endothelium.

After 30–60 minutes of incubation, the cultured cells were able to repopulate and reconstitute a new endothelium over Descemet's membrane (Fig 5–5). The process involved cell adhesion to Descemet's membrane, expansion or spreading out of the cells to cover the surrounding area, and cohesion of the cells to one another to form a continuous monolayer. Cohesion was observed within 1 hour after seeding of the cells, when the cells contacted one another by means of long thin cytoplasmic processes, or filopodia. Occluding junctions were not observed after 1 hour of incubation, but were noted in about one third of the cells after 72 hours.

When corneal buttons seeded an hour before were subjected to trephination and sutured into a rabbit host, the cell layer maintained its integrity 24 hours after keratoplasty. The feasibility of endothelial replacement in keratoplasty appears promising. Continuing studies of the cellular processes involved in formation of the reconstituted endothelium and its attachment to Descemet's membrane are needed. The coating time is much reduced by preserving the innermost layer of Descemet's membrane, which contains laminin, a protein involved in adhesion of endothelial cells to their basement membrane.

▶ [While refractive keratoplasty seems to have caught the imagination of both professional and lay people, endothelial cell replacement has far more important therapeutic implications. If it turns out that endothelial cells can be used from the blood vessels or other tissues of the keratoplasty patients, both the problem of tissue availability and that of rejection would be eliminated. Moreover, eye banking would be changed overnight in ways we cannot, at this time, even guess.] ◀

5–16 **Statistical Analysis of the Rate of Recurrence of Herpesvirus Ocular Epithelial Disease.** Little is known of the rate of recurrence of ocular epithelial herpesvirus disease. Jonathan J. Shuster (Univ. of Florida, Gainesville), Herbert E. Kaufman (Louisiana State Univ., New Orleans), and Anthony B. Nesburn (Univ. of Southern California, Los Angeles) carried out a prospective study of 119 patients who had had at least 2 attacks of ocular epithelial herpes but were free of disease at the beginning of the study. They were receiving human leukocyte interferon, but the low-titer preparation being used is now known to have no influence on the natural recurrence rate. A total of 1,279 months of follow-up was obtained.

Recurrence rates are given in the table. The estimated risk of recurrence within 1 year was about 25%. Recurrences could not be correlated significantly with age or sex, but a short interval between the last 2 recurrences tended to be associated with future short recurrence times. Patients at risk for at least 6 months and who had no recurrence during the study had an average interval between the last 2 documented episodes of 27 months, compared to 13 months for those with a recurrence during the study. Nearly half the patients with a previous interval of less than a year had a recurrence during the study, and all but 1 of these episodes occurred within 15 months after entry into the study.

The interval between attacks of herpesvirus infection must be taken into account in future studies of the recurrence of ocular herpes. Recurrence rates in this study are similar to those reported in previous studies. Estimates of the risk of

ESTIMATED PROSPECTIVE RECURRENCE RATES OF OCULAR
HERPESVIRUS DISEASE IN 119 PATIENTS

Months of Study	Recurrence Rate Estimate (%)	Standard Error (%)	Effective Sample Size	Lost to Follow-up
6	14.4	±3.6	96	20
12	24.5	±4.8	81	13
18	29.1	±5.5	68	3
24	32.9	±6.5	52	1

recurrence will help in planning the management of patients with ocular herpes.

5–17 **Bilateral Herpetic Keratitis.** Keratitis due to herpesvirus is one of the most common causes of unilateral corneal opacification. Involvement of both eyes is unusual, but may be particularly disabling when it occurs. K. R. Wilhelmus, M. G. Falcon, and B. R. Jones (London) reviewed the findings in 30 patients with bilateral herpetic keratitis, among about 1,000 patients having corneal disease due to human herpesvirus. The 21 males and 9 females had an average age of 28 years at the time of initial corneal disease. Ulcerative keratitis was treated with topical antiviral medication, with or without wiping debridement. Progressive stromal or uveal inflammation was controlled with a topical steroid. Keratoplasty was considered in patients with corneal opacity, stromal loss, or refractory inflammation.

Four patients had a systemic illness just before the initial episode of keratitis. Atopy was present in 12 patients. One patient was receiving a topical steroid when keratitis developed in both eyes. In 17 patients the eyes were affected simultaneously. Seven patients had cutaneous vesicles on the face, and 6 had conjunctivitis and preauricular lymphadenopathy. Recurrent ulcerative keratitis developed in 41 eyes, stromal disciform keratitis in 24, and anterior uveitis in 10. Ocular hypertension developed in 4 eyes, and corneal vascularization in 24. A corneal opacity developed in 43 eyes of 26 patients. Keratoplasty was done in 11 patients, bilaterally in 2 of them. Six eyes required repeat keratoplasty. Ten eyes had acuity of 6/60 or worse after the final episode of ocular inflammation. Two patients had such vision in both eyes. In 4 atopic patients, secondary microbial keratitis developed.

The incidence of bilateral herpetic keratitis in this series was about 3%. Patients with bilateral involvement tend to be younger and to be atopic. In some cases viral shedding may be responsible, or immunity to herpesvirus may not develop from initial exposure of one eye. Infection with two different viral variants is another possibility. A high rate of complications occurs in patients with bilateral herpetic eye disease. The factors associated with bilateral herpetic eye disease also apparently predispose to progressive corneal inflammation and opacification.

▶ [The recurrence rate appears to be 25% in the first year, increasing to 33% in the second year, with about 3% of cases bilateral.] ◀

5–18 **Prognostic Indicators of Herpetic Keratitis: Analysis of Five-Year Observation Period After Corneal Ulceration.** Kirk R. Wilhelmus, Douglas J. Coster, Hugh C. Donovan, Michael G. Falcon, and Barrie R. Jones (London) followed 152 patients with herpetic keratitis over a 5-year period. The patients, seen in 1974 with a dendritic or geographic corneal ulceration, were treated with 3.3% vidarabine ointment, 1% trifluridine solution, or mechanical wiping debridement. Antiviral chemotherapy was administered 5 times daily until the epithelial ulcer healed. Topical prednisolone was administered for progressive stromal or uveal inflammation, stromal lysis, corneal neovascularization, inflammatory ocular hypertension, or indolent inflammatory ulceration.

Most of the initial ulcers were dendritic. The mean patient age was 49 years. A topical steroid had been used or was being used at the time of presentation in 46% of the patients. The follow-up findings are summarized in the table. A recurrent herpetic corneal epithelial ulcer was observed in 40% of patients, and 13 had more than 1 recurrence. Recurrences were more frequent in men than in women and in patients with a previous herpetic corneal ulcer. Nearly half of the patients with stromal inflammation had used a topical steroid. One patient had a glaucomatous visual field defect and underwent trabeculectomy. Acuity after 5 years was 6/5 to 6/12 in 73% of patients; 6/18 to 6/60 in 24%; and worse than 6/60 in 3%. Seventeen patients had a final acuity worse than before the ulcer, about half of them because of stromal opacification related to herpetic keratitis. Patients with a large geographic ulceration were especially likely to have visual loss because of stromal opacification.

Recurrence of herpetic keratitis was related to male sex

(5–18) Arch. Ophthalmol. 99:1578–1582, September 1981.

FREQUENCY OF OCCURRENCE OF
SELECTED VARIABLES DURING FIVE-
YEAR OBSERVATION PERIOD OF 152
PATIENTS AFTER ULCERATIVE HERPETIC
KERATITIS

Subsequent Complication	No. (%)
Recurrent ulceration	61 (40)
Disciform stromal keratitis	24 (16)
Irregular stromal keratitis	14 (9)
Corneal opacity	33 (22)
Ocular hypertension	8 (5)
Bacterial keratitis	2 (1.5)

and previous herpetic ulceration in this series, but not to the type of treatment used initially. Stromal disease could not be related to previous use of a steroid. The type of initial treatment did not influence the subsequent occurrence of corneal scarring or decreased visual acuity.

5–19 **Systemic Immunity in Herpetic Keratitis.** The precise means by which the immune system protects the host against herpes simplex virus (HSV) infection is unclear, but cellular immunity apparently has an important role in combating cell-to-cell spread. D. L. Easty, C. Carter, and A. Funk (Univ. of Bristol) examined immune function in 27 patients with dendritic ulcers, 17 of whom also had minimal stromal involvement, and 30 patients with active stromal disease. Ten of the latter patients had disciform disease, 6 had limbal involvement, and 14 had diffuse-type disease. Twelve cases of severe atopic disease with a history of epithelial followed by stromal disease also were evaluated; also in the study were 31 normal subjects, 16 of whom had antibody to HSV.

Six of 12 atopic patients with herpetic keratitis had elevated serum IgE levels. No differences in complement-fixing antibody titers were observed in the patient groups. Patients with stromal disease tended to have depressed cell-mediated immunity to HSV antigen in the whole-blood lymphocyte transformation test with phytohemagglutinin

---

(5–19) Br. J. Ophthalmol. 65:82–88, February 1981.

(PHA). Group differences in macrophage migration inhibition factor production were not observed.

A specific deficit in the cell-mediated immune response to HSV in patients with stromal disease is evident. The whole blood lymphocyte transformation test can be recommended for use as an index of potential risk for stromal disease in patients with early ulcerative disease. Kinetic studies have indicated variation in immune function in primary and recurrent ulcerative disease; recurrent ulcerative disease generally produces a positive response. The corneal surface may be protected during recurrent active disease by local and systemic immunologic factors. More severe forms of stromal disease may occur after steroid therapy is administered.

▶ [It is impossible to read this article and the preceding one without developing serious concern about the use of corticosteroids in herpetic keratitis. Most believe that there are specific indications for corticosteroid use, but great care must be taken.] ◀

5–20 **Thygeson's Superficial Punctate Keratitis** is a disease of unknown cause characterized by episodes of tearing, irritation, and photophobia in a chronic course, with both spontaneous and steroid-induced remissions. Khaalid F. Tabbara, H. Bruce Ostler, Chandler Dawson, and Jang Oh (Univ. of California, San Francisco) reviewed the findings in 45 previously unreported cases of Thygeson's superficial punctate keratitis (SPK) and the results of viral cultures in 10 cases. Follow-up ranged from 6 months to 24 years. The mean age at the onset of ocular symptoms was 29 years. No associated systemic illness or trigger mechanisms were identified. Disease had been active for an average of 3½ years. The corneal lesions consisted of conglomerates of granular white-gray fine intraepithelial dots, occasionally assuming a stellate pattern. Nearly half of the patients had subepithelial opacities. With 2 exceptions, the lesions were predominantly in the visual axis. There was an average of 12 corneal lesions. Disease was bilateral in all but 2 patients.

Topical steroids, usually fluorometholone and medrysone, were used in 32 patients, and controlled exacerbations in about half of cases. Two patients used therapeutic soft contact lenses. Scraping the lesions did not appear to influence the course of disease. Neither idoxuridine nor topical antibiotics altered the course. None of 10 specimens yielded any virus. Thirty-two patients had acuities of 20/30 or better in both eyes at follow-up, whereas 5 patients had acuities worse than 20/50. One of the latter patients had stromal scarring from herpes simplex infection treated with steroids. Three patients with lesions near the limbus had experienced peripheral corneal vascularization.

Thygeson's SPK often begins in the second and third decades and pursues a chronic course. It usually is bilateral, and is not contagious. Steroids should be used sparingly if at all, and in low and infrequent dosage. Idoxuridine should not be used to treat Thygeson's SPK. Therapeutic soft contact lenses may provide symptomatic benefit. The visual outcome is generally good.

5–21 **Clinical Observations on the Corneal Thickness and the Corneal Endothelium in Diabetes Mellitus.** Functional abnormalities in diabetic patients may be detected long before anatomical changes are evident. N. Busted, T. Olsen, and O. Schmitz (Univ. of Aarhus) evaluated corneal thickness and the corneal endothelium in 81 insulin-dependent juvenile-onset diabetic patients with a mean age of 34 years. The mean duration of diabetes was 15 years. Central corneal thickness was measured with a modified Haag-Streit pachometer. The corneal endothelium was photographed by specular microscopy. Control values for corneal thickness were obtained from 49 normal subjects, and specular microscopy was performed on 67 normal subjects.

Of the 81 patients, 11 had background retinopathy and 23 had proliferative retinopathy. The mean corneal thickness was 0.527 mm in the normal group, 0.544 mm in diabetic patients without proliferative retinopathy, and 0.566 mm in those with proliferative changes. Corneal thicknesses were similar in the eyes of patients with unilateral proliferative changes and in those of patients who had received laser treatment on one side only. Corneal thickness could not be related to duration of diabetes, daily insulin dosage, or fasting blood glucose level. Endothelial cell density correlated significantly with the duration of diabetes, but the decrease in density per year was about the same as the normal age-dependence value. Mean cell densities were similar in patients with and without proliferative retinopathy. Folds in the central epithelial layer were found in 13 (16%) diabetic patients, 10 of whom had proliferative retinopathy. The mean intraocular pressure in diabetic patients was 15.3 mm Hg. Tensions did not correlate with corneal thickness and were not related to the presence or absence of retinal complications.

Increased corneal thickness in diabetic patients may be a result of an increased water content or an increased dry weight content of the cornea or both. The presence of small folds in Descemet's membrane may be an indication of increased hydration of the cornea; if this is present, it may be due to abnormal function of the corneal endothelium. Increased corneal thickness may be one of the earliest detectable changes in the eye of a diabetic patient, and it may be an indicator of the risk of retinal complications.

▶ [It is well known that the eyes of diabetic patients, like the rest of their bodies, heal poorly. Cataract surgical wounds do poorly and corneal epithelial defects heal slowly. It is then not surprising that corneal thickness is increased and, indeed, corneal metabolism is depressed as reflected by decreased oxygen utilization. These changes are very early in the course of the disease and their relationship to diabetic retinopathy, if any, is unknown.] ◀

5–22 **Long-Term Changes in Corneal Endothelium Following Intraocular Lens Implantation.** Corneal edema in patients having intraocular lens implantation was shown by Bourne and Kaufman (1976) to result from damage to the endothelium. Gullapalli N. Rao, Richard E. Stevens, Jeffrey K. Harris, and James V. Aquavella (Univ. of Rochester) examined 52 eyes of 48 patients who underwent intracapsular cataract extraction with intraocular lens implantation and 35 eyes of 32 patients who had simple cataract extraction. The mean patient age was 64 and 63.5 years, respectively, and the postoperative interval, 29.5 and 27.4 months. A Worst-Medallion type of lens was used in most instances. Specular microscopy was performed 2–4 weeks, 3–6 months, and 12–15 months postoperatively, and again from 16 months to 43 months after operation.

Postoperative loss of endothelial cell density was more marked in the patients having intraocular lens implantation (Fig 5–6). The 2 groups showed considerable widening of the difference in cell loss over time. Eyes with anterior chamber lenses showed minimal cell loss, but there was no significant difference between eyes with Binkhorst and Worst-Medallion lenses. The mean cell loss 1 year after lens implantation was 43.4% and after simple cataract extraction, 10.1%. Precipitates were noted on the corneal endothelium in about two thirds of the intraocular lens group. A significant change in corneal thickness was observed only in the intraocular lens group.

Endothelial cell loss was greater after intraocular lens insertion than after simple cataract extraction in this series. Progressive deterioration in the corneal endothelium was observed after intraocular lens insertion. This procedure still must be approached cautiously. Use of sodium hyaluronate in anterior segment surgery and use of posterior chamber lenses may reduce the degree of insertional

Fig 5–6.—Difference in degree of cell loss between the intraocular lens group and the simple cataract extraction group. Intraocular lenses produced a greater magnitude of cell loss, and the loss was progressive with time. Worst-Medallion and Binkhorst lenses produced more profound changes in the corneal endothelium than did Choyce-Tennant lenses. (Courtesy of Rao, G. N., et al.: Ophthalmology (Rochester) 88:386–397, May 1981.)

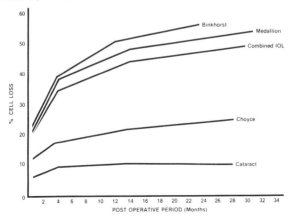

damage to the corneal endothelium. The adverse effects of chronic inflammation may be countered by changes in the composition of implant material, improved quality control, and better sterilization methods.

▶ [We do not know the significance of corneal endothelial cell loss, but we do know that the cells are critical for normal corneal translucency. This study suggests greater cell loss with implants than with standard cataract surgery, and we will have to wait and see what the long-term results will be.] ◀

5–23 **Rheumatoid Scleritis.** Scleritis has been described in about 0.5% of patients with rheumatoid arthritis. Charles C. Barr, Helen Davis, and William W. Culbertson (Univ. of Miami) describe a patient with rheumatoid arthritis and diffuse anterior scleritis with extensive involvement of orbital and adnexal tissues who responded to high-dose systemic steroid therapy.

Woman, 59, with elbow and knee arthritis for 1 year, exhibited symmetric swelling and limited motion of the elbows, wrists, ankles, and fingers and subcutaneous nodules on the forearms. The sedimentation rate was 110, and the rheumatoid titer was 1:5,126. About 3 months later, redness and pain developed in the right eye, and examination showed 5 mm of proptosis and mild ptosis. Also, conjunctival chemosis and palpable nodules were noted. Motility was limited in all fields of gaze.

Computerized axial tomography (CAT) showed a diffuse nonenhancing mass encircling the right globe inferiorly and laterally (Fig 5–7). A smaller mass was noted superotemporally in the left eye. Ultrasonography showed thickening of the episclera and sclera in the inferotemporal region of the right eye. The histologic findings included marked subconjunctival granulomatous inflammation of the substantia propria, palisades of epithelioid cells, and an area of fibrinoid necrosis.

Prednisone, 80 mg daily, was given orally, and 1% prednisolone acetate drops were used in the right eye every 4 hours. Proptosis resolved within 1 month. The patient later became nearly free of symptoms until she died of pneumonia complicating closed head injury 6 months after presentation.

Inflammatory scleritis in patients with rheumatoid arthritis may be either nodular or diffuse and may progress to necrotizing scleritis. Scleromalacia perforans may also develop. Rheumatoid scleritis usually is bilateral. It tends

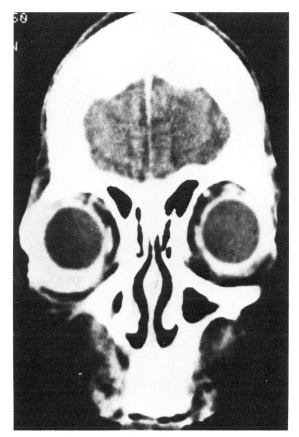

Fig 5–7.—Coronal section. A CAT scan highlights the diffuse scleral thickening inferiorly and laterally in the right eye. (Courtesy of Barr, C. C., et al.: Ophthalmology (Rochester) 88:1269–1273, December 1981.)

to develop in patients with more severe systemic features of rheumatoid vasculitis. Computerized axial tomography is useful in detecting posterior scleritis. Most patients do not respond to topical steroids alone. Either systemic oxyphenbutazone or indomethacin therapy or high-dose systemic prednisone therapy may be necessary.

▶ [The diagnosis of posterior scleritis is difficult, but ultrasound and CAT are definitive, provided the disease is among one's differential diagnostic possibilities.] ◀

6. Glaucoma

Advances in the Management of Glaucoma

JACOB T. WILENSKY, M.D.

Eye and Ear Infirmary,
University of Illinois, Chicago

Doctor Joseph Haas called to my attention that roughly every 20 years a major event occurs. In 1857, Von Graefe began the modern age of glaucoma therapy when he developed peripheral iridectomy. About 20 years later came the beginning of medical therapy of glaucoma with the introduction of pilocarpine. Around the turn of the century fistulization procedures for the surgical management of glaucoma were developed. The year 1920 saw the introduction of the Koeppe gonioscopy lens and the Zeiss slit lamp that almost 20 years after that allowed Otto Barkan to rationalize the diagnosis and therapy of glaucoma by separating it on an anatomical basis into open-angle and angle-closure glaucoma. Approximately 20 years later came the introduction of carbonic anhydrase inhibitors and the development of stable epinephrine preparations. Now, again some roughly 20 years later, another major advancement has occurred. The application of laser surgery techniques has opened a new era in glaucoma therapy.

As is so often the case, the seemingly overnight acceptance of laser therapy of open-angle glaucoma seen during the past year was not a sudden event, but was based on more than a decade of clinical research and experimentation. Among others, Worthen in the United States, Hager in Germany, Ticho in Israel, and Krasnov in Russia had tried various techniques using several different types of lasers. While none of them was overwhelmingly successful, they did report encouraging results that helped stimulate others (most notably Wise) to continue working in this field. The numerous reports published during 1981 have clearly confirmed Wise's work and have contributed to the rapid propagation of this technique.

During the same period, two other forms of laser therapy for glaucoma were gradually gaining widespread acceptance and utilization. Laser iridectomy was attempted as early as 1970 by Zweng and associates, but it was not until 1975, when Abraham published a clinical series, that the utility of this technique was established. Work by Abraham, Pollack, and others refined the technical aspects of laser iridotomy, improving the success rate to around 90%. By 1981, laser iridotomy had replaced surgical iridectomy as the standard method of creating a hole in the iris at most ophthalmic teaching centers.

In the mid-1970s, a number of observers noted a regression of rubeosis iridis in some eyes with neovascular glaucoma treated with panretinal photocoagulation therapy (PRP). Purposeful treatment of patients with rubeosis confirmed the value of PRP in inducing regression or even disappearance of the new iris vessels in a significant percentage of cases. Prospective studies in patients with both diabetes and central retinal vein occlusion indicated the value of PRP as a prophylaxis against the development of rubeosis iridis and neovascular glaucoma. Although disagreements exist as to the precise indications and timing of PRP for rubeosis iridis and neovascular glaucoma, the technique itself is established firmly as a valuable form of glaucoma therapy.

Because open-angle glaucoma accounts for most of the glaucoma seen in western countries, the introduction of laser trabecular therapy has had a much greater impact on the ophthalmic community than did the other two techniques. All three techniques, however, have clearly had a major effect on glaucoma therapy. It seems evident that any ophthalmologist treating glaucoma patients in the future will have to become familiar with the various modalities of laser himself. On the other hand, as the amount of filtering surgery continues to decline, fewer ophthalmology resi-

Chapter 6–GLAUCOMA / 131

dents will be adequately trained in this technique and this procedure, like trabeculectomy, eventually may be performed only by specialists at tertiary care centers.

Most of the advances in the management of glaucoma that we have discussed in this essay have related to glaucoma therapy. Over this 120-year period, we have learned relatively little about the cause of open-angle glaucoma. Let us hope that the next major advance will eliminate the need for these therapeutic modalities.

6–1 **Glaucoma Treatment by Trabecular Tightening With the Argon Laser.** James B. Wise evaluated a safe laser treatment of glaucoma in more than 100 patients, and followed up 66 phakic eyes for up to 3 years. All patients were aged 40 and older, and most were surgical failures or had uncontrolled glaucoma and were candidates for surgery. The procedure was done on an outpatient basis with the patient under topical and subconjunctival anesthesia. A three-mirror contact lens was used with a 50-µ spot focused on the trabecular meshwork and 100-µ spots placed in the pigmented trabecular band using 800–1,000 mW and a 0.1-second exposure time. Synechiae and blood vessels were avoided. Antibiotic drops were instilled postoperatively. Some medical therapy was continued for at least a month. A large reduction in the need for medication was typical even when eyes still required some medication.

Of 66 eyes with phakic open-angle glaucoma, 75% had an intraocular pressure of 20 mm Hg or below 6 months after treatment, and 91% had a pressure of 22 mm Hg or less. The average fall in pressure was 12.5 mm Hg. Medication requirements greatly decreased. Only 2 eyes required further surgery. One fifth of the patients had normal pressures when not receiving medication. Particularly good results were obtained in 5 heavily pigmented eyes in 4 black patients and in an Indian patient. The results remained stable on subsequent follow-up; the outcome at 3 months predicted the future course for at least 3 years. Only 2 significant complications have occurred in 108 treated eyes: a case of endothelial burn injury, and a case of severe uve-

(6–1) Int. Ophthalmol. Clin. 21:69–78, Spring 1981.

itis probably due to anterior segment ischemia when lidocaine with 1:100,000 epinephrine had been used subconjunctivally.

This laser method allows control comparable to that achieved by conventional surgery in white patients, and better than that achieved in black patients. The procedure is simple and safe and apparently reverses the basic pathophysiology of primary open-angle glaucoma. Accurate focus is essential. The effects may take 3 or 4 weeks to appear.

6–2 **Long-Term Control of Adult Open-Angle Glaucoma by Argon Laser Treatment.** James B. Wise (Oklahoma City) has evaluated a new approach to laser therapy of glaucoma, based on reducing the diameter of the trabecular ring and reopening the normal outflow system with multiple small burns spaced 360 degrees around the meshwork. A total of 150 treated phakic eyes in patients aged 40 and older were followed for 6 months or longer. Most had primary open-angle glaucoma. Previous filtering procedures had failed in 8 instances. Nearly all patients had intraocular pressures above 22 mm Hg despite multidrug therapy. Most had progressive optic nerve damage and field loss. An argon laser was used to deliver 100 to 120 burns 50 μ in diameter at 800 to 1,200 mW around the pigmented trabecular band just in front of the scleral spur.

Mean posttreatment intraocular pressures were significantly lower in all groups of eyes (table), and there was no tendency for pressures to rise over the long term. Increased medical therapy was not necessary for the group as a whole. Excellent results have been obtained in blacks and Indians, who often respond poorly to filtering operations. Complications have been minimal. One patient with severe ocular argyrosis had a corneal endothelial burn that resolved. One patient with posttraumatic endothelial dystrophy developed bulbous keratopathy 16 months after laser treatment. Anterior synechiae were seen in one eye and severe uveitis in another. Four eyes developed angle-closure glaucoma after laser therapy and discontinuance of miotics.

Laser trabecular tightening is safe and convenient. If it fails, conventional medical or surgical treatment is still

PRESSURE REDUCTION AFTER LASER TREATMENT*								
Duration of Follow-up	6 mo	12 mo	18 mo	24 mo	30 mo	36 mo	42 mo	48 mo
Number of eyes in interval	150	105	69	59	37	25	13	11
Mean IOP mm Hg, prelaser	28.37	29.69	29.59	29.37	28.91	27.60	29.61	30.40
Mean IOP mm Hg, postlaser	16.11	17.00	18.06	17.92	18.42	16.26	17.25	17.11
Mean decrease in IOP	12.26	12.68	11.53	11.45	10.49	11.34	12.36	13.29

*Mean postlaser intraocular pressure (IOP) and mean IOP drop show no significant change over 4 years.

possible. Control is obtained as often as with trabeculectomy in adults with open-angle glaucoma. In elderly patients and blacks, results are better than those obtained by surgical procedures. Refinements of the technique may preclude the need for lifelong medical therapy in many patients with primary open-angle glaucoma.

6–3 **Argon Laser Trabecular Surgery in Uncontrolled Phakic Open-Angle Glaucoma.** Arthur L. Schwartz, Mark E. Whitten, Bruce Bleiman, and David Martin (Washington, D.C., Hosp. Center) reviewed the results of argon laser therapy in 36 consecutively treated phakic eyes with clinically uncontrolled open-angle glaucoma. All patients had intraocular pressures of 19 mm Hg or above with progressive field loss or disc changes, or both, despite maximally tolerated drug therapy. Twenty-four of the 33 patients followed were black. Twenty-nine eyes had primary open-angle glaucoma, 3 had pseudoexfoliation, 2 had pigment dispersion, and 1 had an angle recession. One hundred burns were applied to the pigmented trabecular meshwork band above the scleral spur over the entire angle (Fig 6–1). A 50-μ spot size, a 0.1-second exposure, and a power setting of 900 to 1,400 mW were used. A corticosteroid was used topically for a week after treatment.

Five treated eyes had a temporary rise in intraocular pressure. At 2 months there was a mean pressure reduction of 9.7 mm Hg in treated eyes, and the decrease persisted throughout 18 months of follow-up (table). The average difference in pressures in 25 pairs of treated and untreated eyes at 6 months was 9.1 mm Hg, a significant effect. The increase in outflow facility in treated eyes was maximal 2

(6–3) Ophthalmology (Rochester) 88:203–212, March 1981.

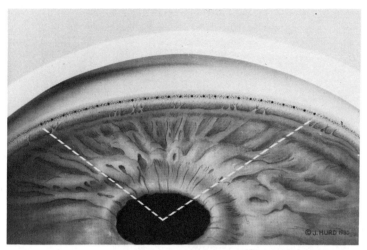

Fig 6–1.—Ninety-degree angle view with 25 evenly spaced laser burns in trabecular meshwork. (Courtesy of Schwartz, A. L., et al.: Ophthalmology (Rochester) 88:203–212, March 1981.)

months after treatment. Transient iritis followed treatment in nearly all cases. Two eyes had a microscopic hemorrhage at the site of treatment. No iris atrophy was observed. Peripheral anterior synechiae developed in 29% of treated eyes. A significant fall in intraocular pressure occurred in these eyes.

Argon laser trabecular surgery holds much promise for use in the management of glaucoma. It can be offered pa-

MEAN CHANGE IN PRESSURES FROM BASELINE IN TREATED AND UNTREATED EYES

	Treated Eye				Untreated Eye			
Time	No. Eyes	Mean mm Hg	Standard Deviation	P Value	No. Eyes	Mean mm Hg	Standard Deviation	P Value *
1–3 weeks	32	−8.0	6.2	<0.001	28	−1.9	3.8	<0.02
1 week	28	−7.7	6.1	<0.001	28	−1.8	5.1	NS
2 weeks	26	−6.9	5.2	<0.001	24	−1.0	3.9	NS
3 weeks	31	−9.6	3.5	<0.001	29	−0.9	4.2	NS
2 months	34	−9.7	4.6	<0.001	33	−0.6	6.5	NS
4 months	30	−10.0	4.2	<0.001	29	−0.3	4.0	NS
6 months	25	−8.7	5.1	<0.001	25	+0.4	4.4	NS
12 months	14	−7.7	4.3	<0.001	9	0.0	2.5	NS
18 months	7	−10.0	2.3	<0.001	3	−2.3	.6	<0.02

*NS: not significant.

tients in clinical trials as an alternative to filtering operations. Laser therapy appears to be especially indicated for patients representing surgical failure, patients who refuse operation, and those at significant surgical risk. It may also be useful for patients whose cataracts might well worsen to the point of visual handicap after filtering operations.

6–4 **Argon Laser Treatment of the Anterior Chamber Angle for Increased Intraocular Pressure.** Pekka Pohjanpelto (Central Hosp. of Päijät-Häme, Lahti, Finland) reviewed the results of laser treatment of the anterior chamber angle for increased intraocular pressure in 65 eyes of 63 patients with a mean age of 68 years. Exfoliation syndrome was present in 35 treated eyes of 34 patients. The initial patients would otherwise have been operated on for elevated pressure and a progressive field defect despite maximal tolerated drug therapy, but the indications later were broadened. A continuous-wave argon laser was used to deliver 70–110 burns to the chamber angle into or just posterior to the pigmented trabecular band. A 50-μ beam diameter, a 0.1-second exposure time, and a starting power setting of 800 mW were used. Dexamethasone was used in the treated eye for 1 week.

Changes in intraocular pressure are shown in Figure 6–2. Nine eyes with exfoliation syndrome, followed up for a year, showed a slightly increased average intraocular pressure, but no general deterioration in control was evident. The pressure increased distinctly in only 1 case. In 12 eyes without exfoliation syndrome that were followed up for a year, the results did not deteriorate in initially successful cases. The average fall in intraocular pressure was slightly less than in exfoliation cases. In both groups, a highly significant pressure fall was observed 3 months after treatment. Outflow improved in eyes in both groups. Intraocular pressure was controlled in 88% of all cases. Gonioscopy showed a decrease in pigment in several cases. Few complications occurred. There were 8 failures of laser therapy.

The results of laser treatment of the chamber angle for increased intraocular pressure have been encouraging. The treatment has generally been effective, and significant

---

(6–4) Acta Ophthalmol. (Copenh.) 59:211–220, April 1981.

136 / OPHTHALMOLOGY

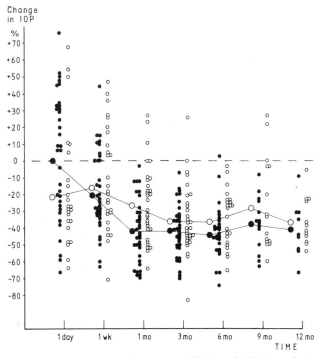

Fig 6–2.—Changes in intraocular pressure *(IOP)* in individual eyes during follow-up after laser therapy. *Large circles,* mean values; *small open circles,* eyes without exfoliation syndrome; *small solid circles,* eyes with exfoliation syndrome. (Courtesy of Pohjanpelto, P.: Acta Ophthalmol. (Copenh.) 59:211–220, April 1981.)

complications have not occurred. Laser therapy now is used when medical management is ineffective and the chamber angle is open. Surgery is performed only if laser treatment is ineffective, and laser therapy has nearly supplanted trabeculectomy.

6–5 **Laser Therapy for Open-Angle Glaucoma.** Jacob T. Wilensky and Lee M. Jampol (Univ. of Illinois) evaluated laser therapy in patients with open-angle glaucoma whose intraocular pressures were inadequately controlled by maximally tolerated medical therapy. A 50-μ spot size and

---

(6–5) Ophthalmology (Rochester) 88:213–217, March 1981.

0.1-second burn were used. Power was initially set at 1,000 mW and increased as needed up to 1,500 mW. Eighty to 100 burns were delivered over the entire arc of the trabecular meshwork. A corticosteroid preparation was used after treatment.

Average intraocular pressure fell from 27.5 to 20.3 mm Hg on follow-up for about 11 months in 22 treated eyes (table). Similar results were obtained in white and black patients, and the outcome was unrelated to angle pigmentation. The course of intraocular pressure in three treated eyes is shown in Figure 6–3. No eye has required subsequent glaucoma surgery. The average facility of aqueous outflow in 13 eyes increased from 0.105 to 0.168 after treatment, and this effect was not an artifact of testing. After treatment, most patients had mild uveitis, which lasted 1 to 2 weeks. Two eyes had more severe uveitis. Most patients examined showed no changes in the angle at gonioscopy after treatment. About one fourth of patients had multiple, small corneal epithelial burns that cleared rapidly and have had no apparent sequelae. Two patients had post-

PRETREATMENT AND POSTTREATMENT INTRAOCULAR PRESSURE

Eye	Initial IOP (mm Hg)	Last IOP (mm Hg)	Change in IOP (mm Hg)	Follow-up (months)	Comments*
1	22	22	0	14	Poor drug compliance
2	32	22	10	14	
3	32	22	10	14	
4	24	22	2	13.5	Less medication
5	23	16	7	13	
6	28	24	4	13	Severe uveitis; PAS; IOP up to 50 mm Hg
7	26	17	9	11	Severe uveitis; PAS; elevated IOP for months
8	25	19	6	13	
9	21	16	5	11	
10	29	26	3	13	Less medication
11	29	22	7	12	Less medication
12	26	18	8	12	Less medication
13	26	22	4	12	Fuchs' dystrophy; corneal edema
14	28	19	9	10	
15	30	18	12	10	
16	28	19	9	11	
17	32	28	4	9	
18	32	18	14	10	Less medication
19	30	24	6	9	
20	28	18	10	8	
21	28	14	14	7	
22	26	21	5	7	Less medication
Mean (±SD)	27.5 ± 3.2	20.3 ± 3.4	7.2 ± 3.6	11.3 ± 2.1	

*PAS: peripheral anterior synechia.

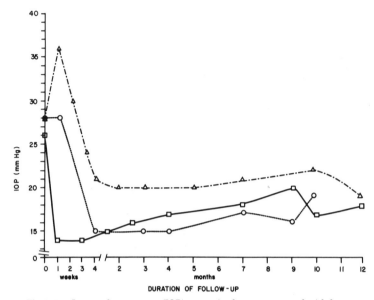

Fig 6–3.—Intraocular pressure *(IOP)* course in three eyes treated with laser goniotherapy. Note posttreatment increase in one eye *(triangles)* and prolonged effect in all three eyes. (Courtesy of Wilensky, J. T., and Jampol, L. M.: Ophthalmology (Rochester) 88:213–217, March 1981.)

treatment corneal edema, which resolved over several weeks.

How laser treatment of the trabecular meshwork lowers the intraocular pressure is unknown; there is no histologic evidence of a trabeculectomy. Thermal contracture of the meshwork may open the adjacent pores, or decreased aqueous production may be responsible for the treatment effect. Further, substances such as mucopolysaccharides that may interfere with aqueous outflow may be broken down by the laser burns. Laser goniotherapy may be a useful addition to glaucoma management, especially in phakic patients with primary open-angle glaucoma who are not well controlled on maximal medical therapy. Preliminary results in cases of exfoliation syndrome and pigmentary glaucoma have been promising. The procedure would not usually be expected to be effective in eyes with pressures exceeding 30 mm Hg.

▶ [Photocoagulation of the trabecular meshwork using an argon laser, in the manner described by Wise and others, is effective in reducing intraocular pressure despite early studies suggesting the contrary. The method is receiving widespread acceptance, and the indications for its use are increasing rapidly. Precisely how the method works, however, is still not completely clear. Indeed, we will probably not know how laser burning of the trabecular meshwork is beneficial until we understand the pathogenesis of open-angle glaucoma.] ◄

6–6 **Trabeculectomy vs. Thermosclerostomy: Randomized Prospective Clinical Trial.** Trabeculectomy is safer than the more classic types of filtering procedure, though it is perhaps slightly less effective in reducing intraocular pressure. Its filtering sclerostomy is covered with a flap of partial-thickness sclera and a flap of conjunctiva and Tenon's capsule, reducing the risks of early flattening of the anterior chamber, prolonged hypotony, late perforation, and endophthalmitis. Pierre Blondeau and Charles D. Phelps (Univ. of Iowa) compared trabeculectomy with thermosclerostomy in a prospective series of 98 eyes of 64 patients with primary open-angle glaucoma, pigmentary glaucoma, or exfoliative glaucoma. Thirty-four patients had each procedure performed in one eye. Fourteen had a trabeculectomy in one eye, and 16 had a thermosclerostomy in one eye only.

Intraocular pressures were usually about 3 mm Hg lower in eyes subjected to thermosclerostomy (Fig 6–4). The procedures were about equally effective in reducing pressures to under 22 mm Hg, and this held true for patients followed for 5 years or longer. More eyes in the thermosclerostomy group required a second operation for glaucoma or cataract. Thin blebs were more frequent in thermosclerostomy eyes and thick blebs or no bleb in trabeculectomy eyes. Over two thirds of eyes in both groups lost acuity, but the loss was generally more rapid and noticeable in the thermosclerostomy group. A hole developed in the conjunctival flap in 1 trabeculectomy and in 4 thermosclerostomies. The rates of hyphema formation were comparable in the two groups. A flat anterior chamber with corneal endothelial contact was more frequent in the thermosclerostomy group. Cataract, late hypotony, and leaking or infected blebs were all much more frequent in the thermosclerostomy group. Retinal de-

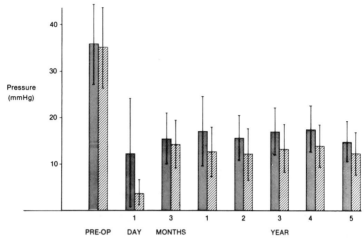

Fig 6–4.—Average intraocular pressures (mean ± SD) preoperatively and at various intervals after trabeculectomy *(stippled bars)* and thermosclerostomy *(hatched bars)*. (Courtesy of Blondeau, P., and Phelps, C. D.: Arch. Ophthalmol. 99:810–816, May 1981; copyright 1981, American Medical Association.)

tachment occurred in one eye in the thermosclerostomy group.

Both trabeculectomy and thermosclerostomy are effective operations for open-angle glaucoma, but there is a much greater risk of vision-threatening complications after thermosclerostomy, and only a slightly greater mean pressure reduction is obtained with this procedure.

6–7 **Trabeculectomy in Black Patients.** Ronald D. Miller and John C. Barber (Univ. of Texas Med. Branch, Galveston) report the largest series of trabeculectomies in black patients in the United States. A total of 122 primary trabeculectomies were performed for glaucoma in 86 black patients who were followed up for at least a year postoperatively. There were 48 women and 38 men in the series. The average age was 52.3 years, and the average follow-up was 26.2 months. Standard trabeculectomies were performed with a partial-thickness scleral flap. Topical steroids and cycloplegics were used postoperatively.

(6–7) Ophthalmic Surg. 12:46–50, January 1981.

Results Reported of Series of Trabeculectomies in Black Patients

Study	Country	Year	No Cases	Follow-Up	Success Without Medication (%)	Success With Medication (%)
Welsh	South Africa	1972	29	Not Stated		65 (total)
Chatterjee	Ghana	1972	24	Up to 12 mo	79	4
Kietzman	Nigeria	1976	221	4 mo (minimum)	74	—
Freedman	USA	1976	64	19 mo (average)	57	25
Ferguson	USA	1977	50	2 yr	76	8
David	South Africa	1977	49	6-30 mo	10	63
Sanford-Smith	Nigeria	1978	51	Not Stated	65	—
Schimek	USA	1977	23	6-36 mo		83 (total)
BenEzra	Israel	1978	100	2-12 mo	79	—
Thommy	Nigeria	1979	111	6 mo (minimum)	95	—
Bakker	Kenya	1979	88	3 mo (minimum)	82	—
Richardson	USA	1979	—	—	30	54
Merritt	USA	1980	23	16 mo (average)		22 (total)
Miller	USA	1980	122	26.2 mo (average)	39	18

A total of 70 eyes were controlled postoperatively; 48 eyes had no medication. Trabeculectomies in 43% of eyes were considered failures. Patients older than age 60 years had the best outcome; no patient younger than age 20 years had successful results. The size of the trabecular block could not be related to the outcome. Failure was invariable when more than 5 sutures were used in the scleral flap. The intraocular pressure was controlled in all patients with filtering blebs. Significant complications were rare. Visual acuity usually decreased little after surgery. Ten patients required extraction of cataracts, and 16 required drainage because of large choroidal detachments with loss of the filtering bleb. In 12 cases the anterior chamber was surgically reformed. Six conjunctival wound leaks had to be repaired. Eighteen hyphemas cleared spontaneously.

These results were compared with those in previous reports of trabeculectomy in black patients in the table. The overall results in this study were similar to those obtained with previous filtering procedures. The primary cause of failure of trabeculectomy has been scarring of the bleb or blocked filtration leading to loss of the bleb. Surgery has given the best results in patients older than age 60 years. The superiority of trabeculectomy over other filtering procedures for black patients who require surgery for glaucoma remains unproved.

▶ [Both this article and the preceding one suggest that trabeculectomy is safer than other surgical procedures used to lower the intraocular pressure (IOP). Trabeculectomy, however, has not been shown to be better at lowering the IOP than other surgical procedures. In general, the procedure is successful only a little more than half the time in blacks. This makes glaucoma surgery in blacks much worse than in whites, who have as high as an 80% to 90% success rate. In general, operation seems very poor for blacks, and new means must be found when the eye requires surgery for glaucoma.] ◀

6–8 **Peripheral Iridectomy: Fifteen Years Later.** Robert C. Drews (Washington Univ., St. Louis) has reviewed the records of 32 patients having peripheral iridectomy before 1964. Twenty-six had iridectomies in both eyes. Average age was 66 years. A simple keratome, forceps, and de Wecker scissors technique was used in all cases, without suturing. Angle closure was diagnosed in 40 eyes, and chronic angle closure in 12. Three eyes had branch vein occlusions before surgery. One eye had had a retinal detachment. Four eyes developed macular degeneration after surgery. Average follow-up after surgery was 8.9 years.

(6–8) Trans. Am. Ophthalmol. Soc. 78:70–87, 1980.

Peripheral iridectomy was done prophylactically in most cases. The only surgical complication, apart from 1 case in which the iris was not penetrated, was hyphema in 3 eyes, 2 in the same patient. Thirty eyes required topical medications after operation, including all those with chronic angle-closure glaucoma. No eye developed visual field loss or showed progressive field loss after operation, and none showed new glaucomatous cupping. Cataract progressed after operation in 28 of 34 eyes, and 15 eyes needed cataract surgery during follow-up. No eye without cataract before operation developed a cataract that reduced vision measurably according to the Snellen test chart.

No significant surgical or long-term postoperative complications resulted from peripheral iridectomy in this series of patients. The question of what level of risk of damage from an acute attack justifies peripheral iridectomy remains unanswered. In the present series, no significant cataract developed in any eye without a cataract before operation. Posterior synechiae have not been observed, but the eyes were not routinely dilated after operation.

6–9 **Complications of Peripheral Iridectomy in Primary Angle-Closure Glaucoma.** Peripheral iridectomy is generally considered to be safe, and it is often performed prophylactically, but it is not entirely without risk. Fu-Jin Go and Yoshiaki Kitazawa (Univ. of Tokyo) reviewed the results of peripheral iridectomy, performed with microsurgical techniques, in 155 eyes of 113 patients with primary angle-closure glaucoma. The 75 women and 38 men had a mean age of 62 years. Operation was indicated when peripheral anterior synechia was present in less than three fourths of the circumference of the angle. Twenty eyes were operated on because of a favorable intraocular pressure response to medical treatment. Thirty-five fellow eyes were operated on prophylactically.

Complications occurred in 17.7% of the eyes that were operated on. Twenty-one eyes had a transient rise in intraocular pressure, 6 had hyphema, and 1 developed malignant glaucoma. The eye with malignant glaucoma responded to intracapsular lens extraction and trabeculectomy. The hyphemas absorbed spontaneously within 1 week after operation, except in 1 eye that required irrigation. Cataract developed later in 13% of eyes, and posterior synechia was seen in 12% of eyes. Medication was necessary to reduce intraocular pressure in one third of eyes. In 6 other eyes the pressure could not be controlled by medical treatment. Failure to obtain control without medication was associated with peripheral anterior synechiae extending over more than half of the circumference of the angle.

The amount of peripheral anterior synechia is a useful guide to selecting an operation for glaucoma and in predicting the postoperative course. Whether peripheral iridectomy precipitates progress of cataract is still controversial. The lack of change in peripheral anterior synechiae in eyes operated on prophylactically and the rarity of serious complications support operation on the fellow eye in patients with unilateral acute, primary angle-closure glaucoma, provided the angle is critically narrowed.

▶ [Minor complications do occur with peripheral iridectomy, but serious problems are very rare. It is interesting to note that in the United States there was a higher rate of fellow eye surgery than in Japan, but all concluded that surgery was relatively safe and beneficial.] ◀

▶ ↓ The author of the following paper discusses argon laser iridotomy. Although there also are some complications with this procedure, they seem even less serious than with peripheral iridectomy. Even if one third of the iridotomies do close off with time, it seems reasonable to use this procedure before resorting to surgery. ◀

6–10 **Laser Iridotomy: Current Concepts in Technique and Safety.** Irvin P. Pollack has performed laser iridotomies on more than 500 eyes. The results in 215 eyes are reviewed here. Argon lasers were used. A total of 148 eyes were followed up for 1 to 4 years. Laser iridotomy was successful in 95% of these cases. The procedure is illustrated in Figure 6–5. In 68% of 77 consecutive cases in which energy levels of 500–2000 mW were used for 0.1–0.5 second, with a 50 to 200-µ spot size, the iris opening remained patent after the first treatment. In no case did closure occur after 6 weeks. When the opening was 50% closed the pigment was dislodged with energy levels of 200–500 mW. The best results were obtained with energy levels of 2 W or less for 0.2 second. A fibrous membrane bridged the defect in 1 case,

Chapter 6—GLAUCOMA / 145

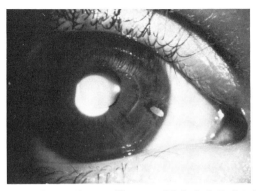

Fig 6–5.—Argon laser iridotomy. (Courtesy of Pollack, I. P.: Int. Ophthalmol. Clin. 21:137–144, Spring 1981.)

and posterior synechiae were seen in another. Tonographic and perfusion studies in rabbits showed no significant change in outflow facility within 5 months after multiple laser iridotomies.

Only about two thirds of laser iridotomies have remained patent. Treatment using a contact lens with a 50- or 100-μ spot and energy levels of under 2 W for 0.2 second is recommended. The success rate depends on iris color and thickness, corneal tolerance, the depth of the anterior chamber, and patient cooperation. It also depends on the operator's experience and proficiency. Patency can be judged by viewing the anterior lens capsule through the iridotomy. Complications include corneal epithelial and endothelial burns, lens opacities due to fragmentation of lens fibers and atrophy of the lens epithelium, and retinal scarring.

Laser iridotomy is a relatively safe procedure without the hazards of intraocular hemorrhage, infection, and wound dehiscence that are incurred with invasive intraocular procedures. The procedure is performed on outpatients, and both eyes can be treated at the same session. Postoperative morbidity is minimal.

Timolol: Canadian Multicenter Study. Timolol, a nonselective β-blocking drug, has been rapidly accepted as an

(6–11) Ophthalmology (Rochester) 88:244–248, March 1981.

antiglaucoma drug, but most previous reports of short-term topical therapy have involved small numbers of patients. R. P. LeBlanc and Gordon Krip evaluated topical timolol maleate therapy in a multicenter study of 382 patients with baseline intraocular pressures exceeding 21 mm Hg. After a washout period, patients received 0.25% timolol drops every 12 hours, and those without control a week later were treated with 0.5% timolol drops for another week. Where necessary, previously used drugs then were added.

Intraocular pressures at 2 and 6 weeks were very significantly different from baseline values in all groups. In most groups, pressures were comparable after 2 and 6 weeks of treatment. Pulse rates were altered significantly in patients who responded to 1 or 2 weeks of treatment, but no significant blood pressure changes occurred.

This short-term study confirmed the efficacy and relative safety of topical timolol maleate therapy for glaucoma.

6–12 **Timolol in Combination with Other Glaucoma Drugs** is discussed by W. Merkle (Univ. of Munich). In 39 selected patients with open-angle glaucoma, in whom pressure regulation with timolol alone was inadequate, success was achieved by using this drug in combination with various other glaucoma drugs for treatment periods of 12–18 months. With timolol alone, the initial median value of 35.4 mm Hg reached an average lowering of intraocular pressure (IOP) of 9.7 mm Hg, or 27.2%. Timolol was given alone to 32 patients during the first 3 weeks, 4 patients from weeks 4 to 7, and 2 patients for 4–6 months, and their IOP could not be lowered to a normal level. In 6 patients (average age 70.3 years) timolol lowered the median pressure from 33.9 to 25.5 mm Hg.

After additional administration of 0.5%–2% pilocarpine, the patients showed a new tension reduction of 7 mm Hg over 15 months of treatment. Similar effects were observed with the addition of carbachol: 13 patients (average age 69.4 years) receiving timolol had their pressure lowered from 33.4 to 25 mm Hg, and with added 0.75%–2.25% carbachol another tension reduction of 6.7 mm Hg was reached over 18 months of treatment. A lesser pressure lowering effect

(6–12) Klin. Monatsbl. Augenheilkd. 178:50–54, January 1981.

was experienced with aceclidine, administered to 8 patients (average age 58.9 years). Their IOP was lowered from 33.4 to 24 mm Hg with timolol and by another 4.4 mm Hg with the addition of 2% aceclidine over a period of 12 months.

For younger patients, needing combination therapy, the pupil is least affected by aceclidine. Adrenalin also has a negligible effect on the pupil and is a beneficial combination drug for lowering the IOP. Six patients (average age 48 years) with an initial IOP of 30.5 mm Hg demonstrated a lowering of 6.4 mm Hg, and with 0.1% adrenalin had another reduction of 6.1 mm Hg over a 12-month period. Acetazolamide was only briefly tested in 6 patients (average age 69.6 years). With 0.5% timolol two times daily, the initial IOP of 50.9 mm Hg was lowered by 20.4 mm Hg and a one-time 250-mg acetazolamide, given 2½ hours after timolol administration, reduced the pressure again by 13.5 mm Hg. Because of systemic side effects, long-term therapy with acetazolamide is not recommended. The reason these patients' IOP under long-term therapy with timolol alone could not reach normal levels has not been established. Almost all these patients, however, had had glaucoma for a long time (average 12.4 years), which could not be regulated by classic therapy.

As an alternative to a risky operative procedure or continuous treatment with carbonic anhydrase inhibitors, a combination therapy is an acceptable treatment for lowering IOP, especially since timolol is very compatible with other antiglaucoma drugs.

Study of the Additive Effect of Timolol and Epinephrine in Lowering Intraocular Pressure. An additive effect of timolol maleate in reducing intraocular pressure would be an important advance in the management of glaucoma. John V. Thomas and David L. Epstein (Harvard Med. School) carried out a double-blind study of timolol and epinephrine in patients with intraocular pressures of 23 mm Hg or above off treatment, open angles, and stable visual fields. The 16 patients had an average age of 62 years; 31 eyes were studied. Initially, patients were treated with 0.5% timolol or 1% epinephrine borate twice daily for 2 weeks;

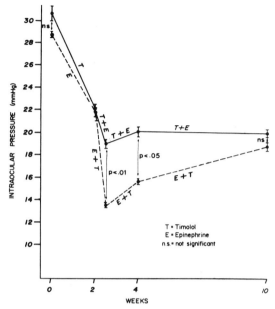

Fig 6–6.—Intraocular pressure measurements in two treatment sequences ($T + E$, timolol supplemented with epinephrine; $E + T$, epinephrine supplemented with timolol). (Courtesy of Thomas, J. V., and Epstein, D. L.: Br. J. Ophthalmol. 65:596–602, September 1981.)

the other agent was then added for 2 weeks of combined treatment.

Outflow pressure fell significantly with timolol alone, and a significant further effect was noted 1 day after epinephrine was added. The additive effect was still present but less marked after 2 weeks, but was not significant after 8 weeks of combined treatment. Epinephrine alone also significantly reduced outflow pressure (Fig 6–6); timolol had a significant additive effect that was less marked after 2 weeks and was absent after an average of 8 weeks of combined treatment. The fall in intraocular pressure when timolol was added to epinephrine was significantly greater than when epinephrine was added to timolol, although no significant difference was evident after 8 weeks of combined treatment. Outflow facility was increased by epinephrine alone and was reduced 2 weeks after timolol was added. Timolol alone increased the facility of outflow; but the addition of epinephrine did not increase the outflow facility.

It appears that epinephrine alone increases the facility of outflow; added timolol blocks this effect but produces a fall in intraocular pressure by decreasing the rate of aqueous inflow. When epinephrine is added to timolol therapy, a temporary fall in intraocular pressure may result from a non-β mechanism. Patients who require both drugs should receive epinephrine alone for several weeks, which should then be supplemented intermittently with timolol.

▶ [To avoid surgery for glaucoma, it is common to use combined drug therapy, but the efficacy of a combination of timolol and epinephrine is still not clear. In the preceding article, epinephrine was helpful when added to timolol with a year of follow-up. In the second study, the combination was initially effective, but after 2 months was no better than one of the drugs alone. Further studies obviously are necessary.] ◀

6–14 **Timolol Maleate and Intraocular Pressure in Low-Tension Glaucoma.** Timolol maleate is useful in reduction of intraocular pressure in many patients with chronic open-angle glaucoma. Its use in patients with low-tension glaucoma has been suggested. W. E. Gillies and R. H. West (Melbourne) evaluated results of timolol maleate administration in 13 patients with glaucomatous optic disc cupping and visual field loss whose intraocular pressures had never exceeded the normal range. All but 1 patient were women. The mean age was 71.6 years. Timolol maleate drops, 0.25% or 0.5%, were applied twice daily, alone or in conjunction with other antiglaucoma medications. Eight patients completed 14 weeks of timolol therapy.

The average initial intraocular pressure was 19.5 mm Hg, which was significantly above that of the general population over age 40 years. A majority of eyes showed a decrease in pressure after 2 weeks of timolol therapy. The average decrease in these 20 eyes was 4.5 mm Hg. The pressure increased in 12 eyes in the next 4 weeks, although usually not to initial levels. Nine eyes showed an increase in pressure while 7 showed a decrease at 7–14 weeks. After 14 weeks, the average reduction from the initial intraocular pressure in 16 eyes was 4 mm Hg.

(6–14) Trans. Ophthalmol. Soc. N.Z. 33:33–35, 1981.

The net decrease in intraocular pressure in these patients after 14 weeks of timolol therapy was considered a useful therapeutic effect in most instances. The initial pressure levels and the response to treatment are more typical of eyes with chronic open-angle glaucoma than of eyes with normal aqueous dynamics. The suggestion that timolol will reduce intraocular pressure to the episcleral venous pressure level in these eyes implies that the outflow facility is normal. The present findings, however, suggest that this is not the case in most patients with low-tension glaucoma.

▶ [Low-tension glaucoma must be defined carefully. In this case, the authors stated that the optic nerve is affected by a normal intraocular pressure. Timolol had a variable effect on the intraocular pressure and it might be reasonable to give the drug a therapeutic trial in these patients who are extraordinarily difficult to manage.] ◀

6–15 **Penetration of Timolol Eye Drops Into Human Aqueous Humor.** Timolol maleate effectively reduces intraocular pressure for both the short and the long term with minimal adverse effects. Calbert I. Phillips, R. Shayle Bartholomew, Ghulamqadir Kazi, Claude J. Schmitt, and Roger Vogel measured timolol levels in the aqueous humor after intillation of eye drops in 20 patients scheduled for cataract extraction. Two drops of 0.5% timolol were instilled, usually 2–3 hours before surgery, and the aqueous humor was aspirated at the start of the operation. Most patients had general anesthesia preceded by administration of diazepam.

Timolol levels in the aqueous humor ranged from about 150 ng/100 mg in the first 1–2 hours to 10 ng toward the end of a 7-hour interval. Levels were on the order of 1/5000th of that in the drops. The logarithm of concentration of timolol was significantly related to the sampling time. Measured values may be slightly underestimated because of the method used to remove the specimens.

An exponential decay of aqueous humor levels of timolol maleate was observed in this study. This presumably results from many factors which include the turnover rate of aqueous humor, tissue uptake, and diffusion or bulk flow of aqueous humor beyond the anterior chamber.

▶ [It is surprising that the clearance of timolol from the anterior cham-

▶ ↓ The following five articles report various complications of timolol. The drug was released by the Food and Drug Administration in a relatively short time and has become a primary drug for the treatment of glaucoma in an even shorter time. Only now are we beginning to see complications and learning to use the drug judiciously. ◀

6–16 **Safety and Tolerability of Timolol Maleate Ophthalmic Solution in Perspective.** Timolol maleate, a β-adrenergic blocking agent with no significant intrinsic sympathomimetic or local anesthetic activity in animals, has been widely used in recent years in the United States to reduce intraocular pressure. Several recent reports of unusual and unexpected adverse effects in patients receiving timolol ophthalmic solution have appeared. Irving M. Katz and Sharon L. Kasdin (West Point, Pa.) summarized data from several sources regarding the safety of timolol ophthalmic solution. Data were taken from 1,001 patients treated for up to 15.5 months in the New Drug Application (NDA) studies and from those who continued treatment for up to 48 months. Data also were obtained from the Drug Experience and Epidemiology Department of Merck Sharp & Dohme Research Laboratories and from the National Registry for Drug-Induced Ocular Side Effects.

Of 704 patients in the NDA data base who received timolol ophthalmic solution alone, 66 (9%) had adverse effects. Reports of symptoms of ocular irritation in controlled studies are summarized in the table. In an investigational program, side effects were documented in 182 (12%) of 1,517 patients treated. About half of the 169 ocular incidents documented by Merck Sharp & Dohme involved ocular irritation, and 46 of the rest were visual or refractive in nature. There were 18 reports of corneal abnormalities. Most of the reported CNS side effects were minor in nature. Most respiratory effects represented bronchospasm. Many reported cardiovascular effects consisted of bradycardia.

Recent findings do not alter the conclusion from initial clinical trials that timolol maleate ophthalmic solution is a safe and highly effective antiglaucoma treatment that is

---

(6–16) Ocular Therapy Surg. 1:76–80, Nov.–Dec. 1981.

INCIDENCE OF SYMPTOMS OF OCULAR IRRITATION
INVESTIGATIONAL STUDIES*

	All Studies (Data Set II)			NDA Studies* (Data Set I)	
	Baseline		Timolol	Timolol	
Symptom	Number Studied	Percent With Symptoms	Percent With Symptoms	Number Studied	Percent With Symptoms
Burning	1,444	9	13	600	16
Tearing	1,444	8	11	600	12
Foreign body sensation	1,443	7	9	600	10
Smarting	1,428	4	8	529	11
Itching	1,444	7	10	600	10
Photophobia	1,444	6	8	600	9
Sore, aching, or tired eyes	1,443	7	10	579	11
Dryness	1,431	3	6	529	6
Blurred vision	1,319	14	20	489	19
Browache	1,443	5	6	579	9
Headache	1,443	6	9	579	11

*Based on direct queries to patients.

well tolerated by the vast majority of treated patients. It is a potent β-blocking agent, however, and all topically applied drugs can be absorbed, dictating caution in the use of timolol in patients with a history of chronic obstructive lung disease or congestive heart failure. Serious side effects from the ocular instillation of timolol are rare, but aggravation of obstructive airway disease, an increase in heart failure, and mental confusion have been described.

6–17 **Corneal Anesthesia After Topical Treatment With Timolol Maleate: A Case Report.** Timolol maleate, a nonselective β-blocking agent, is being increasingly used to treat glaucoma. It is said to lack local anesthetic properties, making it suitable for topical administration, but a few reports of adverse corneal effects have appeared. Berit Calissendorff (Huddinge, Sweden) reports data on a patient in whom corneal anesthesia developed during timolol treatment.

Woman, 58, with primary open-angle glaucoma, was treated with 4% pilocarpine 3 times a day for 6 years. In 1978, treatment was changed to 0.5% timolol maleate once daily. In 1979, only the left eye, which had a glaucomatous disc, was treated with 0.5% timolol twice daily. The right eye was considered to have ocular hypertension. After a year of timolol therapy the left cornea was found to be nearly anesthetic, while the untreated right cornea had normal sensitivity. Slit-lamp examination was negative. Timolol was discontinued, and a week later the difference in sensitivity between the eyes was less marked. Sensitivity was equal in both eyes 3 weeks later, but the intraocular pressure in the left had risen to 32 mm Hg. Sensitivity of the left cornea remained normal after reinstitution of treatment with 0.5% timolol twice daily for 3 weeks, but it was reduced after another 6 weeks of treatment. No other corneal abnormalities were observed. Pilocarpine therapy then was reinstituted.

Timolol was strongly implicated as the cause of corneal anesthesia in this case. The patient was relatively young and was receiving no other treatment. Corneal sensitivity returned when timolol was discontinued and declined again when it was readministered. The mechanism of the change is obscure. Probably individual kinetic factors are contributory. Corneal exposure to timolol and its absorption into the aqueous and plasma appear to vary markedly between individuals.

▶ [Timolol evidently may cause corneal anesthesia as well as ocular irritation. The ocular effects, however, appear fewer than with pilocarpine or epinephrine.] ◀

6-18 **Bronchospasm Precipitated by Ophthalmic Instillations of Timolol** is reported by Stephen D. Lockey, Sr. Timolol maleate (Timoptic) is a widely prescribed ophthalmic solution used for the treatment of simple chronic glaucoma. It is absorbed into the systemic circulation from the eye and has been shown to produce hypersensitivity reactions, visual disturbances, aggravation or precipitation of certain cardiovascular disorders, and attacks of bronchospasm in an unknown percentage of patients with preexisting bronchospastic disease, in about 5–15 minutes after its instil-

(6–18) Ann. Allergy 46:267, May 1981.

lation. Such proved to be the case in the patient described.

Woman, 70, had redness of the right eye for 5 days. On examination she had a visual acuity of 20/20 in the right eye and 20/16 in the left. A subconjunctival hemorrhage was present in the right eye. The clinical appearance of the optic discs suggested advanced glaucomatous damage. The subjunctival hemorrhage was not related to the glaucoma. Timolol maleate drops, 0.25% twice a day in both eyes, was given. Physical examination showed the patient to be agitated, extremely weak, stridulous, and in respiratory distress. Many rhonchi and wheezes were present over the lung fields. The throat was mildly inflamed with no edema. Temperature was 97.8 F. The pulse was 58 beats per minute and irregular. Respirations were 24 per minute and blood pressure was 102/58. The patient was originally treated with epinephrine with no significant improvement in stridor or dyspnea. All symptoms subsided under the influence of oxygen administered by mask and dexamethasone sodium phosphate and aminophylline administered intravenously.

The Food and Drug Administration has received reports of 22 cases of precipitation or aggravation of bronchospasm, in addition to one death from status asthmaticus apparently associated with the administration of timolol maleate eye drops. Allergists and physicians should be aware in prescribing timolol maleate eye drops, a β-adrenergic agent, to patients with preexisting asthmatic conditions and other cardiopulmonary problems.

6–19 **Bronchoconstrictive Side Effect of Timolol Eye Drops in Patients With Obstructive Lung Diseases** was studied by A. Vonwil, M. Landolt, J. Flammer, and H. Bachofen (Univ. of Bern). Today, glaucomas are most frequently treated with local application of β-adrenergic blockers. These drugs ensure an effective lowering of intraocular pressure and offer the patient additional subjective advantages (no miosis, no formation of myopia, and negligible local irritation). The best-known medication at present is timolol maleate (Timoptic). Despite the small dose, the effect on the heart-circulatory system of healthy probands can be substantiated. Individually documented descriptions of acutely aggravated conditions in cardiac and asthmatic patients after timolol therapy lead to the assumption of a causal con-

---

(6–19) Schweiz. Med. Wochenschr. 111:665–669, May 1981. (Ger.)

nection. Not only timolol but also other ophthalmic solutions such as carbachol, can have a bronchoconstrictive effect.

In a double-blind crossover study, 7 patients with chronic glaucoma and obstructive lung disease were selected. Each patient received sequential glaucoma therapy as well as placebo treatments. Timolol 0.5%, 1 drop 2 times daily, or carbachol 3%, 1 drop 3 times daily, was administered. The third treatment consisted of Ringer's solution as placebo, 1 drop 2 times daily. Each substance was instilled bilaterally for 2 dyas and in a random sequence. Five-day treatment-free intervals were arranged between the 2-day treatment periods. Lung function tests were taken at the beginning of the study and after each treatment period.

The comparison of placebo with timolol and carbachol treatment showed the most significant increase of bronchial obstruction after only a short-term timolol treatment. The observation of serious lung function impairment in 3 patients after treatment with carbachol suggests that carbachol is not a safe alternative for patients with obstructive lung disease. The fact that only some and not all asthmatic patients have severe reactions to carbachol could be explained by strong individual differences of hyperreactivity in the bronchial tree. The degree of conjunctival absorption of carbachol also differs from patient to patient.

Whenever a deterioration of airway obstruction occurs in elderly patients or bronchial asthma becomes manifest late in life, topically administered β-adrenergic receptor blocking and cholinergic agents must be considered as causative factors. Optimal communication among all physicians caring for glaucoma patients is essential.

▶ [There have been enough reports of the association of timolol and bronchospasm to warrant the conclusion that the drug is contraindicated in patients with chronic obstructive pulmonary diseases such as asthma, and it may be that the drug also should not be used in patients with congestive heart failure.] ◀

20 **Nail Pigmentation Following Timolol Maleate Therapy.** β-Adrenergic blocking agents such as timolol have been used increasingly in glaucoma therapy because of their efficacy in reducing intraocular pressure in certain condi-

tions, but adverse effects occasionally occur. Vera Feiler-Ofry, Victor Godel, and Moshe Lazar (Tel Aviv) report findings in a patient with open-angle glaucoma in whom unusual nail pigmentation developed during topical timolol maleate therapy.

Woman, 56, with open-angle glaucoma for 5 years, had acuity of 6/9 on the right and 6/12 on the left, with bilateral progressive cupping and field losses. Her disease was not controlled by 4% pilocarpine, epinephrine, and Diamox therapy. Timolol maleate 0.5% was used twice daily, reducing pressures in both eyes to 14 mm Hg. No further loss of the visual fields was noted after 6 months, but brown discoloration appeared in nearly all nails of the hands and feet. The digits had normal temperature, and the pigmentation was not altered by ambient temperature change. There was no pain, numbness and tingling, or swelling. Normally colored nails began growing a month after timolol therapy was discontinued. Intraocular pressures remained at about 20 mm Hg when the previous treatment was resumed.

The unusual pigmentation of the nails was associated with topical timolol maleate therapy for glaucoma in this patient. Propranolol reportedly induces brown discoloration of the tongue. It may be that toxic metabolic products of timolol interfere with the melanocyte system. The pigmentation was reversible after withdrawal of timolol therapy.

6–21 **Neovascular Glaucoma Following Central Retinal Vein Obstruction.** Neovascular glaucoma (NVG) follows central retinal vein obstruction (CRVO) in about 20% of cases. Larry E. Magargal, Gary C. Brown, James J. Augsburger, and Richard K. Parrish, II (Jefferson Med. College, Philadelphia) conducted a prospective study of 155 consecutive patients referred in 2 years with CRVO. Panretinal photocoagulation was performed on 32 eyes with CRVO before iris neovascularization or NVG developed. Twenty-two of these eyes had ischemic CRVO and 1 had hyperpermeable CRVO.

Twenty-one patients had bilateral CRVO. Average patient age was 64 years; 60% of patients were men. Over half the patients were hypertensive, and over one-third had evidence of atherosclerotic cardiovascular disease. Average follow-up of patients who were not operated on was 8 months.

(6–21) Ophthalmology (Rochester) 88:1095–1101, November 1981.

About half the eyes had a hyperpermeable pattern initially, and nearly a third had an ischemic pattern. Neovascular complications were far more common in the ischemic group. Final acuity depended largely on the intensity and duration of macular edema. Neovascular glaucoma developed in 60% of eyes with ischemic CRVO. No patient under age 50 developed NVG. Primary open-angle glaucoma or ocular hypertension was associated with the development of NVG. Neovascular glaucoma was also more frequent in patients with hypertension, atherosclerotic cardiovascular disease, or diabetes. The response of NVG to treatment was better in eyes without extensive angle closure. None of the eyes treated prophylactically by photocoagulation developed NVG during follow-up.

The mechanism by which retinal ischemia leads to NVG is unknown, but diffusion of a vasoactive substance anteriorly through the vitreous has been postulated. In view of the high risk of blindness in advanced cases of NVG that follow ischemic CRVO, maintenance of a comfortable, cosmetically acceptable eye appears to be a realistic goal. Preliminary results with panretinal photocoagulation in eyes with ischemic CRVO suggest the potential benefit of this form of prophylaxis.

-22 **An Approach to Management of Neovascularization of the Iris and Secondary Glaucoma** is presented by Stephen J. Ryan. Indications for treatment of neovascularization of the iris include prophylaxis, treatment of secondary glaucoma to preserve vision, need to reduce intraocular pressure, and analgesia. Retinal detachment with neovascularization and an open angle is managed by reattaching the retina with or without other procedures as indicated. If the media are opaque, a washout procedure or repeat vitrectomy is combined with reattachment. Neovascularization with an open angle and clear media is managed by panretinal photocoagulation with argon laser or xenon arc, and then goniophotocoagulation. If the media are opaque, goniophotocoagulation is carried out, with peripheral cryotherapy and vitrectomy or a washout procedure if indicated. If the angle is closed by synechiae a filtering procedure is performed. Where there is no potential for significant recovery of vision, symptomatic relief can be obtained with medical therapy, retrobulbar alcohol injection, cyclocryotherapy, ciliary ablative procedure, or enucleation.

Patients with iris neovascularization and secondary glaucoma have not had good visual results. Most patients have not done well on medical therapy, but slightly more than 50% of patients responded well to photocoagulation. A significant number of filtering procedures have not yet been performed. The pathogenesis of iris neovascularization is not yet entirely understood. The least risky management offering the greatest benefit is indicated. Patients must be followed very closely during medical therapy, because development of neovascular glaucoma can progress quite rapidly. A detached retina should be reattached. The effects of photocoagulation remain unclear, but a positive response as is seen in proliferative diabetic retinopathy is likely. Peripheral ablation of the retina with cryotherapy can be performed in cases with vitreous hemorrhage, although the treatment can be dangerous. A filtering procedure generally is necessary for patients with neovascular glaucoma and a completely closed angle. In patients with pain and no visual potential, where treatment with retrobulbar alcohol is inadequate, cyclocryotherapy or another means of ablating the ciliary body is indicated.

▶ [There are many causes of neovascular glaucoma, and the success of treatment has always been very poor. Panretinal photocoagulation is beneficial in patients who have neovascular glaucoma associated with central retinal vein obstruction and with diabetic retinopathy. The problem is when the treatment should be carried out. Once the disease has progressed, it is difficult to treat, so a decision must be made at the first sign of angle neovascularization and ocular hypertension. The major problem is that these complications can occur very rapidly, so the patients must be watched closely. Indeed, some would carry out panretinal photocoagulation prophylactically.] ◀

6–23 **Cyclocryotherapy: Experimental Studies of the Breakdown of the Blood-Aqueous Barrier and Analysis of a Long Term Follow-Up Study** is reported by R. Haddad (Univ. of Vienna). Cyclocryotherapy (CTh) of the ciliary body is generally used when conservative or other operative procedures have failed. In most cases, this treat-

---
(6–23) Wien. Klin. Wochenschr. [Suppl. 126] 93:3–18, 1981.

ment leads to a long period of a complaint-free condition, even when the intraocular pressure (IOP) can be regulated only for a short time. The various factors (tip of the cryoprobe and temperature, simple or repeated application, pretreatment with prostaglandin-synthetase inhibitors and phenylephrine, grade of pigmentation, influence of neutral transference of inflammation, and preoperative inflammation of the anterior uvea) were studied, which influence the immediate increase in IOP and the rise in protein concentrations in aqueous humor after the procedure. Early and late histologic findings after CTh were described.

Fifty-two patients (60 eyes) with different types of chronic glaucoma were treated with CTh and were followed up for a period ranging from 7 to 44 months (mean 22.9 months). During this period, IOP was maintained under 22 mm Hg in 60% of all cases. The best results were achieved in patients with open-angle glaucoma (75%) and the worst results, in patients with juvenile glaucoma (50%). However, only 10 eyes with juvenile glaucoma were tested over a short period (average 14.8 months); for these, judgment should be reserved. Cryocoagulation of half of the ciliary body yielded good results in only 35%, whereas cryotherapy of the second half lead to a decrease of IOP in a further 78%. In 20 eyes, only one quadrant of the ciliary body was treated; only in 3 (15%) could a lowering of IOP be observed. By repeating the treatment of the second quadrant, the IOP was regulated in 4 of 7 eyes. Nine eyes developed persistent hypotony; of these, 2 became phthisical. Factors other than extensive coagulation may also contribute to chronic hypotony.

The results of the experimental and clinical observations imply that the treatment schedule (temperature, time and number of applications, dimension of cryode) chosen for these patients is a comparatively safe procedure with regard to the complications and yields good results as far as the reduction of IOP is concerned.

▶ [Almost one fifth of these eyes developed hypotony, but that is still better than most of the previous reports. Indeed, some surgeons would only use cyclocryotherapy in blind, painful eyes in place of enucleation. This relatively optimistic report suggests that perhaps the technique should be investigated further, using controlled clinical trials.] ◀

6-24 **Optic Disc Hemorrhages Precede Retinal Nerve Fiber Layer Defects in Ocular Hypertension.** Small splinter hemorrhages of the optic disc are predictive of visual field defects in glaucoma, and retinal nerve fiber layer (RNFL) defects may precede visual field defects by some years. P. Juhani Airaksinen, Eila Mustonen, and Hannu I. Alanko (Univ. of Oulu) found that disc hemorrhages precede the development and progression of RNFL defects in glaucoma suspects. Over 4,600 pairs of optic disc stereophotographs of 1,548 patients with glaucoma or suspected glaucoma were evaluated for disc hemorrhage. Hemorrhage was found in 90 instances, in 32 of which there were no other pathologic disc changes. Twenty-five patients had no visual field defects on routine perimetry. The 18 women and 7 men had a mean age of 61 years when first seen with suspected glaucoma and a mean age of 64 when disc hemorrhage was first observed.

Eight patients (32%) developed pathologic changes on follow-up (table). Six had a RNFL defect, at the site at which bleeding was observed, with 1 exception. All 8 patients developed notching of the neural rim of the disc or concentric enlargement of the cup. All the changes were evident within about 3 years after initial evaluation. None of 7 patients examined by the Friedmann method developed central field defects. Four patients had glaucomatous field defects within 1 to 2 years after the disc changes and RNFL damage were observed. The changes in 1 patient are shown in Figure 6–7 on page 162.

Small optic disc hemorrhages may precede RNFL defects and extension of existing defects in glaucoma suspects. The hemorrhages are the first detectable evidence of a change from ocular hypertension to glaucoma in at least some instances, and they predict the site of future damage. A diagnosis of ocular hypertension is not consistent with the presence of a definite, irreversible defect of the RNFL.

6-25 **Incidence of Optic Disc Hemorrhages in Chronic Simple Glaucoma and Ocular Hypertension.** Optic disc hemorrhages in glaucoma patients vary in size and intensity and may be missed on ophthalmoscopy, particularly in

Chapter 6–GLAUCOMA / 161

DATA ON 8 OCULAR HYPERTENSIVE PATIENTS IN WHOM OPTIC DISC HEMORRHAGE (ODH) PRECEDED DEVELOPMENT OF GLAUCOMATOUS OPTIC DISC CHANGES, RNFL DEFECTS, AND VISUAL FIELD (VF) DEFECTS

Case No.	Sex	Age at initial visit	Follow-up (mo) prior to ODH	ODH first observed (mo-yr)	Location of the haemorrhage on the disc	Period of time (mo) from ODH until glaucomatous changes were observed in		Period of time (mo) from ODH until	
						Optic disc	RNFL	normal VF was last recorded	glaucomatous VF defect was first recorded
1	M	65	55	4–76	temporal	21	21	27	33
2	F	61	139	9–78	superotemporal	3	3	9	15
3	F	46	135	6–78	superotemporal	30*	30	33	—
4	F	52	65	5–75	inferotemporal	53	–(?)	65	—
5	F	59	68	4–77	inferotemporal	29	–(?)	40	—
6	F	65	33	12–76	inferotemporal	38*	38	43	49
7	F	55	82	4–74	inferotemporal	29	29	0	55
8	F	60	0	5–71	inferotemporal	96	96	0	96

*Narrowing of neural rim was detected only by electronic subtraction method.

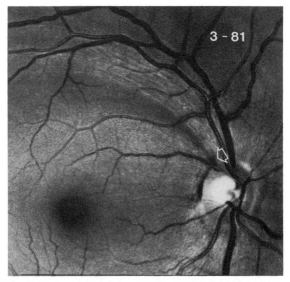

Fig 6–7.—Retinal nerve fiber layer defect and hemorrhage *(arrow)*. (Courtesy of Airaksinen, P. J., et al.: Acta Ophthalmol. (Copenh.) 59:627–641, October 1981.)

patients using miotics. J. Gloster (Univ. of London) reviewed 1,829 optic disc photographs obtained during the examination and follow-up of 320 patients with glaucoma and 169 with ocular hypertension. A total of 2,714 photographs were of adequate quality for a reasonable determination to be made of whether or not a disc hemorrhage was present.

Most hemorrhages were "splinter" hemorrhages, but others had a blotchy, rounded shape. The most common site of hemorrhage was the inferotemporal sector of the disc. The findings in patients with glaucoma are summarized in the table. Hemorrhages were increasingly prevalent with repeat photography. Probably at least a third of glaucomatous eyes showed optic disc hemorrhages at some time. Disc hemorrhage was more prevalent in patients with field defects, but the incidence could not be related to the degree of field loss. The incidence of hemorrhage increased significantly with an increasing vertical cup-disc ratio. Hemor-

INCIDENCE OF OPTIC DISC HEMORRHAGES IN RELATION TO
NUMBER OF OCCASIONS ON WHICH DISC PHOTOGRAPHY WAS
DONE ON GLAUCOMATOUS PATIENTS

Number of occasions on which photographs were taken

	1	2	3	4	5	6	7
Number of eyes photographed (617)	325	113	66	45	32	26	10
Number of eyes with disc haemorrhages (60)							
on 1 occasion	16	16	7	3	4	5	1
on 2 occasions	—	0	1	0	2	2	1
on 3 occasions	—	—	0	1	0	0	0
on 4 occasions	—	—	—	0	0	0	1
Total	16	16	8	4	6	7	3
Incidence of disc haemorrhage	4·9%	14·2%	12·1%	8·9%	18·8%	26·9%	30·0%

rhages were less frequent in ocular hypertension than in chronic simple glaucoma. They were more frequent in low-tension glaucoma than in chronic simple glaucoma. Glaucomatous eyes with lower pressures had more optic disc hemorrhages than those with higher pressures, and this could not be attributed to differences in the frequency of photography.

Optic disc hemorrhages were more frequent in glaucomatous eyes with lower intraocular pressures than in those with higher pressures in this study. Pressures may have been more uniform in eyes during treatment than when maximum pressures were recorded. The higher rate of disc hemorrhage in eyes with lower pressures may reflect the increased vulnerability of the tissues in some glaucomatous eyes, or there may sometimes be an ischemic process that is responsible for hemorrhages in the posterior segment and causes reduced aqueous formation in the anterior segment, limiting the elevation of intraocular pressure.

▶ [We are constantly looking for a means of predicting which ocular hypertensive patients are going to develop glaucoma. The authors of the preceding article suggest that optic disk hemorrhages herald glaucoma in some patients with ocular hypertension. The author of this article found that hemorrhages come and go in at least one third of glaucoma patients, and their frequency of occurrence was less in ocular hypertensives. More studies need to be carried out to elucidate the role of optic disc hemorrhages, ocular hypertension, and glaucoma.] ◀

6–26 **Prophylactic Therapy of Ocular Hypertension: A Prospective Study.** Only a small proportion of patients with ocular hypertension have primary open-angle glaucoma, which is defined by visual field defects. The prognosis in an individual case is not easy. Yoshiaki Kitazawa (Univ. of Tokyo) conducted a prospective study of the efficacy of early or prophylactic treatment of ocular hypertension with the β-blocking agent timolol maleate. The 52 patients in the study had intraocular pressure levels that exceeded 25 mm Hg with no apparent visual field loss or compromise of the angle; 27 patients were followed for a year or longer. Each group of 26 patients included 20 with a higher risk of visual field loss. Study patients received 0.25% timolol twice daily, or 0.5% timolol if the pressure did not fall below 20 mm Hg.

Intraocular pressures declined significantly in timolol-treated patients but remained elevated in patients treated with placebo. The average level of pressure fell from 26.1 to 22.0 mm Hg in the study group. During the study, 2 placebo-treated patients and 1 timolol-treated patient had a glaucomatous field defect in one eye. All 3 cases were categorized by the discriminant function approach as early primary open-angle glaucoma at the outset. No side effects were noted other than an occasional burning sensation when 0.5% timolol was received. No changes in corneal sensitivity or tear secretion were observed.

These preliminary findings appear to indicate that prophylactic treatment of ocular hypertension with timolol is effective and safe. The study will continue for another 2 years. Much more needs to be learned about possible side effects from long-term treatment with timolol.

▶ [The conclusion that ocular hypertensive patients may benefit from timolol treatment seems premature, since glaucoma only develops in a small percentage of these patients. Nonetheless, if it turns out that timolol is essentially benign in systemically healthy persons, its prophylactic use will have to be carefully considered.] ◀

6–27 **Pigment Dispersion Syndrome: A Clinical Study.** Pigment dispersion syndrome is a result of idiopathic atrophy of the pigment layers of the iris with liberation of pig-

---

(6–26) Trans. Ophthalmol. Soc. N. Z. 33:30–32, 1981.
(6–27) Br. J. Ophthalmol. 65:264–269, April 1981.

ment and its deposition along paths of aqueous flow. Harold G. Scheie (Univ. of Pennsylvania) and J. Douglas Cameron (Univ. of Minnesota) reviewed the findings in 799 affected eyes of 407 patients seen in 1946 to 1977 with pigment dispersion syndrome. Demographic features of the group are given in the table. Data on 72 patients with chronic simple glaucoma (143 eyes) also were reviewed. Forty-seven study patients had increased intraocular pressure without typical disc changes or visual field defects, and 104 had glaucoma. There was only 1 case of familial pigmentary glaucoma. Iris colors were similar in the groups with normal and elevated pressure and the group with glaucoma.

The anterior chamber angles were open in all eyes. Most eyes with or without glaucoma showed heavy pigmentation of the trabecula. Retinal detachment was found in 6.4% of all patients, including 7.6% of patients with pigmentary glaucoma. No retinal detachments were found in patients with chronic simple glaucoma. About 75% of eyes with pig-

SEX AND AGE DISTRIBUTION OF PATIENTS WITH PIGMENT DISPERSION SYNDROME		
	Men	*Women*
Pigment dispersion (overall group)		
Patients	204 (50%)	203 (50%)
Average age	46·3 years	49·8 years
Median age	44 years	54 years
Age range	14 to 84 years	19 to 74 years
Pigment dispersion (normotensive)		
Patients	108 (42·2%)	148 (57·8%)
Average age	47·6 years	49·6 years
Median age	44 years	53 years
Age range	14 to 85 years	19 to 75 years
Pigment dispersion (increased pressure)		
Patients	31 (66%)	16 (34%)
Average age	44·6 years	53·5 years
Median age	42 years	54 years
Age range	25 to 72 years	44 to 68 years
Pigment dispersion (glaucoma)		
Patients	65 (62·5%)	39 (37·5%)
Average age	45·8 years	50·2 years
Median age	46 years	53 years
Age range	18 to 84 years	21 to 77 years

mentary glaucoma were controlled medically. A filtering operation was necessary in 48 eyes of 32 patients, and 8 eyes required more than one operation. Surgery was necessary in 21 eyes of 13 patients with chronic simple glaucoma. None of these eyes required more than one operative procedure.

Pigment dispersion syndrome with glaucoma is more frequent in men than in women. Iris color does not appear to be related to pigmentary glaucoma. In asymmetric cases the eye with the higher pressure has a more heavily pigmented chamber angle, indicating that pigment is important in the development of glaucoma. A high rate of retinal detachment was noted in the present series. Medical therapy was somewhat less effective in controlling intraocular pressure in patients with pigmentary glaucoma than in those with chronic simple glaucoma. More patients with pigmentary glaucoma required multiple operations to achieve satisfactory pressure control.

6–28 **A Clinicopathologic Study of Four Cases of Primary Open-Angle Glaucoma Compared to Normal Eyes.** Ben S. Fine (Armed Forces Inst. of Pathology, Washington, D.C.), Myron Yanoff, and Richard A. Stone (Univ. of Pennsylvania) compared 8 eyes obtained at autopsy from 4 patients with chronic open-angle glaucoma to eyes with normal aging changes. In 2 cases the earliest changes were localized to the uveal part of the drainage angle, with compaction of the uveal meshwork and formation of a prominent scleral spur on the original scleral roll, as well as "hyalinization" or atrophy, or both, of the outermost part of the ciliary muscle and associated uveal meshwork. Occasionally, there was mild proliferation of canalicular endothelium into the lumen of Schlemm's canal. In a third case there was distinct atrophy of the uveal meshwork and ciliary muscle, and iris root atrophy in the severely affected eye. Extensive but variable obliteration of Schlemm's canal occurred. The fourth case showed marked endothelial proliferation in Schlemm's canal and only aging changes in the anterior uveal structures.

The histologic changes in primary open-angle glaucoma

may represent exaggerated aging changes that range from excessive involvement of the uveal pathway to excessive involvement of the canal of Schlemm. In 3 of the 4 present cases the changes occurred chiefly within the iris root, uveal meshwork, and anterior ciliary body. In only 1 case were the changes in the area of Schlemm's canal most prominent. Comparison of changes in the two eyes in patients with asymmetric clinical findings suggests that the uveal outflow pathway is the earliest site of histologic abnormality in some patients with chronic primary open-angle glaucoma. Extensive damage to Schlemm's canal may lead to further occlusion in such cases. Uncertainty remains concerning mechanisms of aqueous outflow and the relative contributions of the corneoscleral meshwork-Schlemm's canal pathway and the uveal pathway in both normal and abnormal eyes.

▶ [It would appear that if we live long enough we will all have glaucoma.] ◀

6-29 **An Analysis of Treatment of Congenital Glaucoma by Goniotomy.** Early reports of goniotomy as initial treatment of congenital glaucoma suggested a poor outcome, although most patients were operated on without direct angle visualization. Warren L. Broughton (Natl. Naval Med. Center, Bethesda, Md.) and Marshall M. Parks (Childrens Hosp. Natl. Med. Center, Washington, D.C.) report the results of goniotomy in 50 eyes with congenital glaucoma. All patients were followed up for at least 6 months after initial surgery. The Worst goniolens was used in all instances. Eighteen of the 34 patients operated on had unilateral disease. Four patients had a family history of congenital glaucoma. Two patients were premature, and 1 had Down's syndrome.

Success was defined as a decrease in intraocular pressure to less than 21 mm Hg with no progression of disease for at least 6 months after surgery. All patients were eventually cured surgically, although 6 eyes required other procedures. Nineteen eyes had a second operation. Three of 7 eyes with a recurrence of intraocular hypertension required alternative operations. The overall success rate for goniotomy was 88%. Success rates were not related to the age at onset or age at the time of initial treatment, or to the intraocular pressure level. The mean follow-up from the final surgery was 66 months. The mean intraocular pressure at the last follow-up examination was significantly lower than the initial value. Fifteen of 29 eyes had an acuity of 6/12 or better at last follow-up, and 20 had an acuity of 6/18 or better. No significant postoperative complications occurred. No patient required medical treatment for control of the intraocular pressure after successful surgery.

A visualized goniotomy had a success rate of 74% in this series for reducing intraocular pressure to normal levels for at least 6 months after the initial procedure. The results compare favorably with those of more complicated procedures, although some recurrences will develop and require further surgical treatment. A change toward hypermetropia is a good office indicator of surgical success.

▶ [The success rate is high, but the disease must be recognized. The authors' emphasis on the importance of refractive change toward myopia seems of considerable value.] ◀

6–30 **Unintentional Lens Injury in Glaucoma Surgery** is discussed by Kenneth C. Swan and Thomas W. Lindgren (Univ. of Oregon). Cataract formation often occurs months to years after surgery for glaucoma. The slowly developing lens opacities usually have the morphological features of senile cataract. They should, at most, be considered sequelae to rather than complications of the surgery. Accidental injury to the lens still occurs despite improved surgical methods and the nearly routine use of an operating microscope in the Pacific Northwest. If the capsular defect is small, the opacity may be limited to the site of injury and is readily overlooked. Extensive lens injury usually is followed by widespread opacity, first seen through the iris coloboma and later spreading into the upper part of the pupillary area. Acute cataract formation also is seen, with displacement of the lens and incarceration of lens material in the operative wound. Severe uveitis that complicates glaucoma surgery can result from accidental rupture of the lens capsule.

Accidental injury of the lens is a relatively rare occur-

(6–30) Trans. Am. Ophthalmol. Soc. 78:55–69, 1980.

rence in glaucoma surgery, but it probably is more common than the few reports would indicate. Many clinicans appear to be unaware of the condition. Perforation of the lens capsule should definitely be suspected when a cataract develops within days or weeks after filtration surgery or iridectomy. Early removal of the lens should be considered if a persistent uveitis is present, since this can lead to failure of the operation and also loss of the eye. Angle closure and resultant worsening of the glaucoma have been major factors leading to enucleation after unintentional lens injury.

6–31 **Aqueous-Venous Shunt for Glaucoma: A Further Report.** The aqueous-venous shunt is a microsurgical pro-

Fig 6–8.—Essential steps for aqueous-venous shunt procedure. **A,** vortex vein anterior wall incision. **B,** insertion of collagen tubing into vortex vein with Lee forceps, immobilization of collagen tubing into episclera with four interrupted 9–0 nylon sutures on each corner of Dacron fixation sheet, and 2-mm beveled sclerolimbal incision about 2 mm posterior to limbus. **C,** collagen tube has been inserted into anterior chamber. **D,** double closure of Tenon's and conjunctival flap incision with separated 7–0 collagen suture to prevent late exposure of collagen tubing near corneoscleral limbus. (Courtesy of Lee, P., and Ward, R. H.: Arch. Ophthalmol. 99:2007–2012, November 1981; copyright 1981, American Medical Association.)

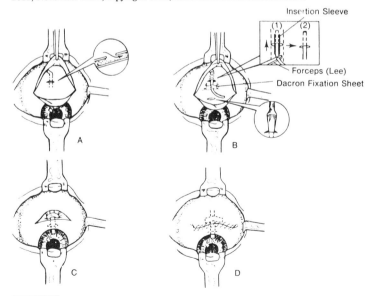

(6–31) Arch. Ophthalmol. 99:2007–2012, November 1981.

Long-Term Results of Aqueous-Venous Shunt Procedure*

Case†	Diagnosis	Previous Surgery	Visual Acuity Preoperative	Visual Acuity Postoperative	Intraocular Pressure, mm Hg Preoperative	Intraocular Pressure, mm Hg Postoperative	Outflow Facility, μL/min/mm Hg Preoperative	Outflow Facility, μL/min/mm Hg Postoperative	Complication	Follow-up, yr	Final Results
1	POAG	PLS + TC	20/40	20/60	20	14	0.07	0.24	Flat AC	6	S
2	POAG	SC + TC	20/25	20/30	18	15	0.10	0.20	None	5½	S + M
3	POAG	None	20/200	20/200	19	22	0.09	0.21	None	2½	S + M
4	POAG	None	HM	CF	26	26	0.13	ND	Flat AC, extrusion of tube	2½	F
5	POAG	SC	20/30	20/40	33	30	ND	ND	None	3	F
6	POAG	TC	HM	HM	32	28	0.09	ND	Flat AC	4	F
7	OAG, trauma	2 TCs, TO, 2 CYLs	LP	? LP	37	7	0.11	0.35	None	3½	S
8	POAG	TC	20/30	20/20	25	25	0.05	ND	Flat AC	2	F
9	POAG	None	20/30	20/30	20	24	0.08	0.18	None	2	S
10	POAG	None	20/25	20/25	32	18	0.06	0.14	None	1	S + M
11 (HK 1)	POAG	SC	LP	LP	37	18	...	...	AC; part of tube fell into angle	5	S + M
12 (HK 2)	Juvenile	PLS	LP	NLP	42	4	...	...	None	6	S
13 (HK 3)	POAG	SC	LP	? LP	31	16	...	...	Cataract	6	S
14 (HK 4)	POAG	PLS	CF	20/400	36	23	...	...	None	6	S + M (silicone)
15 (HK 5)	OAG, trauma	PLS	CF	CF	42	16	...	...	None	5	S + M (silicone)
16 (HK 6)	POAG	SC	20/200	20/100	38	12	...	...	None	1½	S

*Abbreviations: POAG, primary open-angle glaucoma; PLS, posterior lip sclerotomy; SC, sclerotomy with cautery (Scheie); TC, trabeculectomy; CYL, cyclocryotherapy; HM, hand motions; CF, counting fingers; LP, light perception; NLP, no light perception; ND, not done; AC, anterior chamber; S, successful; S + M, successful with medication; F, failure.
†HK 1 through HK 6 refer to case numbers in the Hong Kong series.

cedure used to relieve glaucoma. A microsized collagen or silicone tube is inserted between the anterior chamber and the lumen of the extraocular portion of a vortex vein to establish aqueous drainage. Pei-fei Lee and Robert H. Ward (Albany, N.Y.) evaluated this procedure in 10 patients with advanced glaucoma refractory to medical management. Six had had glaucoma surgery. Six of 15 patients from Hong Kong who had had standard glaucoma surgery also were evaluated. Silicone polycarbonate block copolymer microsized tubing was used rather than microsized collagen tubing in 2 of these 6 cases. Average follow-up after aqueous-venous shunt procedure was 3.8 years. The operation is illustrated in Figure 6–8.

Twelve of 16 eyes benefited from the procedure (table). Further glaucoma medication was necessary in 6 of the 12, but in lower dosage. Tonometric studies showed a substantial reduction in aqueous outflow resistance in eyes with patent shunts. Average decrease was about 25% to 50% of the preoperative value. Intraoperative pressure decreased from 30.4 mm Hg to 18 mm Hg in all eyes after surgery. Tolerance to the tubing was good in all eyes.

Early postoperative complications usually were related to rapid outflow of aqueous humor and poor pupillary dilation. Late complications usually were related to the positioning of the tubing and to the status of the eye before surgery. Late cataract developed in 1 patient. In no case did the implanted tubing migrate into the anterior chamber.

The aqueous-venous shunt operation has given satisfactory clinical results in patients with severe intractable glaucoma. The procedure is relatively simple, of low risk, and is well tolerated. Further study is needed to clearly define the applications and limitations of the aqueous-venous shunt procedure.

▶ [Valve implants have been developed to a stage where the materials and fixation have solved most of the problems of inflammation and migration. The problem, however, is the same as for trabeculectomy: scarring at the conjunctival end. The vortex vein is theoretically ideal because one can easily be sacrificed without choroidal vascular problems, and conjunctival scarring with occlusion should not occur.] ◀

7. The Lens

Lens Implantation, Correction of Aphakia, and Cataracts

EDWARD COTLIER, M.D.
YOG R. SHARMA, M.D.

Department of Ophthalmology and Visual Sciences
Yale University School of Medicine

In the United States, the trend for the past 5 years has produced an increased number of intraocular lens implantations. Results of several series in terms of visual acuity and complications are beginning to appear. The larger series belong to those surgeons with more expertise and do not reflect the eyes operated on by "average" eye surgeons. Nevertheless, in short-term follow-up, Kratz et al.[1] found after phacoemulsification that postoperative visual acuity was 20/40 or better in more than 85% of cases after implantation of two-loop and four-loop Binkhorst lenses, or Choyce Mark VII or Shearing posterior chamber lenses. In this series, the incidence of cystoid macular edema (CME) was highest, 7.3%, with Choyce Mark VII lenses and 4.7% and 3.4% with two-loop and four-loop Binkhorst lenses. In England, however, Percival[2] found a higher incidence of CME; the incidence of persistent CME was 6% in 232 eyes operated on, and his detailed analysis revealed a total incidence of 20% CME including 14% of transient CME as documented by fluorescein angiography. Persistent loss of vision occurred "in 9% of cases which had no other visual defect." Furthermore, he found, "Indomethacin at the time of surgery did not significantly reduce the incidence or severity of clinical CME in intracapsular cases." A slightly higher incidence of permanent CME (6.3%) was found by Shammas and Milkie after secondary lens implantation.[3]

The problems and tribulation associated with the "legalization" of intraocular lenses by the Food and Drug Administration (FDA) is well summarized in the "Update Report on Intraocular Lenses."[4] The impotence of the FDA in regulating medical practice is obvious. This is due to the limited resources of the agency that cannot police an area involving the vested interest of lens manufacturers and aggressive surgical entrepreneurs. The need for well-controlled prospective randomized studies on intraocular lenses and other methods for correction of aphakia has been known since 1966. At that time, a panel that I convened with National Eye Institute support at O'Hare Airport analyzed the problems regarding intraocular lenses. Since then, the problems have been magnified and now the situation is practically out of control. Intraocular lenses and correction of surgical aphakia are a "no man's land" and extremely difficult to legislate.

In a survey of 142 physicians, useful information was gathered regarding photocoagulation in patients with intraocular lenses.[5] Even after an uneventful implantation, there is greater endothelial cell loss as compared with simple cataract extraction,[6] but, disturbingly, this study reported that deterioration of the corneal endothelium after an intraocular lens implant is progressive. As the authors pointed out, this needs further elucidation, and they have suspected that chronic low-grade smoldering uveitis accompanying intraocular lenses may be responsible for endothelial damage. Another study[7] reported, "When combined with intraocular lens implantation, extracapsular lens extraction, even when performed by surgeons inexperienced with extracapsular techniques, caused no greater corneal endothelial damage than intracapsular extraction." Follow-up in this study was 8 weeks.

Girard[8] reported impressive results with pars plana lensectomy with ultrasonic fragmentation and, because of versatility of the method and its applicability to any age group, it may become used more widely in the near future.

What is the best way to correct aphakia? We have intraocular lenses and contact lenses, and keratophakia and the keratomileusis of Barraquer[9] seem to be gaining a deserved place in this armamentarium. This surgery has been performed at certain centers in the United States and the results of Barraquer confirmed and duplicated. In fact, a modification, termed "epikeratophakia," which has the advantage of being reversible, already has been given a prospective clinical trial.[10] Though complete visual recovery is slower as compared with intraocular lenses and contact lenses, the technique of Barraquer has promise; certainly, when intraocular lenses and contact lenses are contraindicated, refractive keratoplasty is an alternative.

Congenital cataracts, especially monocular, continue to present a formidable challenge. In a limited series[11] of 8 neonates with total monocular cataracts, surgery was done at the earliest possible time—1 patient was only 7 hours old! The oldest patient in this series was aged 41 days. Though no binocular vision was attained, in a follow-up exceeding 2.5 years, visual acuity of 20/30 or better was achieved in 5 patients and 20/80 or better in the other 3. There was a cheering note in that 4 eyes with concomitant microphthalmos were not "an insurmountable obstacle to attaining good visual function." Thus, Beller et al. conclude, "Surgery during the neonatal period is not only justified but probably essential in any successful management of monocular congenital cataracts." In another study in infants with complete bilateral cataracts, Rogers et al.[12] indicated the need for early surgery and stressed constant visual correction to obtain normal or near-normal vision. Peyman et al.[13] reported excellent surgical results in 32 eyes with congenital cataracts by pars plicata lensectomy and vitrectomy and "The procedure can be performed in infants as soon as the diagnosis of congenital cataract is made."

Has the transient rise of intraocular tension after cataract extraction bothered you? Two studies show it can be controlled by prophylactically administered timolol[14, 15] or by acetazolamide.[15] If your patient has atherosclerotic vessels and especially had anterior ischemic optic neuropathy in one eye after cataract surgery, it may be worthwhile to use timolol or acetazolamide prophylactically during cataract extraction on the contralateral eye.

There is no absolute consensus on an association between

diabetes mellitus and human cataractogenesis. Skalka and Prchal[16] stated, "We found no evidence to substantiate the general claim that senile cataracts occur more frequently and at an earlier age in diabetic patients." But in another study[17] data derived from two population surveys, the Framingham Eye Study and the Health and Nutrition Examination Survey, a marked excess prevalence of senile cataracts in diabetic patients younger than age 65 years was shown. In a large continuing study[18] of cataract patients and a control population conducted in Scotland, several interesting observations have been made, including an association between high blood sugar concentrations and cataracts. Other observations made in this study include an association between elevated blood pressure and cataracts ($P < .001$), high plasma urea concentrations and cataracts ($P < .0001$), low plasma cholesterol levels and cataracts ($P < .0001$), plasma glutamic oxaloacetic transaminase and glutamic pyruvic transaminase levels and cataracts, and also some association between alcohol consumption and cataracts—total abstainers having a higher prevalence of cataracts and nonabstainers a lower incidence, as compared to the control population ($P < .005$)!

The story between blood sugar and cataracts in animals is different. There is definite correlation between hyperglycemia and cataracts, and thus raised lens sorbitol content and cataracts can be slowed down or prevented by use of aldose reductase inhibitors.[19] Kinoshita et al.[19] state, "The fact that aldose reductase inhibitors can effectively block the progression of the cataract sets the stage for the clinical trial to determine their effectiveness in human diabetic cataracts." Supporting the role of polyol pathway in the human diabetic state is the report of increased motor nerve condition in the human diabetic state by the use of an aldose reductase inhibitor.[20]

Evidence for deceleration of senile cataracts by aspirin was presented in arthritis patients with or without diabetes.[21-25] Further work continues, but the exact mechanism of action remains unknown. "To unravel the aspirin effects would require a clear-cut understanding of senile cataract pathogenesis and etiology which is, as yet, unavailable, but several biochemical anomalies noted in senile cataracts may be prevented or reversed by salicylates.[25] After presenting our aspirin findings to ophthalmologists at the 1980–1981 meetings of the American Academy of Ophthalmologists, it is obvious that a large number of ophthalmologists (and their patients) are interested in medical therapy of cataracts.

REFERENCES

1. Kratz R.P., Mazzocco T.R., Davidson B., et al.: A comparative analysis of anterior chamber, iris-supported, capsule-fixated, and posterior chamber intraocular lenses following cataract extraction by phacoemulsification. *Ophthalmology (Rochester)* 88:56–58, 1981. (Article 7–8 in this YEAR BOOK.)
2. Percival P.: Clinical factors relating to cystoid macular edema after lens implantation. *Am. Intro-ocular Implant Soc. J.* 7:43–45, 1981.
3. Shammas H.J.F., Milkie C.F.: Cystoid macular edema following secondary lens implantation. *Am. Intro-ocular Implant Soc. J.* 7:40–42, 1981.
4. Worthen D.M., Boucher J.A., Buxton J., et al.: Update report on intraocular lenses. *Ophthalmology (Rochester)* 88:381–385, 1981.
5. Patz A.: Photocoagulation of retinal, vascular, and macular diseases through intraocular lenses. *Ophthalmology (Rochester)* 88:398–406, 1981.
6. Rao G.N., Stevens R.E., Harris J.K., et al.: Long-term changes in corneal endothelium following intraocular lens implantation. *Ophthalmology (Rochester)* 88:386–397, 1981.
7. Bourne W.M., Waller R.R., Liesegang T.J., et al.: Corneal trauma in intracapsular and extracapsular cataract extraction with lens implantation. *Arch. Ophthalmol.* 99:1375–1376, 1981.
8. Girard L.J.: Pars plana lensectomy by ultrasonic fragmentation. *Ophthalmology (Rochester)* 88:434–436, 1968.
9. Barraquer J.I.: Keratomileusis for myopia and aphakia. *Ophthalmology (Rochester)* 88:701–708, 1981.
10. Werblin T.P., Kaufman H.E., Friedlander M.H., et al.: Epikeratophakia: The surgical correction of aphakia. *Arch. Ophthalmol.* 99:1957–1960, 1981.
11. Beller R., Hoyt C.S., Marg E., et al.: Good visual function after neonatal surgery for congenital monocular cataracts. *Am. J. Ophthalmol.* 91:559–565, 1981.
12. Rogers G.L., Tishler C.L., Tsou B.H., et al.: Visual acuities in

infants with congenital cataracts operated on prior to 6 months of age. *Arch. Ophthalmol.* 99:999–1003, 1981. (Article 7–15 in this YEAR BOOK.)
13. Peyman G.A., Raichand M., Oesterle C., et al.: Pars plicata lensectomy and vitrectomy in the management of congenital cataracts. *Ophthalmology (Rochester)* 88:437–439, 1981.
14. Haimann M.H., Phelps C.D.: Prophylactic timolol for the prevention of high intraocular pressure after cataract extraction. *Ophthalmology (Rochester)* 88:233–238, 1981.
15. Packer A.J., Fraioli A.J., Epstein, D.L.: The effect of timolol and acetazolamide on transient intraocular pressure elevation following cataract extraction with α-chymotrypsin. *Ophthalmology (Rochester)* 88:239–243, 1981.
16. Skalka H.W., Prchal J.T.: The effect of diabetes mellitus and diabetic therapy on cataract formation. *Ophthalmology (Rochester)* 88:117–124, 1981. (Article 7–3 in this YEAR BOOK.)
17. Ederer F., Hiller R., Taylor, H.R.: Senile lens changes and diabetes in two population studies. *Am. J. Ophthalmol.* 91:381–395, 1981. (Article 7–4 in this YEAR BOOK.)
18. Clayton R.M., Cuthbert J., Phillips C.I., et al.: Analysis of individual cataract patients and their lenses: A progress report. *Exp. Eye Res.* 31:553–566, 1980.
19. Kinoshita J.H., Kador P., Catiles M.: Aldose reductase in diabetic cataracts. *JAMA* 246:257–261, 1981. (Article 7–6 in this YEAR BOOK.)
20. Judzewitsch R., Jaspan J.B., Pfeifer M.A., et al.: Inhibition of aldose reductase improves motor nerve conduction velocity in diabetics. *Diabetes* 30(Suppl. 1):118, 1981.
21. Cotlier E.: Rheumatoid arthritis and cataract surgery: Do salicylates slow down cataract formation? *Int. Ophthalmol.* 23:127–129, 1980.
22. Cotlier E., Sharma Y.R.: Aspirin and senile cataracts in rheumatoid arthritis. *Lancet* 1:338–339, 1981.
23. Cotlier E.: Senile cataracts: Evidence for acceleration by diabetes and deceleration by salicylate. *Can. J. Ophthalmol.* 16:113–118, 1981. (Article 7–5 in this YEAR BOOK.)
24. Cotlier E.: Aspirin effect on cataract formation in patients with rheumatoid arthritis alone or combined to diabetes. *Int. Ophthalmol.* 33:173–177, 1981.
25. Cotlier E.: Aspirin and cataracts: From the laboratory to clinical trials. *Medicine in Transition: Centennial of the University of Illinois College of Medicine,* 1981. pp. 207–213.

7-1 **A Change in Indications For Cataract Surgery? A 10-Year Comparative Epidemiologic Study.** Indications for cataract surgery have widened in the past decade, which might account for the steady increase in cataract extractions. Peter Bernth-Petersen (Univ. of Aarhus) reviewed indications for cataract extraction in groups of patients operated on consecutively in 1970 and 1980. All but 15% of cataract extractions in a population of 1 million are performed in the author's department. A comparison was made of 128 patients operated on in 1970, with a mean age of 70.8 years, and 123 patients operated on consecutively in 1980, with a mean age of 71.8 years. Women predominated in both groups.

Significantly more patients in 1970 had bilateral cataract (73% vs. 54%). No significant differences in the distribution of best-eye or worse-eye acuity were observed. Significantly more monaphakic patients were in the 1980 group. The distribution of acuity in both eyes was comparable in the two groups of monaphakic patients. Monaphakia itself now is considered an indication for surgery by many surgeons. The incidence of unilateral cataract of 2% in 1970 and 6% in 1980 was not a significant difference. In all these cases the indication for surgery was mature cataract.

No changes in indications for surgery are evident in cases of bilateral cataract, but a significantly larger proportion of extractions today are done on second-eye cataracts. Monaphakia itself is a stronger indication for surgery in the second eye than it was a decade ago. Increased activity and mobility of elderly subjects may have increased demands for second-eye cataract extraction. Many patients mistakenly believe that they will benefit visually as much from the second extraction as from the first. In addition, the fear of cataract surgery in general may be declining.

▶ [There are many factors that must be considered in the general increase in cataract operations besides an increase in the number of ophthalmologists, such as increase in age of the population. In this study, the author has demonstrated that more second eyes are being done than in the past.] ◀

(7–1) Acta Ophthalmol. (Copenh.) 59:206–210, April 1981.

7–2 **The Effectiveness of Cataract Surgery: A Retrospective Study.** Although the results of intracapsular cataract extraction usually include improved visual acuity, the problems of aphakia remain unsolved, and visual rehabilitation after surgery often is difficult. Peter Bernth-Petersen (Univ. of Aarhus) evaluated the practical results of cataract extraction in 120 patients with senile cataract who underwent intracapsular cryoextraction without lens implantation in a 4-month period in 1978. Running monofilament nylon wound closure was performed in all cases. Thirty-four patients had a second cataract extraction, and 5 had unilateral cataract. Senile macular degeneration occurred in 15 eyes, and diabetic retinopathy involving the macula occurred in 1 eye.

After a year, 9 patients had visual acuity of 0.05 or less, 54 had an acuity of 0.1–0.33, and 57 had an acuity of 0.4–1.25. Considerable improvement in vision had occurred in 58% of cases, while 14% of patients reported no improvement. A year postoperatively, 77% indicated an improved quality of life. Improved abilities to read and to cope, as well as less need for help, were characteristic of patients with acuities of 0.1 and better. Two thirds of patients used aphakic spectacles at follow-up, and 19% used contact lenses. All of the 7% of patients who were employed reported an improved work capacity after the operation. In all, 56% of patients required help in daily activities.

Cataract extraction successfully improves vision, visual function, and quality of life, although in many cases a discrepancy between visual acuity and visual function exists. Relevant factors include the visual disadvantages of aphakic spectacles, deficient cerebral adaptability, poor optics, use of the fellow eye, and difficult social conditions.

▶ [It is discouraging to learn that such a high percentage of patients are unable to utilize their aphakic vision. We don't know yet if intraocular lenses will improve the situation, and it may be that some sort of rehabilitation help is needed. Perhaps the ophthalmic surgeon is not finished with his patient when the wound has healed.] ◀

7–3 **Effect of Diabetes Mellitus and Diabetic Therapy on Cataract Formation.** An association between cataract and

---

(7–2) Acta Ophthalmol. (Copenh.) 59:50–56, February 1981.
(7–3) Ophthalmology (Rochester) 88:117–125, February 1981.

diabetes is clear in animals, but it has not been well elucidated in man. Harold W. Skalka and Josef T. Prchal (Univ. of Alabama, Birmingham) undertook a prospective, double-blind study of this association in male outpatients at diabetes and hematology-oncology clinics. There were 231 diabetics, excluding patients with diabetes secondary to other disease or corticosteroid therapy and those given corticosteroids topically or systemically at any time. Controls included 58 nondiabetics never given corticosteroid therapy and 47 who had received corticosteroids systemically. The groups were similar in age, race, and socioeconomic background. Most controls had been treated for hematopoietic malignancies.

Diabetes was not significantly associated with cataract formation, but an association approaching significance was found for higher grades of cataract. A highly significant association was evident for posterior subcapsular cataracts, mature lenses, and aphakia grouped together. Duration of diabetes, adjusted for age, was correlated with cataract formation, but age was the chief cataractogenic factor in the diabetic group. Dietary control and insulin use were not significantly related to cataract formation, but use of oral hypoglycemic agents was correlated with lens opacities, particularly with posterior subcapsular cataracts. No association was found between cataract and either fasting blood sugar or red blood cell hemoglobin A_1 concentration in diabetics. Among nondiabetics, systemic corticosteroid use was associated with lens opacities, particularly posterior subcapsular cataracts.

Diabetes appeared in this study to be associated with an increased risk of visually significant lens opacities. Age was the most significant factor in the association. Risk factors for the development of posterior subcapsular cataracts include diabetes, use of oral hypoglycemic agents, and systemic corticosteroid therapy.

7-4 **Senile Lens Changes and Diabetes in Two Population Studies.** Three previous studies of extracted cataract have indicated a positive relationship with diabetes in persons younger than age 70 years. whereas two studies of se-

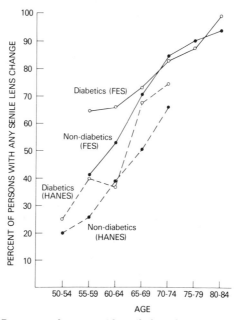

Fig 7–1.—Percentage of persons with senile lens changes in one or both eyes. *FES,* Framingham Eye Study; *HANES,* Health and Nutrition Examination Survey. (Courtesy of Ederer, F., et al.: Am. J. Ophthalmol. 91:381–395, March 1981.)

nile lens changes found no association with diabetes. Sommer (1977) concluded that diabetics are not at an increased risk of developing cataracts, but only of having them removed because they are more likely to come to medical attention. Fred Ederer, Rita Hiller (Natl. Inst. of Health); and Hugh R. Taylor (Johns Hopkins Hosp.) examined this association in subjects in the Framingham Eye Study and those in the Health and Nutrition Examination Survey (HANES). In the Framingham sample, 1,487 subjects aged 52–85 years with senile lens changes were compared with 830 having no such changes. In the Health and Nutrition Examination Survey, 1,234 subjects aged 50–74 years with senile lens changes and 1,413 without such changes were evaluated.

At comparable ages, the proportion of subjects with any lens change was considerably greater in the Framingham series. Senile lens changes were more common in diabetics up to age 69 years in the Framingham series. In the HANES group, lens changes were more common in diabetics in all age groups except that aged 60–64 years (Fig 7–1). In the HANES group for ages 50–64 years, only senile cataract was highly significantly associated with diabetes. In the Framingham series, highly significant associations were found for any lens change; cataract, including aphakia; and precataract. At ages 65–74 years, the HANES group showed significant associations for any lens change and for cataract. The Framingham group showed no significant associations with any types of lens change at over age 64 years. The results for men and women were generally similar.

The present findings fail to support Sommer's hypothesis since they indicate that cataract, whether removed or not, is associated with diabetes in subjects younger than age 70. The apparent decrease in relative risk with advancing age may be due to a smaller proportion of severe diabetics because of higher mortality at earlier ages, or to an increased relative risk of nondiabetic cataract with increasing age.

▶ [There appears to be an association between diabetes and cataracts, but the relationship is complicated and requires careful analysis. This is of considerable importance for the following two studies, because the authors propose using the prospective, randomized, masked clinical trial mechanism to determine the efficacy of salicylates and aldose reductase inhibitors in the treatment of cataracts. These studies will have to be designed with great care because the relationship between diabetes and cataracts is so complex.] ◀

7–5 **Senile Cataracts: Evidence for Acceleration by Diabetes and Deceleration by Salicylate.** Edward Cotlier (Yale Univ.) examined the rate of progression of senile cataract in diabetics, who are known to have accelerated cataract formation, and in patients receiving acetylsalicylic acid because plasma tryptophan levels are increased in cataract patients and acetylsalicylic acid reduces plasma tryptophan by up to 50%. Cataracts studied were collected from the operating rooms of two hospitals. Age of the patient was plotted against degree of opacity of the cataract.

Significantly more advanced cataractous changes were present at earlier ages in diabetic patients. Although rate of progression differed markedly from that in nondiabetics,

---

(7–5) Can. J. Ophthalmol. 16:113–118, July 1981.

age at onset of cataract did not. Distribution of cataracts from patients with systemic hypertension or chronic simple glaucoma did not differ from that for the nondiabetic group. The findings in diabetics taking and those not taking acetylsalicylic acid are compared in Figure 7–2. Similar findings in nondiabetics are shown in Figure 7–3. Progression of cataracts appeared to be markedly delayed by use of acetylsalicylic acid. Also, cataracts appeared later in osteoar-

Fig 7–2 (top).—Mean age of patients with diabetes taking (n = 8) or not taking (n = 45) acetylsalicylic acid *(ASA)* in same population.

Fig 7–3 (bottom).—Mean age of nondiabetic patients taking (n = 246) or not taking (n = 8) ASA in University of Illinois Eye and Ear Infirmary population.

(Courtesy of Cotlier, E.: Can. J. Ophthalmol. 16:113–118, July 1981.)

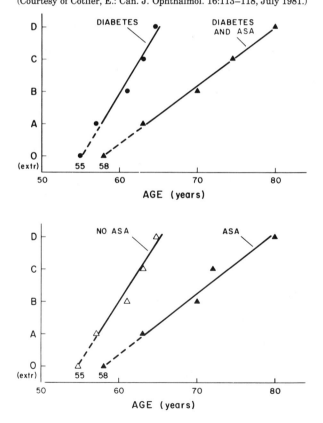

thritic patients taking acetylsalicylic acid than in other arthritic patients.

Diabetes accelerates development of cataracts, but does not significantly alter age at which cataract development begins. Acetylsalicylic acid appears to delay cataract formation. It is possible that reduction in plasma tryptophan is responsible. Available evidence appears to warrant acetylsalicylic acid treatment for early senile cataract, but prospective randomized studies are needed for more definitive conclusions. Use of a microdensitometric method for assessing lens opacities might refine cataract quantitation.

7-6 **Aldose Reductase in Diabetic Cataracts** was investigated by Jin H. Kinoshita, Peter Kador, and Manuel Catiles. An association between cataracts and diabetes in human beings has been suspected for about two centuries. Diabetes produced either by pancreatomy or by chemical destruction of beta cells leads to cataracts in animals. Moreover, the rapidity of cataract development paralleled the severity of the diabetes. An understanding of the development of diabetic cataracts was accelerated by the fact that the process could be duplicated in rats fed galactose.

Histologic studies showed the appearance of hydropic lens fiber cells, which causes swelling of the fibers. As the process continues, the swollen fibers eventually rupture, with the areas appearing to the naked eye as vacuoles. The swelling of these fibers is possibly caused by an increase of electrolytes or an accumulation of abnormal metabolites. Aldose reductase and polyol dehydrogenase are the two enzymes that constitute the polyol pathway. That polyols are responsible for the osmotic change seems reasonable, since these sugar alcohols poorly penetrate biologic membranes, and once formed in the fiber cells, they do not readily leak from the cells.

To study sugar cataracts by organ culture, rabbit lenses were incubated in medium rich in galactose. The lenses quickly accumulated polyol, and the retention of polyol was paralleled by an increase in lense hydration. From the results of this and other experiments, an hypothesis was established depicting the sequence of events responsible for the formation of cataracts. The high sugar level activates aldose reductase that converts the sugar to polyol. Since the lens membranes are relatively impermeable to polyols, dulcitol once formed begins to accumulate, creating a hypertonic condition. To maintain osmotic equilibrium, water is drawn into the lens fibers. The increase in hydration substantially affects membrane permeability, resulting in loss of amino acids and potassium ions and a gain in sodium ions. Another and more pronounced increase in lens hydration results from an accompanying increase in electrolytes.

The most convincing proof for the polyol osmotic theory emerged from experiments with aldose reductase inhibitors. Alrestatin is the latest aldose-reductase inhibitor. Sorbinil, a potent inhibitor, was used to treat diabetic rats at a dose of 60 mg/kg daily, which eventually abolished the synthesis of lens sorbitol. That aldose-reductase inhibitors can effectively block the progression of the cataract sets the stage for the clinical trial to determine their effectiveness in human diabetic cataracts. The use of sorbinil to block conversion of glucose to sorbitol in 31 human diabetics led to a reversible increase in motor nerve conduction velocity, supporting a role for the polyol pathway as a contributory factor in diabetic polyneuropathy.

7-7 **Professional Standards Review Organization Studies Length of Stay for Cataract Extraction in District of Columbia Hospitals.** Mervin H. Zimmerman, Paul Schlein, Norman A. Fuller, and Elizabeth Carrier (Natl. Capital Med. Found., Inc., Washington, D.C.) reviewed the findings in a study done to determine why the length of hospital stay for various conditions including cataract extraction was longer in the District of Columbia than in other PSRO areas. A large migration of patients from Maryland and Virginia into the District for specialty procedures such as cataract extraction was discovered, nearly doubling the rate of extraction in the city and lowering it in surrounding PSRO areas. Lengths of stay in several areas are compared in the table. Data for 1977 to 1979 showed a marked decrease in average length of stay and average preoperative

LENGTH OF STAY FOR ALL MEDICARE RESIDENTS IN STANDARD
METROPOLITAN STATISTICAL AREA (SMSA) ADMITTED FOR
LENS EXTRACTION IN 1976

SMSA area	Days of care per 1,000 enrollees	Average length of stay
San Francisco	44.2	4.3
Pittsburgh	55.8	4.9
Washington, D.C.	44.8	5.6
Philadelphia	57.4	5.7
Cleveland	69.3	6.2
Chicago	64.8	6.4
Detroit	65.0	6.5
Newark	71.0	6.5
New York	72.9	7.1
Baltimore	53.4	8.4

stay in 1979 for Medicare and Medicaid patients with a single diagnosis of cataract.

Caution is needed when nonanalyzed data are used to set program objectives. Length of stay profiles for cataract extraction have been distributed to physicians and hospitals. Physicians may be encouraged to do prehospitalization workups and to perform short-stay cataract extraction. They also should be encouraged to plan the time of discharge, when indicated.

7–8 **A Comparative Analysis of Anterior Chamber, Iris-Supported, Capsule-Fixated, and Posterior Chamber Intraocular Lenses Following Cataract Extraction by Phacoemulsification.** Richard P. Kratz, Thomas R. Mazzocco, Bernard Davidson, and D. Michael Colvard (Univ. of Southern California, Los Angeles) report a series of 1,367 cases of intraocular lens implantations after phacoemulsification, excluding cases with vitreous loss or vitrectomy. All lenses were implanted under air or balanced saline solution. Topical antibiotics were used for a week postoperatively and topical steroids, for 3–5 weeks. Follow-up ranges from 3 months to 5 years. The Rayner Choyce Mark VIII lens was used as an anterior chamber lens, the Binkhorst four-loop lens as an iris-supported lens, the Binkhorst two-loop lens as a capsule-supported lens, and the Shearing lens

TABLE 1.—POSTOPERATIVE VISUAL ACUITY RESULTS FOR EACH LENS TYPE*

Vision	Two-loop (n = 320)	Four-loop (n = 209)	Choyce VIII (Rayner) (n = 82)	Shearing (n = 756)
20/20	15.6%	22.0%	9.8%	36.5%
20/25	18.8%	20.1%	17.1%	24.3%
20/30	26.5%	27.7%	40.2%	19.2%
20/40	24.4%	16.8%	25.6%	11.0%
20/70	7.2%	7.2%	4.9%	5.4%
20/100	2.8%	.5%	1.2%	1.5%
20/200 or less	4.7%	5.7%	1.2%	2.1%
	100.0%	100.0%	100.0%	100.0%
20/25 or better	34.4%	42.1%	26.9%	60.8%
20/40 or better	85.9%	86.6%	92.7%	91.0%

as a posterior chamber lens. The average patient was about 71 years old.

Visual acuity results are given in Table 1 and complications in Table 2. The proportion of patients with 20/40 or better acuity was good with all types of lenses, but more patients with posterior chamber lenses had acuities of 20/25 or better. Iritis was most frequent in patients with anterior chamber lenses, as was clinical cystoid macular edema. Hyphema also was most frequent in this group. Retinal detachments were comparably frequent in all the groups. Lens subluxation was most frequent in patients with capsule-supported lenses, particularly where metal loop lenses were used. Metal two-loop Binkhorst-type lenses were most often associated with corneal decompensation and were most often removed. Persistent intraocular hypertension was infrequent. Shearing lenses tended to be used most often in patients with preexisting glaucoma.

Exceptionally good vision occurred most often in patients in this study who received Shearing-type posterior chamber lenses. Several complications were most frequent with anterior chamber lenses. The Binkhorst two-loop lens subluxed most frequently. Medically controlled glaucoma appears not to contraindicate intraocular lens implantation after phacoemulsification.

▶ [Hardly a month goes by without the introduction of a new kind of intraocular lens. The authors have compared several types and conclude that, in their hands, the posterior chamber lens is best. Phacoemulsifi-

TABLE 2.—COMPLICATIONS FOR EACH LENS TYPE

	Two-loop	Four-loop	(Rayner) Choyce VIII	Shearing
Iritis	2.5%	3.35%	7.3%	3.3%
Hyphema	0.0%	0.0%	4.9%	0.1%
Cystoid Macular edema	4.7%	3.4%	7.3%	2.1%
Retinal detachment	1.3%	1.9%	3.6%	1.3%
Subluxation	3.4%	1.9%	0.0%	0.4%
Lens removal	3.8%	1.0%	0.0%	0.3%
Corneal decompensation	0.9%	0.5%	0.0%	0.0%
Postoperative glaucoma	0.0%	0.5%	0.0%	0.4%

cation is not universally done, but of more interest is the fact that a standard procedure without an implant was not included in their study. The critical study is the comparison between cataract extraction with and without an implant and correction with continuous-wear contact lenses and, more recently, refractive keratoplasty. These questions must be answered with care if our patients are not to be compromised during the evolution of new techniques.] ◄

7-9 **A Histopathologic Study of the Position of the Shearing Intraocular Lens in the Posterior Chamber.** Some surgeons attempt to place the supporting loops of the Shearing posterior-chamber intraocular lens in the bag of residual lens capsule and peripheral cortex, whereas others prefer to place them in the region of the ciliary body sulcus. J. Brooks Crawford (Univ. of California, San Francisco) examined 3 human eyes that had had Shearing intraocular lenses successfully implanted 9, 19, and 28 months previously.

In 1 case the superior loop of the lens extended through the pigment epithelium of the pars plicata of the ciliary body in the ciliary sulcus and was embedded in the ciliary body close to a major artery. The inferior loop was firmly fixed in the residual capsular sac. In the second case the superior loop was firmly held by adhesions in the ciliary body sulcus and the inferior loop was within the peripheral iris. In the third case the superior loop was embedded deep within the pars plicata of the ciliary body close to a major vessel, and the inferior loop was fixed in the residual bag of lens capsule and the peripheral cortex. In the first and third cases, a few epithelioid cells and giant cells surrounded the loops embedded in the ciliary body.

Neither of the eyes with the superior loop of the Shearing lens close to a major artery in the ciliary body had intraocular bleeding. Only these loops provoked minimal inflammation, but this did not destroy a significant part of the loop material. If such a lens must be removed, the best suggestion might be to cut it from its supporting loop and leave the loop in place.

7–10 **Extracapsular Cataract Extraction and Pseudophakos Implantation in Primates: A Clinicopathologic Study.** Alexander R. Irvine examined the effects of cataract extraction and implantation of the Binkhorst iris-plane lens, the Choyce anterior chamber lens, and the Shearing posterior chamber lens in rhesus monkeys, using techniques employed in human beings. The Binkhorst four-loop iris fixation lens was implanted in 2 eyes, the Binkhorst two-loop iridocapsular lens in 9, the Choyce Mark VIII anterior chamber lens in 7, and the Shearing lens in 4. All extracapsular extractions were done by the phacoemulsification technique. Intracapsular extractions in animals that had Binkhorst iris fixation lenses implanted were attempted using α-chymotrypsin and mechanical stripping of zonules. Most Binkhorst lenses used had titanium loops. The animals were killed from 4 to 28 months after surgery.

Synechiae were seen with all lens types. The corneas were clear within a few days after surgery. Intraocular pressures were not elevated except in 2 cases of pupillary block in animals with Choyce lenses in place. No lens dislocations, retinal detachments, or cases of endophthalmitis occurred. The corneal endothelia were surprisingly normal at the time when the animals were killed, and the corneal wounds were well healed 4–6 months postoperatively. In most eyes the wounds were free of incarcerated tissue and the angles were open. There was little evidence of iris inflammation. The Choyce lens often produced marked distortion of the iris root. The trabecular meshwork was free of acute inflammation. Most eyes with extracapsular extraction showed

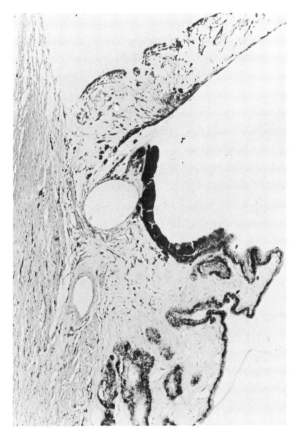

Fig 7–4.—Human eye obtained post mortem a year after Shearing lens implantation shows erosion of loop into the ciliary body identical to that in monkeys in this study. Note proximity of long ciliary artery; reduced from ×28. (Courtesy of Irvine, A. R.: Trans. Am. Ophthalmol. Soc. 78:780–807, 1980.)

some peripheral opacity and Soemmering's cataract. Late opacification of the posterior capsule was noted in some eyes as the result of fibrous metaplasia of the lens epithelium. Tight fibrotic bands had formed where the anterior lens capsule was absent. The ciliary body and the choroid were free of inflammation. One eye showed an area of apparent lattice vitreoretinal degeneration. No optic nerve head cupping was observed.

The findings in 1 human eye (Fig 7–4) confirm the applicability of the present findings to results of clinical cases. The implants in monkeys were well tolerated clinically and showed remarkably little inflammation on histologic study. If a Shearing lens is implanted, every effort should be made to ensure that both loops lie in the capsular envelope.

▶ [This study and the preceding one, plus the fact that there are many new loop configurations, emphasize that intraocular lens fixation is still evolving. Moreover, where the posterior chamber lens loops end up seems problematic.] ◀

7–11 **Increased Incidence of Cataracts in Male Subjects Deficient in Glucose-6-Phosphate Dehydrogenase.** Glucose-6-phosphate dehydrogenase (G6PD) deficiency is expressed not only in the red blood cells but in other tissues, including the lens, and a relation with cataract has been suggested. Nicola Orzalesi, Rolando Sorcinelli, and Gustavo Guiso (Univ. of Cagliari) reviewed 210 consecutive cases of idiopathic, presenile, and senile cataract in men seen between 1975 and 1977. The rate of G6PD deficiency was compared with that in 672 men without cataract seen in the same period. Mean ages of the study and control groups were 71.6 and 54.4 years, respectively. All subjects were of Sardinian origin.

Deficiency of G6PD was identified in 27.6% of cataractous subjects and in 11.6% of controls, a highly significant difference. The latter figure is close to that expected from larger surveys of males of mixed Sardinian origin. In the cataract group, enzyme deficiency was more frequent with decreasing age. The incidence in patients aged 40 to 60 years with presenile cataract was 48.5%.

The earlier and more frequent cataractogenesis observed in G6PD-deficient subjects might be related to the role of this enzyme in lens metabolism. A deficiency reduces the amount of ribose available for nucleic acid synthesis and decreases the renewal of lens proteins. Further, the nicotinamide adenine dinucleotide supply needed for protection of reduced glutathione against oxidation is cut off, enhancing loss of solubility of lens proteins. More epidemiologic studies are needed of the relation between metabolic defects of red blood cells and cataract formation.

(7–11) Arch. Ophthalmol. 99:69–70, January 1981.

7-12 **Cataract: The Ultraviolet Risk Factor.** Near ultraviolet light can induce lens opacity, probably through photoxidation of aromatic amino acids, especially tryptophan. The effect appears to be cumulative and is inhibited by physiologic concentrations of ascorbate and glutathione. Fred Hollows and David Moran (Univ. of New South Wales) evaluated the eyes of 64,307 Australian aborigines and 41,254 nonaborigines during a 3-year field work study of trachoma and ocular health. The Australian mainland was divided into five ultraviolet zones.

A significant correlation was found between climatic ultraviolet radiation and prevalence of cataract. Subjects aged 40 to 59 years showed a disproportionate increase in cataract prevalence with increasing ultraviolet radiation. Aborigines older than age 60 who had cataract were much likelier to be blind or to have poor vision if they lived in a high-ultraviolet zone. Nonaborigines of this age were less likely to be blind or to have poor vision. The overall prevalence of cataract in this group was just under two thirds of that for aborigines. Among younger subjects, nonaborigines had one-fifth to one-sixth the prevalence of cataract as aborigines. Cataract in nonaborigines was associated with less visual loss. Among nonaborigines, cataract prevalence could not be correlated with ultraviolet zone. No significant sex differences were observed.

Solar ultraviolet radiation increases the prevalence of cataract in Australian aborigines, but little is known of other factors that may influence the prevalence of cataract in this population. Cataract develops earlier and has more marked visual consequences in areas of high ultraviolet radiation. Prevention of cataract may be another reason to provide good housing in tropical and arid regions. The use of sunglasses by persons at risk may also be beneficial.

13 **Frequency of Cataract in Atopic Dermatitis.** Atopic cataract has been described in up to a fifth of patients with atopic dermatitis. Jens Dahl Christensen (Copenhagen) attempted to determine the practicality of routinely screening all patients with atopic dermatitis ophthalmologically. Fifty-one patients with atopic dermatitis for at least 5 years

---

(7–12) Lancet 2:1249–1250, Dec. 5, 1981.
(7–13) Acta Derm. Venereol. (Stockh.) 61:76–77, 1981.

and involvement of at least 10% of the skin surface were evaluated in a 3-month period. The 33 female and 18 male patients had a mean age of 24.6 years. None of the patients had atopic cataract, but 17 had ocular disorders. One had bilateral, probably congenital cataracts. Three patients had conjunctivitis, and 13 had refractive errors.

Descriptions of atopic cataract have specified the bilateral occurrence of yellowish opacities and flattened vacuoles at the posterior pole of the lens just in front of the capsule, followed by anterior subcapsular opacities, and eventually opacity of the entire cortex. The changes in the 1 case of cataract in the present series of patients with atopic dermatitis did not resemble those described in cases of atopic cataract. The present findings suggest a certain incidence of atopic cataract, but routine ophthalmologic screening of all patients having atopic dermatitis is not indicated.

▶ [There continues to be a concentrated effort to find and treat biochemical defects associated with cataract formation. Such a relationship appears to exist between lens opacities and glucose-6-phosphate dehydrogenase deficiency. Although enormously difficult to prove, ultraviolet light exposure appears to be associated with cataracts. Finally, patients with atopic dermatitis may have associated cataracts, although the authors conclude that screening large numbers is probably not justified. There is, of course, a long list of factors associated with cataracts, but they only become important when the means of prevention is relatively easy.] ◀

7–14 **Management of Cataract in Patients With Glaucoma: A Comparative Study.** The occurrence of cataract and glaucoma together creates many problems, including the timing of various surgical procedures. George L. Spaeth (Thomas Jefferson Univ., Philadelphia) has reviewed experience with 129 patients who had primary open-angle or chronic primary angle-closure glaucoma with visual field defects and elevated intraocular pressure, as well as reduced acuity from cataract. All were thought to have progressing glaucoma despite maximal tolerated medical therapy. Patients underwent glaucoma surgery initially, usually by trabeculectomy, followed in about 3 months by cataract extraction, or they had intracapsular cataract extraction with simultaneous trabeculectomy, partial-punch sclerectomy, iridencleisis, or cyclodialysis. In most pa-

COMPLICATIONS ASSOCIATED WITH COMBINED CATARACT-GLAUCOMA SURGERY

Intracapsular cataract extraction

Surgery	Post filtration		With trabeculectomy		With partial-punch sclerectomy		With iridencleisis		With cyclodialysis		Alone	
	No.	Per cent	No.	Per cent	No.	Per cent	No.	Per cent	No.	Per cent	No.	Per cent
No. of cases	15		24		30		24		20		16	
Complications												
Significant hyphaema — Mild	3	20	7	30	10	33	4	17	10	50	3	19
Significant hyphaema — Marked	1	7	4	17	2	7	2	8	6	30	2	13
Flat anterior chamber — Mild	0		1	4	0		0		0		0	
Flat anterior chamber — Moderate	0		2	8	3	10	1	4	0		0	
Flat anterior chamber — Re-formation needed	0		1	4	2	7	1	4	0		0	
Corneal oedema	0		2	8	0		1	4	0		0	
Pupillary block — Transient Laser iridectomy needed	0		0		1	3	0		3	15	1	6
Continuing inflammation	0		0		0		6	25	2	10	1	6
Unplanned extracapsular extraction	1	7	0		0		0		0		0	
Sterie hypopyon	0		0		0		0		0		1	6
Total complications	5		17		19		15		21		8	

tients, except those having iridencleisis, two or three peripheral iridectomies were performed. Complications are listed in the table.

No single approach to combined glaucoma and cataract treatment is superior to others. A large elevation in intraocular pressure is more likely to occur in patients having combined cataract extraction and trabeculectomy than in those having extraction combined with partial-punch sclerotomy or extraction after trabeculectomy. Trabeculectomy and sclerectomy are more likely to be associated with a flat anterior chamber than are routine cataract extraction or extraction with cyclodialysis. Astigmatism is more of a problem with procedures designed to leave a leak at the time the cataract is extracted. Persistent inflammation is most frequent in patients having cataract extraction with iridencleisis or cyclodialysis. Hyphema has been most troublesome in patients having extraction combined with cyclodialysis or trabeculectomy.

The goals in a given case should be matched with the most appropriate surgical management. The stage of glaucoma is more important than the state of intraocular pressure control. Wherever possible, cataract extraction should probably be avoided in glaucomatous patients.

▶ [This article should be read in its entirety by ophthalmic surgeons caring for patients with combined glaucoma and cataract. Spaeth has outlined a fine systematic approach to the management of such patients, based on his considerable experience and the careful analysis of a large number of patients.] ◀

7-15 **Visual Acuities in Infants With Congenital Cataracts Operated on Prior to 6 Months of Age.** Gary L. Rogers, Carl L. Tishler, Brian H. Tsou, Richard W. Hertle, and Rae R. Fellows (Columbus, Ohio) determined the visual acuity of 23 infants, 16 normal infants and 7 operated on before age 6 months for complete bilateral congenital cataracts. A modified preferential looking method was used to test vision. Psychological development was assessed using the Bayley Scale of Infant Development. Three infants had congenital hereditary cataracts; no cause was apparent in the other cases. The cataract group had a mean age of 35 weeks and normal infants, 32 weeks.

The 3 infants operated on before age 8 weeks appeared to have normally developing vision, with acuities equal to those of control infants. The others showed a substantial visual lag, with acuities less than 6/60. Similar results were obtained using a checkerboard pattern and bars and checks. Children operated on before age 8 weeks had Bayley test scores within the normal range, whereas those operated on after age 10 weeks exhibited an increasing lag in development.

Both visual acuity and overall development were best in infants with bilateral congenital cataracts operated on before age 8 weeks in this series. All the children were operated on within the first 6 months of life and were fitted with an extended-wear contact lens within 2 weeks after surgery. The critical period for restoring vision remains to be determined, but early surgery is necessary, as is constant visual correction, in order to obtain normal or nearly normal vision.

8. The Uvea

Update on Sympathetic Ophthalmia

HOWARD H. TESSLER, M.D.

Eye and Ear Infirmary, University of Illinois, Chicago

Sympathetic ophthalmia still occurs. Articles describing cases associated with trauma and surgery continue to appear.[1,2] At the University of Illinois Eye and Ear Infirmary, in a 1½ year period between 1978 and 1979 we saw 7 new cases, 3 of which were histologically confirmed. Lubin and Albert feel there is no current reduction in the incidence of sympathetic ophthalmia and that an increased incidence has actually occurred because of the new heroic surgical procedures that can salvage traumatized eyes.[3]

Sympathetic ophthalmia presents itself as a spectrum of disease. It does not always appear as a bilateral granulomatous panuveitis. Sympathetic ophthalmia can occur as a mild nongranulomatous iridocyclitis. It is probable that without enucleation, mild cases of sympathetic ophthalmia may be undiagnosed.

Four patients have been described with a histologic picture of sympathetic ophthalmia in which the remaining eye showed no clinical evidence of inflammation.[4,5] It is probable that these patients had subclinical inflammation in the remaining eye. Thus, sympathetic ophthalmia may occur without clinical evidence of a sympathizing eye.

When sympathetic ophthalmia is clinically suspected, histopathology is classically the method to confirm the diagnosis. However, Stokes and Zimmerman could histopathologically confirm a clinical diagnosis of sympathetic ophthalmia in only 39 of 180 suspected cases after penetrating injury.[6] It is possible that some of the other 141 patients might still have sympathetic ophthalmia despite the negative histopathology. Corticosteroids can modify the inflammatory reaction and, in consequence, the histopathology.[7] In one recent article, when conventional histopathology was only suggestive but not certain of sympathetic ophthalmia, additional flat mounts of the choroid were necessary to find "ill-defined nests of epithelioid cells" to support a diagnosis of sympathetic ophthalmia.[2]

There are no immunologic tests at present that will predict the development of sympathetic ophthalmia before it occurs. There are no immunologic tests that will absolutely make the diagnosis of sympathetic ophthalmia after it has begun.[8] To summarize, the diagnosis of sympathetic ophthalmia is not always certain clinically or even histopathologically.

We still do not have the answer to the cause of sympathetic ophthalmia. Recently, "S" antigen, a soluble polypeptide found in the retina, has been used to create a model of sympathetic ophthalmia. Recent evidence indicates that S antigen may be rhodopsin kinase.[9] In guinea pigs, a histopathologic picture virtually identical to sympathetic ophthalmia can be created by the single injection of 5 to 10 µg of purified guinea pig S antigen in complete Freund's adjuvant into the footpad. Approximately 12 to 15 days after injection, uveitis appeared. If more antigen were injected initially, a severe endophthalmitis occurred. If less S antigen were used (1 µg), a nonspecific nongranulomatous uveitis occurred.[10] It is tempting to speculate that in cases of suspected clinical sympathetic ophthalmia where histopathology is nonspecific, that a less than optimal sensitizing dose of S antigen or another antigen was available. The amount of sensitizing antigen available may also explain the variable course of sympathetic ophthalmia.

Nussenblatt and associates have recently used S antigen to produce uveitis in primates.[11] They emulsified the antigen with complete Freund's adjuvant and injected it into the monkey's neck. Bilateral uveitis occurred in 3–4 weeks. At the dosage of S antigen used, the histology did not resemble sympathetic ophthalmia. The authors speculate that S antigen may not be the whole story in sympathetic ophthalmia, but that it may play a nonspecific initiating or propagating role.

Evidence that S antigen may be involved in other entities is supplied by work that shows cellular and humoral cellular immunity against S antigen in patients with ocular toxoplasmosis, sarcoidosis, and other diseases.[12, 13] Even after laser photocoagulation in diabetics, levels of antibody against S antigen increase.[12] Thus, much of the reactivity we see in uveitis to S antigen may be an epiphenomenon secondary to retinal damage. This may explain the rationale of using corticosteroids even in infectious diseases such as toxoplasmosis.

The best therapy of sympathetic ophthalmia remains prophylaxis. Enucleation before day 7 or 8 is usually protective. Enucleation after day 14 even if the sympathizing eye shows no clinical inflammation may not always be prophylactic.[14-16] Lubin and colleagues feel that enucleation within 2 weeks of clinical inflammation will promote a better prognosis.[3, 7] Thus, if the exciting eye is hopeless, early enucleation is indicated even after sympathetic ophthalmia has occurred. The thought that enucleation is of no value once inflammation is present only holds if the inflammation has been present for longer than 2 weeks.

Prophylactic therapy with corticosteroids will not prevent sympathetic ophthalmia.[15] However, 65% of patients will do well with corticosteroid therapy, so blindness is not the inevitable result it once was.[7] About 20% of cases of sympathetic ophthalmia run such a mild course that low doses of corticosteroids will quiet the disease. These mild cases tend to be of short duration and not recur.[14, 18] Thus, a mild course of inflammation does not rule out sympathetic ophthalmia.

For the 25% of cases that respond poorly to corticosteroids, immunosuppressive agents such as chlorambucil hold real promise.[19] The risk of these drugs is well known, but their ability to salvage otherwise hopeless cases and to avoid long-term corticosteroid toxicity makes them a viable alternative in selected cases.

REFERENCES

1. Dreyer W.B., Zegarra H., Zakov Z.N., et al.: Sympathetic ophthalmia. *Am. J. Ophthalmol.* 92:816–823, 1981.
2. Croxatto J.O., Galentine P., Cupples H.P., et al.: Sympathetic ophthalmia after pars plana vitrectomy-lensectomy for endogenous bacterial endophthalmitis. *Am. J. Ophthalmol.* 91:342–346, 1981.
3. Lubin J.R., Albert D.M.: Sympathetic ophthalmia: Ample room for controversy. *Surv. Ophthalmol.* 24:137–140, 1979.
4. Ikui H.: A case of sympathetic ophthalmia without the sympathizing eye. *Folia Ophthalmol. Jpn.* 21:732–737, 1970.
5. Marak G.E.: Recent advances in sympathetic ophthalmia. *Surv. Ophthalmol.* 24:141–156, 1979.
6. Stokes J.A., Zimmerman L.E.: Clinical pathological studies in cases of suspected sympathetic ophthalmia. Presented at the 7th Annual Military Medico-Dental Symposium, Philadelphia, Oct. 1956.
7. Lubin J.R., Albert D.M., Weinstein M.: Sixty-five years of sympathetic ophthalmia: A clinicopathologic review of 105 cases (1913–1978). *Ophthalmology (Rochester)* 87:109–121, 1980.
8. Rahi A., Morgan G., Levy I., et al.: Immunologic investigations in past traumatic granulomatous and nongranulomatous uveitis. *Br. J. Ophthalmol.* 62:722–728, 1978.
9. Shichi, H.: Possible identity of experimental uveitogenic antigen (S antigen) with rhodopsin kinase. *Jpn. J. Ophthalmol.* 25:306–311, 1981.
10. Rao N.A., Wacker W.B., Marak G.E.: Experimental allergic uveitis: Clinicopathologic features associated with varying doses of S antigen. *Arch. Ophthalmol.* 97:1954–1958, 1979.
11. Nussenblatt R.B., Kuwabara T., deMonasterio F.M., et al.: S Antigen uveitis in primates: A new model for human disease. *Arch. Ophthalmol.* 99:1090–1092, 1981.
12. Gregerson D.S., Abrahams I.W., Thirkill C.E.: Serum antibody levels of uveitis patients to bovine retinal antigens. *Inv. Ophthalmol. Vis. Sci.* 21:669–680, 1981.
13. Nussenblatt R.B., Gery I., Ballintine E.J., et al.: Cellular immune responsiveness of uveitis patients to retinal S antigen. *Am. J. Ophthalmol.* 89:173–179, 1980.
14. Brauninger G.E., Polack F.M.: Sympathetic ophthalmitis. *Am. J. Ophthalmol.* 72:967, 1971.
15. Kay M.L., Yanoff M., Katowitz J.A.: Development of sympathetic uveitis in spite of corticosteroid therapy. *Am. J. Ophthalmol.* 78:90, 1974.

16. Jay H.H.: Survey of cases of sympathetic ophthalmia occurring in New York State. *N.Y. J. Med.* 36:85, 1936.
17. Makley T.A., Azar A.: Sympathetic ophthalmia: A long-term follow-up. *Arch. Ophthalmol.* 96:257–262, 1978.
18. Woods A.C.: *Endogenous Inflammations of the Uveal Tract.* Baltimore, Williams & Wilkins Co., 1961.
19. Godfrey W.A., Epstein W.V., O'Connor G.R., et al.: The use of chlorambucil in intractable idiopathic uveitis. *Am. J. Ophthalmol.* 78:415, 1974.

8–1 **Ocular Immunology: Review.**—*Part I.*—W. Bruce Jackson and Norbert J. Gilmore (McGill Univ.) point out that allergic or immunologic mechanisms long have been implicated in a variety of ocular diseases. The organization of the immune system is illustrated in Figure 8–1. The eye has been referred to as a local lymph node, because it forms antibody and responds to antigenic challenge with cell-mediated immune responses. Antigen presumably diffuses into the venous circulation or the conjunctival lymphatics and then is carried to central lymphoid organs. Protective immune reactions may result in severe, even lethal damage to the host. Mast cells are abundant in the conjunctiva, and histamine has been shown to be present in normal tears.

Ocular conditions thought to be mediated by anaphylactic, or type I, hypersensitivity include acute atopic conjunctivitis, or hay fever conjunctivitis, with attacks precipitated most often by pollens, and chronic atopic conjunctivitis, which may result from continued exposure to small amounts of allergen. Reactions to topical ophthalmic medications also can produce type I hypersensitivity reactions. In vernal conjunctivitis, a type I hypersensitivity reaction may be combined with another immune process, probably cutaneous basophil hypersensitivity. Similar immunopathologic features have been observed in giant papillary conjunctivitis. Other type I hypersensitivity reactions include the atopic keratoconjunctivitis associated with atopic dermatitis and parasitic infections such as those caused by *Toxocara canis.*

Acute and chronic atopic reactions respond well to treatments designed to remove or avoid antigen, including desensitization. Vernal conjunctivitis and atopic keratocon-

---

(8–1) Can. J. Ophthalmol. 16:3–9, January 1981.

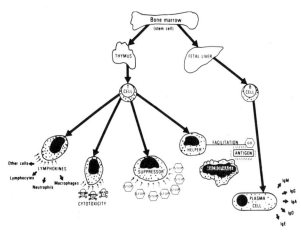

Fig 8–1.—Organization of immune system in human beings. (Courtesy of Jackson, W. B., and Gilmore, N. J.: Can. J. Ophthalmol. 16:3–9, January 1981.)

junctivitis, however, show little response to such management. Topical vasoconstrictors help reduce vascular permeability. Oral antihistamine therapy may be of value in chronic atopic conjunctivitis. Instillation of epinephrine into the conjunctival sac leads to symptomatic improvement in acute atopic attacks. Sodium cromoglycate may be useful prophylactically. Topical and systemic corticosteroid administration may be necessary in the treatment of vernal conjunctivitis and atopic keratoconjunctivitis.

8–2 *Part II.*—Jackson and Gilmore observe that cytotoxic, or type II, hypersensitivity is characterized by the combination of antigens on cell surfaces with IgG or IgM antibodies, resulting in complement activation with cell lysis and in antibody-dependent cell-mediated cytotoxicity. Pemphigus vulgaris, in which ocular lesions are rare, and cicatricial pemphigoid, which affects the mucosae of the mouth and eyes, probably are mediated by type II hypersensitivity reactions. Other conditions in this category include drug-induced ocular pseudopemphigoid and Mooren's ulcer, a chronic, painful corneal ulceration that probably has an autoimmune basis. Immune corneal graft rejection involves

---

(8–2) Can. J. Ophthalmol. 16:59–65, April 1981.

humora (type II) as well as cellular (type IV) mechanisms.

Immune complex disorders, or type III hypersensitivity reactions, involve antigen and antibody, the antigen not being fixed to cell membranes. The complexes may cause platelet aggregation, microthrombus formation, and local ischemia. Scleritis and scleromalacia probably are mediated by type III hypersensitivity reactions. A peripheral corneal gutter or furrow may occur in patients with rheumatoid arthritis. Corneal infiltrates and peripheral catarrhal ulcers associated with staphylococcal blepharoconjunctivitis have been associated with type III hypersensitivity reactions. Uveitis may occur in patients with immune complex diseases such as rheumatic diseases, Wegener's granulomatosis, and Behçet's disease.

Cell-mediated, or type IV, hypersensitivity reactions require sensitized T lymphocytes, which when in contact with a specific antigen may transform into killer cells that attack cell-bound antigens and either cause cell death or release soluble factors that mediate inflammation. Ocular diseases probably mediated by type IV hypersensitivity reactions include contact dermatoconjunctivitis and corneal graft rejection. Phlyctenulosis is considered to be a delayed hypersensitivity response to organisms present elsewhere in the body. A cell-mediated response to herpes simplex virus may be responsible for the stromal infiltration and edema seen in herpetic stromal keratitis. Type IV reactions have a role in many diseases characterized by granulomatous inflammation, such as histoplasmosis, tuberculosis, and sarcoidosis.

8–3 **Iridocyclitis in Black Americans: Association With HLA B8 Suggests an Autoimmune Etiology.** The histocompatibility antigen HLA B27 has been associated with ankylosing spondylitis in whites, and more than half of white Americans with anterior uveitis have been reported to have HLA B27. Robert B. Nussenblatt (Nat'l. Inst. of Health) and Kamal K. Mittal (Food and Drug Administration, Bethesda, Md.) have examined the phenotypic frequencies of HLA antigens in black Americans with recurrent iridocyclitis and no evidence of rheumatologic disease. Forty-two

---

(8–3) Br. J. Ophthalmol. 65:329–332, May 1981.

Comparison of HLA-B8 Positive and Negative Black Americans With Iridocyclitis.

		HLA B8 Positive n=10	HLA B8 Negative n=31
Sex	Male	3	15
	Female	7	16
Visual acuity*	20/20–40	5	7
	20/50–80	3	15
	20/100–LP	2	9
Age at onset	1–20 yr	1	1
	20–40 yr	9	30
Uveitis	Bilateral	10	27
	Uniocular	0	4
	Nongranulomatous	10	23
	Granulomatous	0	8
Disease association	None	0	27
	Sarcoid	0	4

LP = perception of light.
*Best visual acuity in poorer eye.

patients were compared with 129 control blacks. Four patients with iridocyclitis also had a diagnosis of sarcoidosis. The frequency of HLA B8 was increased greatly in the patient group, with a relative risk of 5 to 4. An increased incidence of HLA Aw36 and HLA Bw58 also was observed. The frequency of B27 was nearly identical in the patient and control groups. No patients, but 9% of controls, had HLA B15. No DR antigen was significantly more frequent in the patient group. Female patients predominated among those who were B8 positive. These patients tended to have bilateral, nongranulomatous disease and no systemic disease associations (table).

The HLA B8-associated iridocyclitis seen in black Americans is clearly distinct from the anterior uveitis seen in white Americans in association with B27. This is the first report of an association between B8 and intraocular inflammatory disease. The role that B8 may have in the pathogenesis of autoimmune disease remains unclear. Further studies are needed to better define the immunologic and nonimmunologic characteristics of both B8-associated and nonassociated uveitides.

▶ [The etiology of uveitis is now thought to be primarily autoimmune, and histocompatibility testing has furnished evidence of the association in several types of the disease.] ◀

8-4 **Melanomas of Eye: Stability of Rates** is discussed by Daniel Strickland and John A. H. Lee (Univ. of Washington, Seattle). About 10% of malignant melanomas occur in the eye. Both cutaneous and ocular melanomas are more prevalent in white than in black populations, but ocular melanomas do not exhibit the marked latitude gradient in the United States found for cutaneous melanomas. The incidence of and mortality from cutaneous melanomas are in-

INCIDENCE AND DEATH RATES* FROM TUMORS OF EYE IN PERSONS AGED 15 AND OLDER AS A SURROGATE MEASURE FOR MELANOMAS OF EYE: ANNUAL PERCENT CHANGES IN THESE AND RATES FOR SKIN MELANOMAS

	Mean annual no. of events (standard deviation)	Rates per time period					Annual % change	
							Eye	Skin
		Incidence						
		1950–	1955–	1960–	1965–	1970–74		
Connecticut								
Male	9.0 (1.9)	6.8	11.6	10.1	8.2	8.2	−0.1	+4.2
Female	8.0 (1.8)	9.2	6.8	10.5	6.7	6.8	−1.2	+3.8
		1948–	1953–	1958–	1964–	1968–72		
Denmark								
Male	14.6 (1.9)	13.1	12.7	14.0	16.6	16.7	+1.5	+4.5
Female	11.7 (1.4)	10.0	11.0	11.5	13.7	12.3	+1.2	+5.5
		Mortality						
		1951–	1956–	1961–	1966–	1971–75		
England and Wales								
Male	64.9 (10.3)	3.4	3.6	3.7	3.9	3.9	+0.7	+2.9
Female	70.0 (14.2)	2.8	2.8	2.9	3.1	3.5	+1.1	+2.9
Canada								
Male	20.5 (4.8)				3.6	4.1		+3.5
Female	16.8 (5.0)				2.7	2.9		+3.3
US whites								
Male	151.7 (13.4)	3.6	3.4	3.0	2.8	2.7	−1.5	+3.0
Female	145.6 (12.9)	2.9	2.8	2.4	2.3	2.1	−1.7	+1.9
		1955–	1960–	1965–	1970–	1975–77		
Australia								
Male	11.1 (4.1)	2.8	3.7	3.5	3.3	3.9	+1.1	+2.9
Female	10.8 (3.8)	2.9	2.8	2.3	3.3	2.8	+0.2	+1.8
		1955–	1960–	1965–	1970–	1975–76		
New Zealand								
Male	3.4 (1.4)	4.1	5.3	5.8	4.2	3.9	−0.6	+3.9
Female	2.7 (1.8)	2.8	2.6	3.3	3.5	3.1	+1.0	+2.5
		1956–	1961–	1966–	1971–	1976–78		
Japan								
Male	9.3 (3.6)	0.5	0.4	0.4	0.5	0.5	−0.5	+5.2
Female	10.7 (4.3)	0.5	0.4	0.2	0.4	0.4	−1.8	+5.7

*Rates per million per year age adjusted to the International Union Against Cancer (UICC) standard European population. Annual percent changes are the slopes of lines fitted to period rates divided by the means of the period rates for each population and multiplied by 100. Each of the trends of eye tumor rates is unlikely to be the same as the corresponding skin melanoma trend.

(8–4) Am. J. Epidemiol. 113:700–702, June 1981.

creasing rapidly, for reasons that are not apparent. In contrast, reported rates of ocular melanoma have declined from 1947–1948 to 1969–1971. Ocular tumors at age 15 and older can be used as a surrogate measure for ocular melanomas (table). Incidence and mortality rates for malignant ocular melanoma have changed very little in Europe, North America, Australasia, and Japan, in contrast to the rapid rise in rates for malignant cutaneous melanoma in the same populations. Only small, inconsistent changes in rates for ocular melanoma are observed over time, and no consistent sex pattern is evident.

Whatever is causing the current rise in incidence of malignant melanoma of the skin is not affecting the incidence of ocular melanomas in the same manner. It is not clear whether high socioeconomic status, a major factor in cutaneous melanoma, also influences ocular tumors. The similarity of temporal trends for ocular and cutaneous melanomas in Japan to those in white populations is of interest in view of the low rates for both types of tumor and the large proportion of cutaneous melanomas in Japan that are of the acral lentiginous type.

8–5 **Metastatic Disease From Uveal Melanomas: A Review of Current Concepts With Comments Concerning Future Research and Prevention** is presented by Lorenz E. Zimmerman (Armed Forces Inst. of Pathology, Washington, D.C.). Unless an intraocular melanoma invades the sclera anteriorly, lymphatic spread is highly unlikely. Prompt enucleation of uveal melanomas is reasonable only if preservation of life is considered; however, overall improvement in survival after enucleation leaves much to be desired. Smaller lesions are less likely to be true malignant melanomas and not all small tumors will grow to become large ones. The natural history of uveal melanoma is still not well understood. There is some evidence that enucleation hastens the hematogenous dissemination of uveal melanomas. These tumors are not relatively homogeneous lesions. Some lesions have mitotic activity restricted to relatively small areas (Fig 8–2). Melanomas may not grow exponentially, and the growth rate of metastases may differ

---

(8–5) Trans. Ophthalmol. Soc. U.K. 100(Pt. 1):34–54, April 1980.

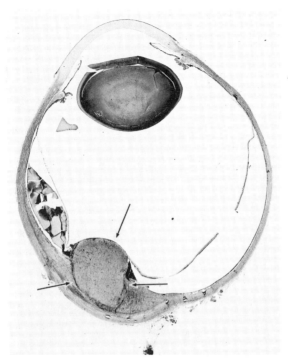

Fig 8–2.—Choroidal melanoma, 13 × 9 × 5 mm, containing a centrally located discrete nodule *(arrows)* that has ruptured Bruch's membrane; reduced from ×8. (Courtesy of Zimmerman, L. E.: Trans. Ophthalmol. Soc. U.K. 100(Pt. 1):34–54, April 1980.)

from that of the primary tumor, and at different metastatic sites.

Because uveal melanomas typically spread long before they become symptomatic, enucleation is not likely to influence overall patient survival. Early treatment should reduce the chance of dissemination. Mortality in the first several postoperative years can be reduced by decreasing preoperative and intraoperative manipulation of the eye and avoiding fluctuations in intraocular pressure. Attempts to improve the prognosis through surgical modifications and radiotherapy should be encouraged. Central registries of well-documented cases of untreated uveal melanoma should be established. A concerted effort is needed to elucidate the natural history of uveal melanoma.

▶ [Zimmerman has stimulated everyone to reevaluate their thinking about uveal melanomas. He has accomplished this primarily by suggesting that enucleation may actually cause metastases and shorten survival. This abstract is of Zimmerman's fine lecture at the Centenary Meeting of the Ophthalmological Society of the United Kingdom. He not only suggests that new techniques for enucleation should be devised, but that the natural history of the tumor is unknown and should be studied. Many ophthalmologists are now waiting for growth of small uveal melanomas before considering enucleation.] ◀

8–6 **Uveal Melanoma in Children and Adolescents.** Charles C. Barr (Univ. of Miami), Ian W. McLean, and Lorenz E. Zimmerman (Armed Forces Inst. of Pathology, Washington, D.C.) reviewed data on 78 patients who were younger than age 20 years at the time of enucleation or excision of a uveal melanoma. The survival rate of patients with choroidal and ciliary body tumors was lower than that of patients with tumors of the iris (Table 1). Thirteen of the 42 patients with melanomas arising from the choroid or ciliary body, or both, died of metastasis a median of 4 years after enucleation. Median follow-up of the surviving patients was 15 years. Both the incidence and mortality of choroidal tumors increased with advancing age. The most significant factors in risk of death from metastatic melanoma were a clinically advanced tumor or a large tumor. Four of 36 patients with tumors of the iris died of metastatic melanoma; the rest were well after a median of 16 years. Increasing tumor size appeared to worsen the outcome in this group as well. All 4 patients who died were

TABLE 1.—ACTUARIAL SURVIVAL OF PATIENTS WITH MALIGNANT MELANOMAS*

Location of Tumor	No. of Cases†	No. of Deaths	% Survival		
			5 yr	10 yr	15 yr
Choroid and ciliary body	51	13‡	79	79	75
Iris	40	4	92	92	87

*Adjusted by exclusion of deaths unrelated to primary tumor.
†Includes 13 cases unavailable for follow-up within first 5 years.
‡Three deaths occurred more than 15 years after enucleation.

TABLE 2.—CELL TYPES IN IRIS AND
CHOROIDAL TUMORS*

	Iris Tumors	Choroidal and Ciliary Body Tumors
Nevus	9	0
Spindle	17	12
Mixed	9	26
Epithelioid and necrotic	1	4
Total	**36**	**42**

*$\chi^2 = 19.5; P = .005.$

among the 14 with invasion to the level of Schlemm's canal or the aqueous veins.

Uveal melanomas in children and adolescents resemble their counterparts in adults, apart from their relative rarity. Pediatric patients in the present series with choroidal and ciliary body melanomas did less well than those with tumors of the iris. The iridic tumors were of a more benign cell type than the choroidal and ciliary body tumors (Table 2). Choroidal tumors more often consisted of mixed, epithelioid, or necrotic cells rather than nevus and spindle cells. In addition, iridic tumors usually were treated when they were much smaller than choroidal tumors because they were more readily recognizable. Treatment of children should not differ significantly from that of adults with uveal melanoma, but prospective trials of enucleation and more conservative measures are needed to determine the best method of treating all patients with uveal melanoma.

▶ [Zimmerman et al. continue to question established thinking about uveal melanomas and press for clinical trials to assess the efficacy of enucleation.] ◀

8–7 **Prognosis in Metastatic Choroidal Melanoma.** Agop Y. Bedikian, Hagob Kantarjian, Sue E. Young, and Gerald P. Bodey (Univ. of Texas, Houston) reviewed the records of 73 patients who were treated in 1973–1979 for primary melanoma of the choroid and ciliary body with metastasis. These patients were among 109 patients seen in this period

---

(8–7) South. Med. J. 74:574–577, May 1981.

with primary ocular melanoma arising in the choroid or ciliary body. The 43 women and 30 men had a median age of 58 years at diagnosis of the primary melanoma. Primary treatment was enucleation in 71 cases. Two patients who had systemic metastases were treated primarily with chemotherapy.

The clinical features at the time of recurrence are shown in the table. Weight loss was the most common symptom. Biopsy confirmation of recurrent melanoma was obtained in 51 cases. The liver was the most common site of metastasis, followed by the bone marrow, lung, and skin. A total of 44 patients had liver metastasis that was diagnosed at the time of tumor recurrence, and in 24 cases the liver was the only organ involved. An elevated lactic dehydrogenase level was the most sensitive indicator of hepatic metastasis. Brain metastasis occurred in 6 patients. Four patients had orbital recurrences, and all of them had distant

Symptoms and Signs at Recurrence of Melanoma

Symptoms	Percentage
Weight loss	65
Abdominal pain	37
Generalized weakness	24
Anorexia	17
Subcutaneous nodules	14
Chest pain	13
Nausea/vomiting	13
Bone pain	11
Fever	3
Other	6
Asymptomatic	11
Signs	
Hepatomegaly	58
Subcutaneous nodules	18
Lymphadenopathy	8
Jaundice	4
Neurologic abnormalities	4
Abdominal masses	3
Others	3
Normal physical examination	17

metastases despite orbital exenteration. The median interval from primary resection to the detection of systemic metastasis was 43.5 months. The median survival from the time of diagnosis of ocular melanoma was 52 months, with a 5-year survival of 43%. Patients younger than age 45 at diagnosis lived longer than older patients. The median survival from the time of development of systemic metastasis was 7 months, with a 1-year survival rate of 29%. Only 7 of 46 patients who had chemoimmunotherapy showed tumor regression, and no complete responses were observed.

Patients with ocular melanoma are at a high risk of recurrence after enucleation, and the prognosis is poor once metastases appear. Chemoimmunotherapy might be beneficial to these patients. Other possible treatments include adjuvant systemic chemotherapy, intrahepatic arterial infusion of antitumor agents, and immunotherapy.

8–8 **Small Malignant Melanoma of the Choroid With Extraocular Extension.** Apparently stationary choroidal melanomas are capable of extensive extraocular extension, and tumor cell dissemination apparently may occur early in the disease. R. Michael Duffin, Bradley R. Straatsma, Robert Y. Foos, and Barry M. Kerman (Univ. of California, Los Angeles) describe a patient with a relatively small intraocular choroidal melanoma but wide extraocular extension and peripapillary invasion.

Woman, 58, had had dense black pigmentation of the right eye since birth and a gradual decline in acuity in the past 3 years. There was a blue nevus on the right side of the forehead, and the skin of the right eyelid was hyperpigmented. Black episcleral pigmentation and a hyperipigmented iris were seen. A dense, 10-degree central scotoma was discovered. A relative flat, yellow-orange, disciform lesion 3.5 mm in greatest dimension extended from the temporal disc margin into the fovea. Subretinal hemorrhage was seen in the macula 3 years later. Five years after presentation, the disciform lesion was about 4.5 mm in diameter and was minimally elevated. Echography, done 2 years later, suggested a subretinal mass about 3.4 mm thick. An increase in lesion thickness to 5.4 mm was observed the next year, with more prominent orbital shadowing, and enucleation was performed.

A prominent extraocular extension was seen in the macular region during enucleation. No disease has been apparent for 2 years

---

(8–8) Arch. Ophthalmol. 99:1827–1830, October 1981.

since operation. An epithelioid-type melanoma was found, with peripapillary scleral infiltration, focal invasion of the juxtalaminar optic nerve, and tumor cells in the subarachnoid space. There was no significant optic nerve invasion. The marked uveal hyperpigmentation was consistent with melanosis oculi.

The incidence of extraocular extension generally increases with the size of choroidal melanomas. Such extension affects the prognosis adversely. Preoperative knowledge of possible extraocular tumor extension is needed by the surgeon. A thorough search for metastasis is an important part of initial evaluation of the patient.

▶ [Reports like these of small tumors extending extraocularly without apparant intraocular growth make judgment about if and when to enucleate extraordinarily difficult.] ◀

First Experiences With Serial Computed Tomography in Choroidal Melanomas are recorded by R. Guthoff, M. Heller, D. Hallermann, and J. Hagemann (Univ. of Hamburg-Eppendorf). Along with sonography, computer tomography is being used in diagnosing soft tissue and osseous orbit pathology as well as intraocular structures. The development of computer tomography led to improved resolving power and significant reduction of scanning time.

Twenty-two patients with intraocular lesions were examined by serial computed tomography after a bolus injection of contrast medium. In 2 patients with a tumor volume under 20 mm, a projecting 1-mm pseudotumor with a volume of 8 mm was found on the initial film but could not be shown with computer tomography. No injection of a contrast medium was given. A projecting 2-mm melanoma was diagnosed on the initial film but showed no measurable increase of density after bolus injection (Fig 8–3). In the group with up to 150-mm tumor volume, changes could be seen on the initial film. In tumors over 150 mm, an increase in density was found in 8 of 9 examinations. The changes in x-ray density of the tumor areas were compared with those of the vitreum and of brain tissue; storage and enhancement of the contrast medium in melanoma were clearly evident.

Evaluation of the serial computed tomograms was sometimes made difficult by three factors: (1) Unless the serial

(8–9) Ophthalmologica 183:154–161, 1981. (Ger.)

Chapter 8–THE UVEA / 215

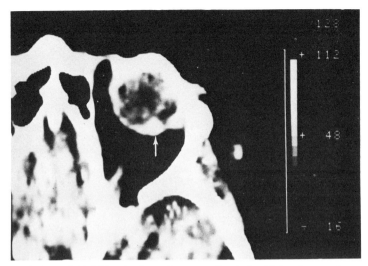

Fig 8–3.—Initial film showing a 2-mm prominent choroidal melanoma. Layer thickness, 2 mm. (Courtesy of Guthoff, R., et al.: Ophthalmologica 183:154–161, 1981.)

pictures are taken in totally identical bulbus position, the tumor will slide within the measuring field and the density–time diagrams will be unreliable. (2) In investigation of small tumors, the partial volume effect obstructs the sharp boundary opposite the vitreum on one side and the bulbus wall and muscle insertion on the other. The density enhancement within the tumor area then cannot be separated clearly from the surrounding structures. (3) A reduced blood supply to the bulbus, caused by increased intraocular pressure, can produce a false negative result.

Based on the authors' first experiences, choroidal melanomas exceeding 2 mm in prominence are identified as highly vascularized areas in which contrast enhancement common to certain brain tumors is seen. Differentiation from large pseudotumors seems to be possible.

–10 **Are Most Iris "Melanomas" Really Nevi? A Clinicopathologic Study of 189 Lesions.** Frederick A. Jakobiec and Glenn Silbert reviewed the findings in 189 cases of iris

(8–10) Arch. Ophthalmol. 99:2117–2132, December 1981.

and ciliary body lesions initially diagnosed as melanomas. The ciliary body was involved in 86 cases and the iris only, in 103 cases. Follow-up clinical data were available in 73% of cases; the mean follow-up was 11 years. The mean patient age was 47 years. There were no black patients in the series. A large majority of patients had asymptomatic lesions.

The pathologic findings are summarized in the table. Cell types could not be correlated with age, sex, the duration or location of lesions, or symptoms. Pupillary distortion and ectropion uveae did not distinguish between benign and malignant lesions. Of 22 patients with a unilateral intraocular pressure elevation, 8 had malignant lesions. Five of 11 patients with ring melanomas of the iris and ciliary body had malignant cytologic findings. The 7 patients with lesions that had a tapioca appearance had predominantly benign cytologic findings. Six of 138 patients followed up had recurrences after local excision. Both benign and malignant lesions in the iris alone and in the iris and ciliary body recurred. Only 12 of 44 patients who initially had enucleation had malignant cytologic findings. Excluding these cases, only 6 of 42 patients with evidence of incomplete excision had recurrences, 3 were associated with lesions having malignant cytologic features.

Patients with iris stromal lesions may be observed for rapid growth; slow growth over many years is compatible

CATEGORIES OF HISTOPATHOLOGIC DIAGNOSES

Lesion Group	Definition	Iris Lesions	Iris and Ciliary Body Lesions	Total(%)
1	Melanocytosis	1	3	4(2)
2	Melanocytoma	5	5	10(5)
3	Epithelioid cell nevus	5	0	5(3)
4	Intrastromal spindle cell nevus	17	25	42(23)
5	Spindle cell nevus with surface plaque	58	16	74(38)
6	Borderline spindle cell nevus	11	19	30(16)
7	Spindle cell melanoma	1	11	12(7)
8	Mixed spindle and epithelioid cell melanoma	3	5	8(4)
9	Epithelioid cell melanoma	2	2	4(2)
Total	...	103	86	189(100)

with a benign progressive nevus. Lesions that involve the iris and ciliary body, especially those producing glaucoma, and lesions with a ring configuration more often have malignant cytologic features and must be watched more closely. However, automatic enucleation in patients with glaucoma is not recommended. If a lesion continues to be worrisome, an excisional biopsy may be performed; extensive lesions require multiple biopsies. An extensive, incompletely excised malignant tumor should be managed by immediate enucleation unless it involves an only eye.

▶ [The treatment of iris melanomas, just like choroidal tumors, is being reevaluated with a more conservative view.] ◀

8–11 **Von Recklinghausen's Neurofibromatosis: Incidence of Iris Hamartomas.** Recent work indicates that iris nodules may be a common and perhaps a pathognomonic feature of neurofibromatosis. The hamartomatous lesions, or Lisch nodules, typically are bilateral dome-shaped, clear to yellow or brown gelatinous elevations on the iris surface (Fig 8–4). Richard Alan Lewis and Vincent M. Riccardi (Baylor College of Medicine, Houston) reviewed the ocular findings in 77 patients from 52 families with a diagnosis of neurofibromatosis. There were 44 female patients with an average age of 20 years and 33 male patients with an average age of 20.6 years.

Lisch nodules were observed in 59 (77%) of the patients and were bilateral in all but 4. Of 61 patients aged 6 years and older, 56 (92%) had Lisch nodules. The number of nodules appeared to increase with advancing age. Iris involvement was observed in 44 (80%) of 55 patients for whom a hereditary pattern of neurofibromatosis was established. No unaffected relatives had Lisch nodules. Presence of nodules could not be correlated with other features of neurofibromatosis apart from age effects. Half of the white patients had choroidal hamartomas, but none of the black patients had such lesions. Two white patients had choroidal lesions without Lisch nodules.

In this series, more than 90% of the patients with neurofibromatosis aged 6 years and older had Lisch nodules on their irides. Lisch nodules seem to be the most common

(8–11) Ophthalmology (Rochester) 88:348–354, April 1981.

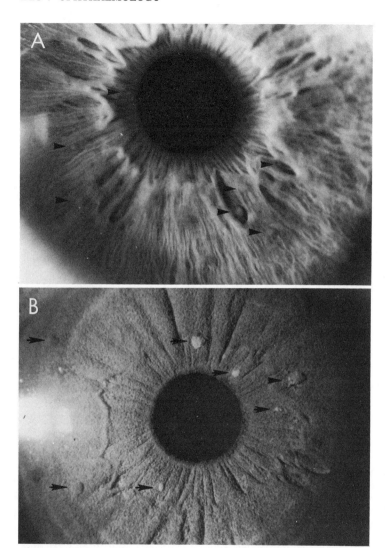

Fig 8–4.—Photographs of the iris of a white woman, aged 29 years (**A**), and of a black woman, aged 32 years (**B**), with neurofibromatosis. Note dome-shaped Lisch nodules *(arrows)* protruding above the iris surface. (Courtesy of Lewis, R. A., and Riccardi, V. M.: Ophthalmology (Rochester) 88:348–354, April 1981.)

clinical evidence of ocular involvement in neurofibromatosis. The finding of Lisch nodules in a patient with café au lait spots only establishes the diagnosis of neurofibromatosis. If an adult relative has no other features of neurofibromatosis, the absence of Lisch nodules indicates that the diagnosis is very unlikely. In possible sporadic cases in postpubertal subjects with café au lait spots only, the finding of Lisch nodules establishes the diagnosis, but their absence does not exclude it.

8-12 **Benign Peripheral Nerve Tumor of the Choroid: Clinicopathologic Correlation and Review of the Literature.** Jerry A. Shields, George E. Sanborn, George H. Kurz, and James J. Augsburger (Thomas Jefferson Univ., Philadelphia) recently encountered a patient diagnosed as having a malignant melanoma of the choroid, but found to have a benign peripheral nerve tumor, presumably a neurilemoma.

Man, 30, gradually developed a "pinwheel of light" in the left eye, and a choroidal tumor was observed. The yellow mass measured about 7×6 mm through its base, was 3.5 mm thick, and extended temporally from the fovea in the left eye. Irregular choroidal vessels were seen in the superficial part of the tumor. The lesion was slightly larger 2 months later. Acuity was diminished after another 3 months, and there was an increase in subretinal fluid and a shallow retinal detachment extending beneath the fovea. The patient refused enucleation and elected to have radiotherapy with a ^{60}Co plaque. The incisional ^{32}P test was borderline positive. At follow-up 6 months later, visual acuity was much reduced in the affected eye, the choroidal tumor was much larger, and extensive serous retinal detachment was present. The patient then consented to enucleation. The prominent choroidal vessels seen at fluorescein angiography were somewhat atypical for choroidal melanoma, but both A-scan and B-scan ultrasonographic studies were highly suggestive of choroidal melanoma.

Examination of the tumor showed spindle cells with long, oval nuclei arranged in fascicles, suggesting the Antoni type A pattern seen with neurilemoma. Deeper parts of the tumor exhibited changes suggestive of the Antoni type B pattern of neurilemoma. Electron microscopic studies failed to show melanin granules. Findings were consistent with those

REPORTS OF SOLITARY UVEAL NERVE SHEATH TUMORS UNASSOCIATED WITH NEUROFIBROMATOSIS

Case	Author(s)	Year	Patient Age	Sex	Tumor Location	Estimated Tumor Size(mm)	Author Diagnosis	Comments
1	Callender & Thigpen	1930	37	F	Ciliary body & choroid	8 · 8 · 5	Neurofibroma	Two solitary tumors in one eye
2	von Papolczy	1932	43	M	Entire globe and orbit		Neurinoma	
3	Freeman	1934	—	—	Choroid		Neurofibroma	
4	Stough	1937	21	M	Choroid	14 · 14 · 10	Neurofibroma	Blind painful eye
5	Trevor - Roper	1944	4	F	Choroid, orbit	20 · 20 · 20	Neurofibroma	
6	Francois	1947	44	F	Choroid	20 · 20 · 20	Schwannoma	Large tumor; no vision
7	Guillaumat & Loisillier	1952	61	F	Choroid	—	Neurilemoma	
8	Donovan	1956	68	F	Ciliary body	10 · 10 · 6	Neurilemoma	
9	Hogan & Zimmerman	1952	—		Ciliary body	10 · 8 · 5		
10	Swan	1964	32	F	Choroid	12 · 12 · 10	Neurilemoma	Acute glaucoma
11	Ferry	1964	—	—	Ciliary body	—	—	—
12	Brewitt et al	1976	44	F	Choroid	7 · 7 · 5	Neurilemoma	
13	Harada et al	1977	33	F	Choroid	12 · 12 · 8	Neurilemoma	Electron microscopy confirmation
14	Packard & Harry	1981	43	F	Choroid		Neurilemoma	Growth documented
15	Shields et al (present case)	1981	30	M	Choroid		Neurilemoma	Present case

of a benign peripheral nerve tumor, and several consultants believed that neurilemoma was the likeliest diagnosis, although a neurofibroma could not be entirely excluded.

Reports of solitary uveal nerve sheath tumors not associated with neurofibromatosis are described in the table. It can be very difficult to distinguish a choroidal neurilemoma clinically from several other choroidal tumors. The ultrasound findings in the present case were identical to those observed with melanomas of comparable size. The ^{32}P test showed an uptake of 91% in this case. These studies and fluorescein angiography probably are of little value in distinguishing a peripheral nerve tumor from an amelanotic melanoma of the posterior uvea. If neurilemoma were suspected, an intraocular needle biopsy could establish the diagnosis.

8–13 **Malignant Metastatic Disease of the Eye: Management of an Uncommon Complication.** Salitha Reddy, Virendra S. Saxena, Frank Hendrickson, and William Deutsch (Chicago) reviewed 24 cases in 1964–1975 of metastatic cancer of the eye; 6 cases involved both eyes. The

(8–13) Cancer 47:810–812, Feb. 15, 1981.

RESPONSE OF SYMPTOMS TO IRRADIATION			
Symptom	Complete response	Partial response	No response
Proptosis	6/9 (66.6%)	3/9 (33.3%)	—
Pain, heaviness	1/4 (25%)	3/4 (75%)	—
Retinal detachment (choroidal metastasis)	4/10 (40%)	4/10 (40%)	2/10 (20%)
Ptosis	1/4 (25%)	1/7 (14%)	5/7 (71%)

average age of the 19 women and 5 men was 68 years. The breast was the primary site of cancer in 17 cases. Ten patients had choroidal metastases, most often at the posterior pole of the eye. Retinal involvement was secondary to choroidal lesions. The other patients most often had proptosis, visual loss, or ptosis. All patients had widespread metastases elsewhere in the body, and most were receiving systemic treatment. All patients received palliative supervoltage radiotherapy for the ocular symptoms.

Ten of 30 affected eyes recovered completely and 11, partially. The average interval from the appearance of symptoms to treatment of the eye was 12½ weeks. Patients with complete responses had been symptomatic less long than the others. Proptosis, pain, and retinal detachment responded significantly to treatment (table). Of 15 eyes that responded and were followed up, all but 1 remained free of symptoms until death. The mean survival from the time of radiotherapy was 6½ months.

The breast was the most common primary site of cancer in this series of patients with ocular metastatic disease. Radiotherapy caused little morbidity, and more than half of the treated eyes responded to a moderately low dose. Irradiation of the anterior chamber was avoided when possible. The patients had limited survival but most of those who responded maintained their response with distinct improvement in the quality of life until they died.

▶ [Because there is essentially no reason to enucleate an eye with metastatic carcinoma, careful ocular diagnosis with extensive systemic workup is essential before considering surgery in the case where ocular diagnosis is uncertain.] ◀

8–14 **In Vivo and In Vitro Measurements of ^{32}P Uptake in Ocular Tissue in Cases of Malignant Melanoma.** J. Wollensak and M. Heinrich (Free Univ. of Berlin) investigated the value of ^{32}P in the diagnosis of intraocular tumors. Forty-eight hours after intravenous injection of 750 µCi of ^{32}P as sodium phosphate, 28 eyes were enucleated. Histologic examination yielded a diagnosis of malignant melanoma of the choroid in 27 cases and an undifferentiated, extremely necrotic epithelial tumor in 1. Because of the small number of cases, only two groups were used for statistical assessment: (1) spindle cell and fascicular melanomas and (2) mixed and epithelioid cell melanomas (with and without necrosis). A higher degree of malignancy was ascribed to group 2. The spindle cell group showed an increased rate of in vivo phosphorus uptake over the tumor areas: 74%–369% (mean value, 228%). The mixed and epithelioid cell group showed corresponding values between 168% and 263% (mean value, 225%). The difference is not statistically significant. The smallest amounts of intravenously injected ^{32}P were found in the vitrous body, lens, sclera, and cornea. The components of the uveal tract showed approximately equivalent levels, and high activities were also found in the retina. As expected, the highest radioactivity was found in tumor tissue. Accordingly, it was possible to calculate the increased ^{32}P uptake in the melanomas as compared with other tissues, particularly the choroid.

The results of both in vivo and in vitro measurements show no correlation between cell type and extent of increased phosphorus uptake in this study. This phosphorus test yields no cell-specific and, consequently, no prognostic data. In vivo measuring procedures involve many uncertainties whereas more precise data on the specific radioactive uptake activity of individual tissue structures can be gained by in vitro measurements.

It should be emphasized that the ^{32}P uptake test does not reflect the degree of malignancy of an individual tumor. Its validity is no greater than that of other examination methods involving less discomfort, such as fluorescence angiog-

---

(8–14) Albrecht Von Graefes Arch. Klin. Exp. Ophthalmol. 217:35–44, 1981.

raphy and ultrasonography. A positive ^{32}P test result can help in the diagnosis of eye conditions but of itself is never enough to justify enucleation.

▶ [There remains debate about the value of the ^{32}P test in uveal melanoma, and further clinical studies seem warranted.] ◀

8–15 **Choroidal Detachment: Clinical Manifestation, Therapy, and Mechanism of Formation.** Choroidal, or ciliochoroidal, detachment (CD) occurs when fluid collects between the uvea and the sclera during or after operation or in association with trauma, local or systemic inflammation, or nanophthalmos. The clinical course is variable. A. Robert Bellows, Leo T. Chylack, Jr., and B. Thomas Hutchinson (Boston) reviewed findings in 112 eyes requiring surgical drainage of a postoperative CD. The indications for drainage of suprachoroidal fluid included a flat anterior chamber with lens-cornea touch for over 12 hours; progressive corneal edema with a shallow or flat anterior chamber; a flat anterior chamber with an inflamed eye and apparent failing bleb; suspected hemorrhagic CD; a persistent wound leak with CD and a flat anterior chamber; and possible concurrent pupillary block. The procedure is illustrated in Figure 8–5.

Seventy-five of the 103 patients studied had had glaucoma filter operations and 22 had had cataract operations alone. Few complications followed posterior sclerotomy for removal of suprachoroidal fluid. Three patients developed sterile hypopyon postoperatively and 1, endophthalmitis. One third of the 75 patients who had had glaucoma operations developed a cataract mature enough to require extraction within 2 years. None of these eyes required further glaucoma surgery, although in some, medical treatment was reinstituted.

When specific indications are present, evacuation of the suprachoroidal space and re-formation of the anterior chamber can restore normal ocular relations and reduce the complications of a flat anterior chamber. There are few operative or postoperative complications. All 4 patients in this series who developed serious inflammation have retained functional vision. Presently an ultrafine filter is used

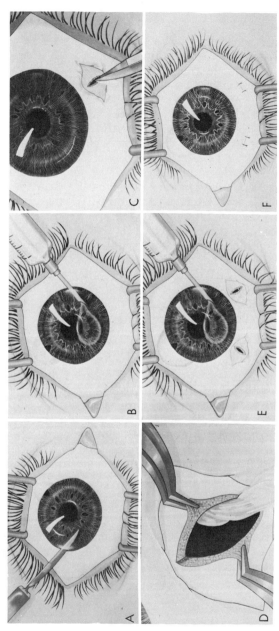

Fig 8–5.—Operative evacuation of suprachoroidal fluid and re-formation of anterior chamber. **A,** clear corneal limbic paracentesis with blade directed toward 6 o'clock meridian. **B,** re-formation of anterior chamber. **C,** circumferential conjunctival incision with radial posterior sclerotomy centered 4 mm from visible limbus. **D,** evacuation of suprachoroidal fluid by lifting, and alternately lifting and depressing scleral wound. **E,** repeated re-formation of anterior chamber with enlarging filtering bleb. Nasal and temporal sclerotomies to enhance more complete drainage. **F,** sclerotomies are not sutured, and conjunctiva is closed with interrupted 10–0 nylon. (Courtesy of Bellows, A. R., et al.: Ophthalmology (Rochester) 88:1107–1115, November 1981.)

whenever solutions are irrigated into the anterior chamber. Whether hypotony or serous effusion occurs first is uncertain, but rapid accumulation of suprachoroidal fluid during operation suggests that hypotony is the initial event.

▶ [The authors suggest that hypotony may be the primary cause of choroidal detachment with fluid collection between the uvea and sclera. Almost all cataract extractions are accompanied by some degree of choroidal detachment, and the longer microscopic intraocular procedures with implants may increase the incidence of complications.] ◀

8–16 **Vitiliginous Chorioretinitis** is characterized by a multifocal pattern of depigmented chorioretinal patches, usually seen in middle-aged or older women. J. Donald M. Gass (Univ. of Miami) reviewed the findings in 8 women and 3 men, aged 42 to 63 years, with this syndrome. They were seen a median of 56 months after onset of the condition. All patients but 1 had floaters in one or both eyes. Four had photopsia also. Most patients considered themselves to be healthy, although 6 had allergies and 3 had skin disease. Two patients developed pigmented white patches on the extremities after the onset of visual symptoms. One patient had 2 children with vitiligo.

All patients but 2 had acuity of 20/40 or better in at least one eye. Only 1 was legally blind at final evaluation. The 5 patients tested with Amsler's grids had some metamorphopsia in one or both eyes. Four of 5 patients had some constriction of the peripheral field. Most patients had evidence of separation and extensive vitreous degeneration in the posterior part of the vitreous cavity. Occasionally inflammation was much more severe in one eye than in the other (Fig 8–6). Yellow-white or faintly orange or pink patches of depigmentation were scattered in the postequatorial part of the fundus. The macular region was relatively spared in all but 2 patients. Six patients had cystoid macular edema. Mild optic disc pallor was present in most patients. Many hypopigmented patches failed to show significant change in the background of choroid fluorescence in the early phase of fluorescein angiography. Electroretinography indicated moderately or severly abnormal rod and cone function in both eyes of all 10 patients examined. Electro-oculograms were generally subnormal.

(8–16) Arch. Ophthalmol. 99:1778–1787, October 1981.

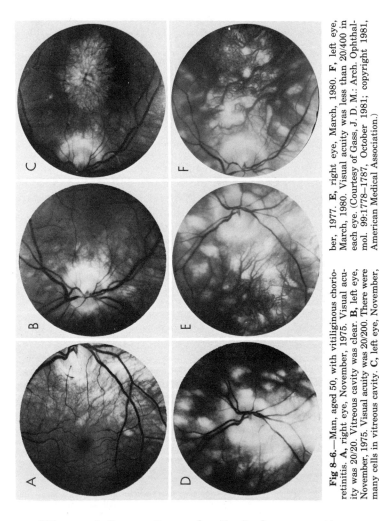

Fig 8-6.—Man, aged 50, with vitiliginous chorioretinitis. **A**, right eye, November, 1975. Visual acuity was 20/20. Vitreous cavity was clear. **B**, left eye, November, 1975. Visual acuity was 20/200. There were many cells in vitreous cavity. **C**, left eye, November, 1975. Cystoid macular edema. **D**, right eye, November, 1977. **E**, right eye, March, 1980. **F**, left eye, March, 1980. Visual acuity was less than 20/400 in each eye. (Courtesy of Gass, J. D. M.: Arch. Ophthalmol. 99:1778–1787, October 1981; copyright 1981, American Medical Association.)

Vitreous inflammation and retinal edema sometimes responded to oral or sub-Tenon corticosteroid administration, but in general the treatment was relatively ineffective. Some features of vitiliginous chorioretinitis are similar to those of Vogt-Koyanagi-Harada disease and sympathetic uveitis.

Chapter 8—THE UVEA / 227

Vitiliginous chorioretinitis may prove to have a cause and pathogenesis similar to those of idiopathic senile vitritis.

8–17 **Choriocapillary Occlusion in Moschcowitz's Disease.** G. Coscas, A. Gaudric, P. Dhermy, J. P. Vernant, and C. Cordonnier (Créteil) report on 2 cases of thrombotic thrombocytopenic purpura, a clinical and biologic entity characterized by a hemolytic anemia, thrombopenia, fever, varied and fluctuating neurologic manifestations, occasionally with renal insufficiency.

The first patient, a woman aged 24, in the 6th month of an uneventful pregnancy, was hospitalized for a petechial purpura and severe anemia in the acute stage, with severe findings including retinal detachment, profound yellow

Fig 8–7.—Angiogram showing alternation of depigmentation and hyperpigmentation in patches of Elschnig spots after the patient's recovery from Moschcowitz's disease. (Courtesy of Coscas, G., et al.: J. Fr. Ophtalmol. 4:101–111, 1981.)

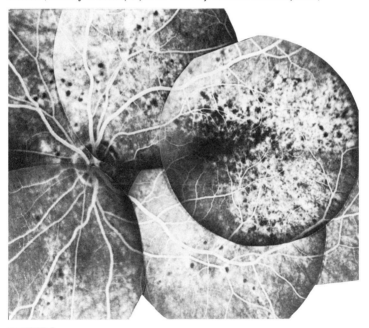

patches and dye leakage in the subretinal space. Histologic examination revealed multiple choriocapillary occlusions and foci of pigmentary epithelial necrosis.

The second patient, a man aged 27, was seen at the sequellar stage, with numerous Elschnig spots well documented by angiography.

These two new cases of choroidal occlusions during the course of Moschcowitz's disease well illustrated the two phases of choriocapillaris occlusion. The acute phase is characterized by severe retinal detachment due to partial necrosis of the pigmentary epithelium opposite the arterioles of the thrombosed choriocapillaris. The retinal detachment occurs due to rupture of the barrier of the pigmentary epithelium that releases the interstitial fluid of the choroid. In the sequellar phase the retina is reattached but the pigmentary epithelium appears abnormal: its continuity is reestablished, but marked by zones of fibrosis, depigmentation, and pigmentary migrations analogous to the patches described by Elschnig during the course of malignant arterial hypertension (Fig 8–7).

▶ [It is surprising that these patients did not have systemic hypertension because the serous detachments of the retina with choriocapillaris occlusive disease rarely occur without an elevation in blood pressure.] ◀

9. Vitrectomy

Treatment of Endophthalmitis

GHOLAM A. PEYMAN, M.D.

Eye and Ear Infirmary, University of Illinois, Chicago

Endophthalmitis is considered one of the worst complications of intraocular surgery and penetrating ocular trauma. The course of the disease depends on the virulence of the organisms' exotoxin and endotoxin. Because of the presence of a blood-retinal barrier, systemic, topical, and subconjunctival administration of antibiotics do not achieve bactericidal levels inside the eye. Thus, the bacteria can grow uninhibited and destroy the delicate ocular structures.

Three large series have reported good results with intravitreal injection of antibiotics to manage endophthalmitis.[1-3] Also to improve the course of the disease, vitrectomy has been advocated. Vitrectomy should work like draining of an abscess in other parts of the body. Endophthalmitis produces severe inflammatory response in the eye with migration of inflammatory cell reactions. Even if the eye survives infection, it is not able to rid itself of cellular debris. The question is when to perform vitrectomy. If endophthalmitis is diagnosed and managed in very early stages, prior to complete opacification of the vitreous, the vitreous may stay clear if the ocular inflammation is halted. To evaluate the timing of vitrectomy, four experimental studies have been performed.[4-7] Using a rabbit model and *Pseudomonas aeruginosa* or staphylococcal epidermidis, Peyman et al.[4] could not demonstrate significant differences between eyes treated with vitrectomy and antibiotics and those treated with simple intravitreal injection. Eyes treated 24 hours after bacterial innoculation were uniformly lost. These findings were reconfirmed using a less virulent organism[5] and *Candida albicans*[6] endophthalmitis. The only significant difference between the intravitreal injection and the vitrectomy groups was the clarity of media. The eyes treated with vitrectomy had clearer media than those treated with intravitreal antibiotic injection. In another study by Cottingham and Forster[7] using rabbits as the experimental model and vitreous culture, more eyes remained culture negative when treated with vitrectomy than those treated with intravitreal injection. The authors did not state if the vitrectomy had an effect on the survival of the eye or the clarity of the media. Unfortunately, most of these studies are inconclusive because the volume of rabbit vitreous is only 1.4 ml. In human beings, in whom the vitreous volume is 4 ml, more inflammatory reaction can be accumulated; therefore, vitrectomy may be able to save eyes that could not be saved by simple intravitreal injection. This issue, however, cannot be resolved by randomized trial, because (1) human endophthalmitis is not a uniform condition produced by a single species of organism, (2) not all endophthalmitis cases are detected within a specified period, and (3) not all cases are treated at the same interval after diagnosis.

We feel that when the ocular media are still clear, a suspected endophthalmitis should be treated with intravitreal injection of antibiotics after vitreous tap for culture has been performed. The technique of intravitreal injection is of great importance to prevent toxicity to the retina. Nontoxic doses of antibiotics should be injected slowly behind the anterior hyaloid membrane. Presence of pus in the vitreous is an indication for vitrectomy. After material for diagnosis has been taken, a nontoxic dose of broad-spectrum antibiotic should be added to the vitrectomy infusion fluid to treat bacterial endophthalmitis. In our hands, the use of intravitreally administered steroids in conjunction with antibiotics has been beneficial in reducing intraocular inflammation.[8]

REFERENCES

1. Peyman G.A., Vastine D.W., Raichand M.: Symposium: Postoperative endophthalmitis: Experimental aspects and their clinical application. *Ophthalmology (Rochester)* 85:374–385, 1978.
2. Forster R.K., Abbott R.L., Gelender H., et al.: Management of infectious endophthalmitis. *Ophthalmology (Rochester)* 87:313–318, 1980.
3. Diamond J.G.: Intraocular management of endophthalmitis: A systematic approach. *Arch. Ophthalmol.* 99:96–99, 1981.
4. Peyman G.A., Paque J., Meisels H.: Postoperative endophthalmitis: A comparison of method for treatment and prophylaxis with gentamicin. *Ophthalmic Surg.* 6:45–55, 1975.
5. Huang K., Peyman G.A., McGetrick J.: Vitrectomy in experimental fungal endophthalmitis: Part I. Fungal infection. *Ophthalmic Surg.* 10:84–86, 1979.
6. McGetrick J.K., Peyman G.A.: Vitrectomy in experimental endophthalmitis: Part II. Bacterial endophthalmitis. *Ophthalmic Surg.* 10:87–92, 1979.
7. Cottingham A.J., Forster R.K.: Vitrectomy in endophthalmitis. *Arch. Ophthalmol.* 94:2078–2081, 1976.
8. Graham R.O., Peyman G.A.: Intravitreal injection of dexamethasone: Treatment of experimentally induced endophthalmitis. *Arch. Ophthalmol.* 92:149–154, 1974.

9–1 **Stability of Pars Plana Vitrectomy Results For Diabetic Retinopathy Complications: A Comparison of 5-Year and 6-Month Postvitrectomy Findings** was made by George W. Blankenship (Univ. of Miami) in 164 diabetic eyes in 152 patients. The mean duration of reduced vision preoperatively was 18 months. More than 60% of eyes had preoperative visual acuities that ranged from hand movements to light perception. Rubeosis iridis was present in 16 eyes. Twenty-one eyes were aphakic, and 35 patients had major opacities. The most common indication for vitrectomy was the presence of dense, nonclearing vitreous cavity hemorrhages. The lens was removed from 94 eyes at the time of vitrectomy, 5 eyes had scleral buckling procedures, and 8 had both lensectomy and scleral buckling. Major vitreous hemorrhage occurred during surgery in 3 eyes, and retinal holes were produced in 31 eyes. Elevated intraocu-

---

(9–1) Arch. Ophthalmol. 99:1009–1012, June 1981.

	VISUAL ACUITIES AFTER VITRECTOMY*				
	6-mo Visual Acuity, No. (%)				
5-yr Visual Acuity	6/6-6/12 (N = 17)	6/15-6/60 (N = 61)	6/90-1/60 (N = 23)	HM-LP* (N = 51)	NLP* (N = 12)
6/6-6/12	13(77)	11(18)	2(9)	0	0
6/15-6/60	4(23)	36(59)	6(26)	1(2)	0
6/90-1/60	0	10(16)	9(39)	1(2)	0
HM-LP*	0	3(5)	0	17(33)	0
NLP*	0	1(2)	6(26)	32(63)	12(100)

*HM indicates hand movements; LP, light perception; and NLP, no light perception.

lar pressure occurred in 38 eyes between follow-up studies, and 32 eyes required steroid therapy.

The course of visual acuity is shown in the table. Stability of or improvement in visual acuity between examinations was characteristic of younger patients with loss of vision for at least 2 years preoperatively because of dense vitreous hemorrhage, who were found at surgery to have attached maculae. Eyes with traction macular detachments tended to have deterioration of vision between follow-up examinations. Only 11 eyes developed rubeosis iridis after the 6-month examination. Nine eyes required cataract extraction during this interval. Most eyes with elevated intraocular pressure at 6 months had normal or low pressures at 5 years. Of 21 eyes with opaque vitreous cavities at 6 months, 15 showed further deterioration at 5 years. Eleven of 14 eyes with macular detachment at 6 months showed further degenerative changes.

General stability of the results of pars plana vitrectomy was shown in this study. More than 80% of eyes with 6/60 or better visual acuity at 6 months continued to have as good or better vision 5 years postoperatively.

▶ [Vitrectomy in eyes with long-standing vitreous cavity hemorrhage has a high rate of long-term success. We do not know if early vitrectomy is more efficacious, with fewer long-term complications, but studies are under way.] ◀

9–2 **Cystoid Macular Edema in Vitreoretinal Traction.** The relation between vitreous traction and cystoid macular

(9–2) Ophthalmic Surg. 12:900–904, December 1981.

edema (CME) remains unclear. J. Reimer Wolter (Univ. of Michigan) reports data on a case of CME associated with definite vitreoretinal traction in a patient with diabetic neovascularization and a preretinal membrane attached to a shrinking vitreous.

Man, 60, with diabetes for about 30 years, developed early proliferative retinopathy in the right eye at age 55, and there was neovascularization arising on the disc. Partial occlusion of the central retinal vein was diagnosed at age 57 years, with a reduction in vision to finger counting at 1 ft. Rubeosis developed a year later, and the eye became blind and painful and was removed. The vitreous was stretched from its base on the pars plana to the optic nerve head and was detached from the rest of the retina. The vitreous remained attached to a posterior preretinal membrane overlying the optic nerve head. This membrane was formed by neovascularization and secondary mesodermal scarring (Fig 9–1), and had firm connections to the retracting vitreous. The foveal retina showed advanced cystoid changes, particularly in the region of pull of the preretinal membrane. The rest of the retina

Fig 9–1.—Vitreous *(v)*, preretinal membrane *(p)*, large cystoid spaces *(c)*, retroretinal serous exudate *(e)*, and fovea *(f)* are seen in membrane formed by neovascularization and secondary mesodermal scarring. Hematoxylin-eosin; ×100. (Courtesy of Wolter, J. R.: Ophthalmic Surg. 12:900–904, December 1981.)

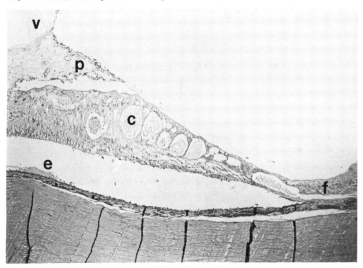

showed atrophy of the inner layers and thickened, hyalinized arteriolar walls. The optic nerve was rather atrophic.

Early vitreous detachment and vitreous retraction were associated with diabetic preretinal neovascularization in this case. Cystoid retinal change appeared to be directly related to the vitreous traction. Cystoid macular edema is largely a nonspecific reaction of the central retina associated with a variety of causes, including traction on the central retina.

▶ [In most cases, however, cystoid macular edema is not related to the vitreous body.] ◀

9–3 **Traction Retinal Detachment: A Cell-Mediated Event.** The chief reason for loss of vision from penetrating injuries of the posterior segment of the eye is development of traction retinal detachment. Jutta H. Ussmann, Elias Lazarides, and Stephen J. Ryan devised an experimental model of traction retinal detachment secondary to posterior penetrating injury in rabbits. A scleral incision through the rabbit pars plana was followed by vitreous prolapse. Prolapsed vitreous was excised and the wound closed microsurgically. Autologous blood then was injected into the vitreous cavity. The eyes were opened at intervals from 3 to 21 days after injury.

Membrane specimens removed 3 and 6 days after injury consisted mainly of condensed vitreous, blood breakdown products, and engorged macrophages. The wound was infiltrated by leukocytes and macrophages. Immunofluorescence tests were negative. Fibroblastic proliferation was evident at 12 days and became progressively prominent, in association with increasingly strong immunofluorescence. Fibrous ingrowth from the wound was prominent at 21 days. Abundant actin filaments were detected within myofibroblasts by immunofluorescence. The highest concentration of intracellular actin correlated with the largest population of myofibroblasts and with the development of traction retinal detachment in the rabbit eye.

Fibroblasts proliferating within the vitreous of the injured rabbit eye contain bundles of intracellular actin filaments, characteristic of myofibroblasts. Increased myofibroblastic proliferation within the vitreous cavity corre-

---

(9–3) Arch. Ophthalmol. 99:869–872, May 1981.

lates temporally with an increase in intracellular actin filaments, and the highest concentration of intracellular contractile protein appears to coincide with the onset of traction retinal detachment. It appears that traction detachment in the rabbit eye is mediated by the contraction of myofibroblast-type cells in a process analogous to wound healing and wound contraction elsewhere.

9–4 **Vitreous Surgery for Macular Pucker.** Patients with visual loss due to localized epiretinal membranes on the macula sometimes can be treated by vitreous surgery. Ronald G. Michels (Johns Hopkins Univ.) reviewed the results of operation in 50 consecutive patients with localized epiretinal membranes. Eyes in which removal of epiretinal tissue would be expected to result in improved vision and in which spontaneous improvement was unlikely were selected for vitreous surgery if the risk of complications was outweighed by the potential visual benefit. The central part of the vitreous gel and the posterior vitreous surface are excised when a posterior vitreous separation is present. All intravitreous opacities are removed from the axial part of the vitreous cavity, and any vitreous sheets causing vitreoretinal traction are divided. Parts of the anterior vitreous gel are spared in phakic eyes.

Fig 9–2 (left).—Idiopathic epiretinal membrane covers macula with linear zone of white opacity *(arrow)* within inner retinal layers. White opacity is probably result of obstruction of axoplasmic flow.

Fig 9–3 (right).—Five months after removal of epiretinal membrane. Linear intraretinal opacity disappeared within 7 days after vitrectomy.

(Courtesy of Michels, R. G.: Am. J. Ophthalmol. 92:628–639, November 1981.)

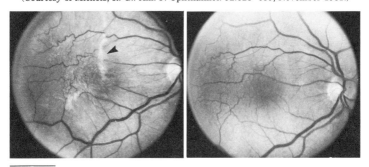

The 34 male and 16 female patients operated on had a median age of 57 years. The epiretinal membrane was present after otherwise successful operations for rhegmatogenous retinal detachment in two thirds of eyes. Visual acuity improved by at least two lines on the Snellen chart in 90% of the eyes that were operated on. A case is illustrated in Figures 9–2 and 9–3. On an average follow-up of 1 year, a sizable amount of epiretinal tissue recurred in 2 cases, but never to the extent present preoperatively. No posterior retinal breaks occurred. Four eyes showed postoperative retinal detachment. Progressive lens opacities occurred postoperatively in 12 of 33 phakic eyes; they were usually nuclear sclerotic changes.

The wrinkled, distorted retina regained a more normal appearance and location within a month after vitreous surgery in these cases. Visual acuity usually improved during this time. Progressive lens opacities were a significant problem, but generally a cataract can be removed successfully. Retinal damage is the most common serious complication, but posterior retinal breaks are infrequent. The low incidence of recurrent macular pucker is encouraging.

9–5 **Pseudo Vitreous Hemorrhage: New Intraoperative Complication of Sodium Hyaluronate** is described by Verinder S. Nirankari, James Karesh, and Vinod Lakhanpal (Univ. of Maryland). Over the past several years, sodium hyaluronate has been used in various intraocular procedures. The major side effect associated with its use has been a transient rise in intraocular pressure in the immediate postoperative period. Earlier reports have attributed this to its viscoelastic nature, resulting in coating and plugging of the trabecular meshwork. Another previously unreported complication is described.

Woman, 77, underwent evaluation for bilateral Fuch's dystrophy and senile cataract OD. She had had extracapsular cataract extraction OS, which was followed by corneal decompensation. Six months later, an 8-mm penetrating keratoplasty with an anterior vitrectomy was performed. A postoperative cystoid macular edema was resolved after 6 months and visual acuity OS is 20/30. Several months after surgery OS, the right cornea developed stromal thickening and epithelial edema with bullous changes. A pene-

(9–5) Ophthalmic. Surg. 12:503–504, July 1981.

trating keratoplasty and an intracapsular lens extraction was performed OD. Considerable bleeding occurred at iridotomy sites, but this was cleared by irrigation. There was considerable bulging of the intact vitreous face after the procedure. Sodium hyaluronate, 0.4 cc, was used to fill the anterior chamber and push the vitreous face back. Postoperative examination the next day showed that the corneal graft was clear and the anterior chamber was deep. However, the pupillary space was completely black with no red reflex visible. Topical and systemic steroids were administered. Over the next 10 days the pupillary space started to clear gradually, and it became evident that the patient had not had a vitreous bleed. Two weeks after surgery, a fundus examination showed clear vitreous without any hemorrhage, retinal tear, or detachment.

Among the sources of bleeding seen after intraocular surgery, expulsive hemorrhage and vitreous hemorrhage are the most serious threats to visual function. The described case showed that, when sodium hyaluronate was used to push the bulging hyaloid face back, the hemorrhage was caught between the intact vitreous and the sodium hyaluronate, and as it clotted it darkened, completely obscuring the posterior segment and mimicking a vitreous hemorrhage. The physical properties of sodium hyaluronate led to this picture of a pseudo vitreous hemorrhage. Although composed of 98% water, sodium hyaluronate is highly viscoelastic. This property makes it extremely useful for reforming the anterior chamber and pushing the anterior hyaloid back. As the use of sodium hyaluronate in intraocular surgery increases, additional complications will be recognized and the surgeon must be aware of them. If a black pupil is observed, the differential diagnosis must include pseudo vitreous hemorrhage.

▶ [The use of sodium hyaluronate is rapidly increasing because it has been shown to help form the anterior chamber and protect the corneal endothelium. As with any new technique, there is still much to be learned about its use. Too much sodium hyaluronate will abnormally expand the posterior chamber, as well as cause transient ocular hypertension. It is hard to distinguish from vitreous, and it may loculate air as well as blood, making visualization difficult.] ◀

10. Retina

Usher's Syndrome

GERALD A. FISHMAN, M.D.

Eye and Ear Infirmary, University of Illinois, Chicago

INTRODUCTION

Usher's syndrome simultaneously combines a congenital, nonprogressive, sensorineural hearing impairment of variable severity with the progressive night blinding disorder retinitis pigmentosa.

Patients afflicted with this double neurosensory impairment require early and accurate diagnosis to receive appropriate guidance for education and better understanding of their disease (with prognosis for visual function), as well as genetic counseling.

The following discussion reviews the pertinent literature on Usher's syndrome and briefly describes current data that support the idea that this syndrome shows clinical and presumed genetic heterogeneity.

The earliest report of the simultaneous occurrence of retinitis pigmentosa and congenital deafness is that of Von Graefe from Berlin in 1858; he found the syndrome in 3 of 5 siblings.[1] While a familial incidence of retinitis pigmentosa and deafness was noted by Liebreich[2] as well, Usher, a British ophthalmologist, was the first in 1914 to emphasize the familial nature of the syndrome and to suggest that it constituted a specific entity.[3] Among 69 unselected patients with retinitis pigmentosa, Usher described 11 with deaf-mutism and an additional 19 patients with "some degree of deafness." Bell,[4] in 1933, found 96 cases of retinitis pigmentosa associated with congenital deafness (variable degree of residual hearing ability with at least some speech facility) or deaf-mutism (profound loss of hearing with unintelligible speech), a prevalence of 10.4% in her total series of 919 cases. Congenital deafness occurred in 22% of cases with autosomal recessive retinitis pigmentosa.

Usher's syndrome is an autosomal recessive disease in which hearing impairment and retinitis pigmentosa represent pleiotropic manifestations of the same gene. There is almost complete penetrance of both traits. The prevalence of the syndrome has been estimated in various countries to be between 1.8 and 3.5 cases per 100,000 in the general population. The prevalence of carriers has been estimated to be between 1/100 to 1/300 persons in the general population. This syndrome is estimated to account for 3% to 6% of congenital deafness and for approximately 50% of those of deaf-blindness.

OCULAR MANIFESTATIONS

Patients with Usher's syndrome characteristically complain of difficulty with night vision, generally within the first or, most frequently, second decade of life. Most will manifest some degree of retinal pigmentary abnormality, which initially consists of nonspecific mottling of the retinal pigment epithelium in a somewhat salt-and-pepper fashion. These alterations are most apparent within the midperipheral retina. Even when pigmentary changes are almost or completely inapparent by ophthalmoscopy, the electroretinogram (ERG) will show amplitude abnormalities of the scotopic (dark-adapted) a- and b-waves. Thus, the ERG should be administered to hearing-impaired children with pigmentary changes of the retina, in whom the diagnosis of auditory and ocular changes (such as rubella) cannot be determined with certainty. In time, most patients will show migration of retinal pigment in the form of a bone spicule-like pigmentation. Retinal vessels ultimately become attenuated, followed by a waxy-appearing atrophy of the optic discs. Fishman and co-workers[5] noted that approximately 44% of patients will show a lesion within the fovea that varies from an atrophic change (29%) to cystoid macular edema (13%). Some degree of posterior subcapsular lens opacity is apparent in most patients by age 45.

Although ERG changes are apparent early in the disease course, initial results of visual field testing may be normal in some patients. Most frequently, midperipheral or partial ring scotomas are apparent. In time, most patients experience a marked depression in peripheral visual fields. The ERG cone and rod responses become progressively diminished, and ultimately nondetectable, as the problems with night vision and peripheral vision become progressively more severe. Fishman and co-workers[5] noted that visual acuity can vary greatly. Most patients retain vision of 20/60 or better until their mid-30s. Although frequently similar, the ophthalmoscopic features (pertaining to extent of pigmentary changes), as well as degree of visual impairment (visual field and central acuity loss), may vary within a given family.

HEARING IMPAIRMENT

The hearing impairment in Usher's syndrome is of the cochlear type. It is bilateral, nonprogressive, and often has a mild to moderate preservation of the low frequencies (from 125 to 500 Hz). Although the hearing loss is congenital, it may not be recognized until the patient is aged 1 or 2 years. Most frequently, the impairment is severe or moderately severe. In some pedigrees, affected members will show a profound deafness and mutism, whereas in others, members will manifest considerably less hearing loss and have surprisingly good speech facilities. Nonetheless, the level and pattern of hearing impairment tend to exhibit a significant positive family correlation. Pedigrees with, as well as those without, profound hearing impairment with deaf-mutism are, to me, acceptable for classification within the rubric "Usher's syndrome," since both types of patients were described among Usher's original 30 unknown deaf patients with retinitis pigmentosa.

Vestibular System Abnormalities

Unresponsiveness or marked hypoactivity of the vestibular organ occurs in patients with Usher's syndrome who manifest profound hearing impairment in association with deaf-mutism. This defect of the vestibular system may be accompanied by disturbances of balance, including an ataxic gait. This occurred in a high percentage (87.6%) of the 177 Usher's syndrome patients described by Hallgren.[6] His study was biased, however, by an underrepresentation of affected persons with ability to hear words, because his cases were culled from schools for the deaf.

As with hearing impairment, there is a familial similarity with respect to the normal or abnormal findings on vestibular testing.[7] In our experience, families in which deaf-mutism is not apparent show normal sensitivity of vestibular function to caloric stimulation, which is in contrast to the marked abnormality in sensitivity in families with deaf-mutism.

Mental Retardation, Psychosis

Usher's syndrome has been reported in association with both psychosis (most frequently of the schizophrenic variety) and mental retardation.[8] Mental deficiency occurred in 22% of Hallgren's[6] series, a remarkably high prevalence possibly reflecting a bias of ascertainment. Hallgren thought that the psychotic behavior, which in 16% of the cases was schizophrenic-like, was related to the double neurosensory deprivation and was not genetically determined. Mental deficiency was noted in 41 of the 172 affected patients (24%) described by Hallgren. He thought that this deficiency was possibly a manifestation of the gene for Usher's syndrome. Hallgren's findings contrast with the 133 cases of Usher's syndrome reported by Nuutila,[9] in which psychotic disturbances were not apparent in a great majority of deaf-blind patients. Further, Nuutila felt that mental deficiency should not be included among the pleiotropic effects of Usher's syndrome. My experience leads to a similar conclusion.

HETEROGENEITY

Genetic heterogeneity provides one possible explanation for the clinical variation observed in patients with Usher's syndrome. Possibly, mutations of different genes or different mutations of the same gene may result in phenotypes that are all classified as Usher's syndrome because they cannot, as yet, be clearly distinguished from one another by genetic or biochemical criteria. In my experience, distinct differences in clinical expressivity provide indirect evidence for at least two genetically different forms of Usher's syndrome. These distinct differences in clinical expressivity also have been noted by other investigators. Merin and co-workers[10] described four clinical types of Usher's syndrome based on their studies of 35 patients with Usher's syndrome from 20 families. Nuutila[9] similarly noted differences in clinical expressivity among patients with Usher's syndrome. In one group (92% of patients), symptoms of pigmentary retinal dystrophy (nyctalopia and poor peripheral vision) were apparent prior to age 10. These patients tended to have profound hearing impairment and disturbances of vestibular function. In a second group (8%), symptoms of retinal dystrophy began after age 20. Hearing was less impaired than in the first group. Patients were able to understand speech, at least to some extent. Davenport and Omenn[11] similarly separated different types of Usher's patients on the basis of onset of nyctalopia and severity of hearing impairment. Fishman and co-workers[12] have completed otologic and ophthalmic investigations on 70 patients with Usher's syndrome. Two distinct types of clinical expressivity were apparent. Twenty-four patients (type I) showed a profound hearing impairment with mutism, a vestibular system nonresponsive or markedly hypoactive to caloric stimulation, and onset of nyctalopia within the first or beginning of the second decade of life. Ataxic-mobility was only occasionally seen, while all patients showed a marked impairment in peripheral visual field. Forty-six (type II) showed variable degrees of hearing impairment that varied from moderate to occasionally severe. All had intelligible speech and showed normal vestibular sensitivity to caloric stimulation. None showed an ataxic gait. Symptoms of nyctalopia generally became apparent first in the latter part of the second decade or the beginning of the third decade of life. Visual field loss varied from no peripheral field loss to marked loss similar to patients within type I. As a group, patients with type II had a lesser degree of peripheral field impairment than patients with type I Usher's syndrome. Further, ERG responses were nondetectable in patients with type I, whereas patients with type II frequently showed residual cone responses and infrequently showed rod responses. Of note, we were unable to discern any differences in central visual acuity loss between types I and II. In both groups, most eyes tended to maintain vision of 20/80 or better until about age 40.

Of the 24 patients with type I Usher's syndrome, four families (9 patients) had 2 or more siblings who were affected. All showed the same degree of ocular, cochlear, and vestibular impairment. In the 46 patients with type II Usher's syndrome, seven families (16 patients) had 2 or more affected siblings. In these patients, severity of ocular and hearing impairment was generally quite similar within the same family, although in some instances the level of hearing impairment and the extent of peripheral field loss showed significant intrafamilial variability. Nevertheless, all members showed normal vestibular sensitivity to caloric testing, even when hearing impairment was occasionally marked in severity.

This review of an important cause of deaf-blindness in our society is intended to rekindle the interest and acumen of the ophthalmic practitioner. Although most patients with Usher's syndrome ultimately experience significant visual impairment, the visual course is not uniformly bleak in all instances. Nevertheless, when, or perhaps before, significant visual impairment becomes apparent, appropriate counseling for future vocational and educational needs is mandatory. Decisive evidence for genetic heterogeneity will await the finding of definitive biochemical or other pathophysiologic differences between types I and II. Nevertheless, compelling differences in the clinical heterogeneity of expressivity strongly suggest genetic heterogeneity within Usher's syndrome, which has important implications for genetic counseling of deaf-blind couples.

REFERENCES

1. von Graefe A.: Exceptionelles verhalten des gesichtsfeldes bei pigmententartung der netshaut. *Albrecht Von Graefe's Arch. Klin. Exp. Ophthalmol.* 4:250, 1858.
2. Liebreich R.: Abkunft aus ehen unter blutsverwandten als grund von retinitis pigmentosa. *Dtsch. Klin.* 13:53, 1861.
3. Usher C.H.: On the inheritance of retinitis pigmentosa, with notes of cases. *R. Lond. Ophthalmol. Hosp. Rep.* 19:130, 1914.
4. Bell J.: Retinitis pigmentosa and allied diseases, in *The Treasury of Human Inheritance*. London, Cambridge University Press, 1933, vol. 2.
5. Fishman G.A., Vasquez V., Fishman M., et al.: Visual loss and foveal lesions in Usher's syndrome. *Br. J. Ophthalmol.* 63:484, 1979.
6. Hallgren B.: Retinitis pigmentosa combined with congenital deafness; with vestibulocerebellar ataxia and mental abnormality in a proportion of cases: A clinical and geneticostatistical study. *Acta Psychiatr. Scand.* [Suppl.] 138:5, 1959.
7. DeHaas E.B.H., Van Lith G.H-M., Rijnders J., et al.: Usher's syndrome: With special reference to heterozygous manifestations. *Doc. Ophthalmol.* 28:166, 1970.
8. Vernon M.: Usher's syndrome: Deafness and progressive blindness: Clinical cases, prevention, theory, and literature survey. *J. Chronic Dis.* 22:133, 1969.
9. Nuutila A.: Dystrophia retinae pigmentosa-dysacusis syndrome (DRD): A study of the Usher or Hallgren syndrome. *J. Genet. Hum.* 18:57, 1970.
10. Merin S., Abraham F.A., Auerbach E.: Usher's and Hallgren's syndromes. *Acta Genet. Med. Gemellol. (Roma)* 23:49, 1974.
11. Davenport S.L.H., Omenn G.S.: *The Heterogeneity of Usher Syndrome*, publication 426. Excerpta Medica Foundation, International Congress Series, abstract 215, 1977, pp. 87–88.
12. Fishman G.A., Kumar A., Joseph M.: Unpublished data, 1982.

▶ ↓ Following are four articles in which authorities discuss diabetic retinopathy. There are several salient points. The most important may be that a great number of nonophthalmologists are unaware of the efficacy of panretinal photocoagulation and that many are not very good at evaluating the retinopathy in the first place. Another general point is that while there are a number of very reasonably sounding theories for the pathogenesis of the disease, there is no hard evidence proving any of them. Finally, and disturbingly, while the essentially destructive techniques of photocoagulation and vitrectomy are helpful, the disease remains a major cause of blindness. Clinical trials of burning and cutting will not solve the problem until basic research has discovered the cause and treatment of the disease. ◀

10–1 **Diabetic Retinopathy, Present and Future,** is discussed by George W. Blankenship (Univ. of Miami). Previous criticisms about deficiencies in the criteria for diagnosis of diabetes mellitus are not applicable to reports given by experienced ophthalmologists who selected the patients from their practices. The increasing occurrence of retinopathy from 50% at 7 years to 90% at 17 years emphasizes the importance of detailed examinations and photography in patients with juvenile-onset diabetes. The 26% incidence of proliferative diabetic retinopathy (PDR) at 26 years, with its associated risk of blindness, further stresses the importance of periodic examinations. The findings show background diabetic retinopathy is slowly progressive without a serious threat of catastrophic visual loss, but advanced PDR is much more serious, and when associated with severe vitreous hemorrhage and traction, retinal detachment often progresses to blindness. Increasing laboratory data and clinical observations support a strong and direct relationship between good diabetic control and minimum retinopathy. Metabolic and biochemical changes start with hyperglycemia stimulating alterations of plasma proteins, causing red blood cell and platelet aggregation and capillary basement membrane thickening. This produces reduced capillary perfusion with retinal ischemia and results in diabetic retinopathy.

Almost all of the recent theories on the development of diabetic retinopathy have been based on retinal ischemia. Fluorescein angiography has confirmed capillary obstruction as an important component of diabetic retinopathy and allows identification of the ischemic areas. The findings of the National Eye Institute's Collaborative Diabetic Retinopathy Study identified several fundus changes that progressed to severe loss of vision when not treated with panretinal photocoagulation.

Pars plana vitrectomy is becoming the standard operative procedure for advanced complications of diabetic retinopathy. As a result of this surgery, substantial improvement of visual acuity has been reported.

Because of the increasing number of known diabetics and

(10–1) Ophthalmology (Rochester) 88:658–661, July 1981.

improvements in research capabilities, there will be significant improvements in general diabetic care. Miniature insulin infusion pumps are rapidly becoming used, and pancreas transplantations are being performed. The Diabetic Retinopathy Vitrectomy Study is evaluating the role of pars plana vitrectomy in diabetes and will establish whether it is better to perform the surgery shortly after the onset of vitreous hemorrhaging or to defer vitrectomy for a year. The Early Treatment Diabetic Retinopathy Study is evaluating the role of laser photocoagulation and aspirin therapy. The most promising basic science research presently being performed is the isolation and identification of vasoformative and vasosuppressive factors from the ischemic retina and vitreous. This work will markedly increase our understanding of the disease process and improve our ability to treat this problem and reduce the loss of vision in diabetic patients.

10–2 **Recent Advances in Diabetic Retinopathy** are reviewed by Lawrence I. Rand (Joslin Clinic). Photocoagulation has provided the only effective treatment of diabetic retinopathy to date. "Scatter" panretinal treatment with the argon laser, avoiding the macula and other vital structures (Fig 10–1), is followed by focal treatment of new vessels. There is impressive evidence that photocoagulation both prevents severe visual loss and slows the progress of retinopathy. It may act by destroying hypoxic retina that produces a vasoproliferative substance or by permitting the choroid to supply a greater proportion of retinal metabolic needs. Vitreous surgery is another major advance in the management of diabetic retinopathy, but it is risky and should be cautiously applied. Hypophysectomy carries an unfavorable risk-benefit ratio. No medical treatment, except perhaps insulin, has been shown to improve the course of diabetic retinopathy. Medical means may be devised to alter the metabolism of retina and choroid, replacing photocoagulation. Should sorbital accumulation in retinal cells prove to be involved, aldose reductase inhibitors might be useful.

The pathogenesis of microvascular changes in diabetic

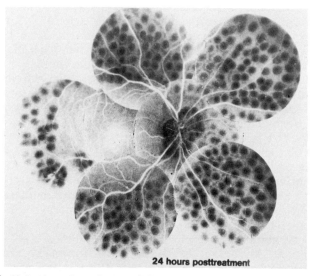

Fig 10–1.—Argon laser photocoagulation according to Diabetic Retinopathy Study protocol. Photograph from Department of Ophthalmology, University of Wisconsin, Madison. (Courtesy of Rand, L. I.: Am. J. Med. 70:595–602, March 1981.)

retinopathy is unclear, but the retinal capillary or precapillary endothelial cell is a logical target. Osmotic mechanisms may be implicated in endothelial cell damage. Vitreous fluorophotometry may prove to be useful in assessment of various diabetic interventions by demonstrating normalization of vitreous fluorescein leakage. If a predisposition to increased flow through radial peripapillary capillary beds is important, their closure by glaucoma or other means could be therapeutic. No specific angiogenic substance has been identified, but recent attempts appear to be promising. A multifactorial risk factor study is being conducted at the Joslin Clinic. The degree of retinopathy may be closely related to survival in diabetes, strengthening the role of retinopathy as an index of microvascular status.

10–3 **Serious Retinopathy in Diabetic Clinic: Prevalence and Therapeutic Implications.** Diabetic retinopathy is the

(10–3) Lancet 2:520–521, Sept. 5, 1981.

most common cause of blindness in persons aged 50–64 years in England and Wales, but photocoagulation now is used effectively to treat diabetic maculopathy and new vessel formation. I. N. Scobie, A. C. MacCuish, T. Barrie, F.D. Green, and W. S. Foulds (Glasgow) reviewed the findings in 1,000 patients evaluated consecutively at a large diabetes clinic. The optic fundi were examined at least once a year by observers trained in identifying diabetic eye disease. Insulin was being used by 36% of the sample, and 35% took oral hypoglycemic agents.

Evidence of diabetic retinopathy was obtained in 26.7% of patients, and a similar proportion had nondiabetic types of eye disease. Serious diabetic retinopathy was seen in 9.5% of patients, with exudative retinopathy in or near the macula in 38, proliferative retinopathy in 38, and signs of retinal ischemia in 19. Most of the patients with proliferative retinopathy, and all of those with ischemic changes, were asymptomatic at the time of study. About half of the patients with serious diabetic eye disease underwent laser photocoagulation.

Serious diabetic retinopathy is relatively frequent in the population attending a large diabetic clinic. The condition may be nearly asymptomatic in a significant number of individuals, making regular examination of the fundi in all diabetics necessary. Special training in ophthalmoscopy is necessary for physicians who screen diabetics for retinopathy. The average time needed for ophthalmic evaluation in this study was 20 minutes, and 40 minutes when fluorescein angiography was added.

Visual Outcome in Moderate and Severe Proliferative Diabetic Retinopathy. Photocoagulation has prevented severe visual loss in eyes with advanced background or early proliferative retinopathy, but those with moderate or severe proliferative diabetic retinopathy (PDR) have not responded as well to modern treatment methods. Rand Spencer, J. Wallace McMeel, and Edward P. Franks reviewed findings in 400 eyes affected by moderate or severe PDR in 330 patients who initially had good vision. Follow-up was made of 103 eyes for 6–23 months, and of

297 eyes for 24–196 months; mean follow-up was 44.3 months.

Initial visual acuities ranged from 20/15 to 20/100. All eyes were managed by conventional methods used before 1977. Twenty-nine of 103 eyes in the shorter follow-up group lost acuity to 5/200. The cause was traction retinal detachment of the macula in half of these patients, and severe vitreous hemorrhage alone in most of the rest. The overall rate of severe visual loss was 35%. Of 286 eyes with an initial acuity of 20/40 or better, 28% declined to an acuity of less than 5/200. The rate of loss for 114 eyes with an initial acuity of 20/50 to 20/100 was 51%.

Severe visual loss was observed in about one third of eyes in this series with moderate or severe PDR and initially good vision, over a mean follow-up of about 3½ years. Conventional management by observation, photocoagulation, or pituitary ablation is suggested for eyes with only flat neovascularization, no evidence of traction retinal detachment, and excellent visual acuity. Eyes with PDR should be evaluated at least every 2–3 months. Vitreous surgery should be considered as an adjunct to conventional management in eyes with decreasing visual acuity or traction retinal detachment. Changes in acuity over time are important prognostic indicators in eyes with moderate or severe PDR.

10–5 **Unilateral Proliferative Diabetic Retinopathy: II. Clinical Course.** Unilateral proliferative diabetic retinopathy (PDR) is common in patients with nonproliferative diabetic retinopathy (NPDR) in the fellow eye. James A. Valone, Jr., J. Wallace McMeel, and Edward P. Franks (Boston) report the findings in 136 patients who had PDR in one eye and NPDR in the other and were followed up for 3 months or longer. Eleven eyes were treated for only 3 months, and follow-up was interrupted by treatment in 47 others. Average follow-up was 34.5 months.

In 58% of the eyes, PDR developed during follow-up, in an average of 24 months; in 42% NPDR remained during follow-up for an average of 26 months. Sixty-four percent of patients who developed bilateral proliferative disease did so within the first 2 years of follow-up. Proliferative changes developed significantly more often in diabetics younger than age 40 years than in those older than age 60. Poor visual prognosis in eyes that initially had NPDR was associated with advanced angiopathy or exudation on initial examination. Neither the development of PDR nor the final visual acuity could be correlated with vascular disease outside the eye, degree of PDR in the fellow eye, or presence of higher intraocular pressure in the eye with NPDR initially.

Over half the eyes with initial NPDR in this series developed changes of proliferative diabetic retinopathy, usually in the first 2 years of follow-up. Relatively young age was associated with a poorer prognosis, as were advanced angiopathy and exudation on initial assessment. The findings support the view that diabetic retinopathy tends to become symmetric, and that the better eye follows the course of the poorer eye. In the present study, increased intraocular pressure did not prevent the development of PDR or visual loss. Thus, the role of asymmetric intraocular pressure may be less important than was previously thought.

▶ [Blinding proliferative retinopathy eventually is bilateral. This sad fact does make it possible to carry out clinical trials using the patient as his own control, but the implications for the younger patient are dreadfully serious.] ◀

10–6 **Clinical Correlation Between Rubeosis Iridis and Optic Disc Neovascularization.** M. Bonnet, M. Jourdain, and N. Francoz-Taillanter (Lyons) reviewed clinical findings and fluorescein angiograms of 293 eyes affected by proliferative diabetic retinopathy, with specific focus on a possible correlation between rubeosis iridis and localization of the new vessels in the ocular fundus. Rubeosis iridis was present in 49% of eyes with optic disc neovascularization (Fig 10–2), compared to 5.5% of eyes afflicted with proliferative retinopathy not associated with new vascular formations in the optic disc. Among the 97 eyes affected by rubeosis iridis, 91 (93.8%) were found to have optic disc neovascularization.

The significant correlation found between rubeosis iridis

(10–6) J. Fr. Ophtalmol. 4:405–410, 1981. (Fr.)

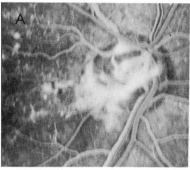 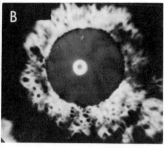

Fig 10–2.—Neovascularization of rubeosis iridis. **A,** fluorescein angiogram of optic disc. **B,** fluorescein angiogram of iris. (Courtesy of Bonnet, M., et al.: J. Fr. Ophtalmol. 4:405–410, 1981.)

and optic disc neovascularization in diabetic retinopathy has both practical and theoretic importance. It permits recognition of high risk for developing rubeosis iridis in eyes affected by proliferative diabetic retinopathy, and on the theoretic level it supports the hypothesis that the new vessels of rubeosis iridis may be a consequence of uveal hypoxia associated with retinal hypoxia.

▶ [Another hypoxia theory is not very helpful, but it is of interest that panretinal photocoagulation is of proved value for optic disc neovascularization and appears helpful for rubeosis iridis.] ◀

10–7 **Efficacy of Argon Laser Photocoagulation in the Treatment of Circinate Diabetic Retinopathy.** Frederick Reeser, Jay Fleischman, George A. Williams, and Arnold Goldman (Med. College of Wisconsin, Milwaukee) have evaluated argon laser photocoagulation in a series of 115 eyes of 105 diabetic patients exhibiting circinate deposits that involved or threatened the macula. The circinate rings consisted of hard intraretinal exudates encompassing at least 300 degrees. None of the eyes showed proliferative retinopathy initially. Sixty-eight eyes of 61 patients had argon laser photocoagulation to leaking vessels, primarily in the center of the circinate ring. Follow-up averaged 2.4 years. Average age at treatment was 58 years. Twenty patients

CLINICAL RESULTS OF ARGON LASER PHOTOCOAGULATION IN TREATING CIRCINATE DIABETIC RETINOPATHY

Years Followed and Treatment Group	No. of Eyes	Visual Acuity Improved		Visual Acuity Stabilized		Worse		Circinate Resolved	
		No.	%	No.	%	No.	%	No.	%
One year									
Treated	68	10	15	47	69	11	16	51	75
Untreated	47	0	—	26	55	21	45	5	11
Two years									
Treated	45	8	18	27	60	10	22	37	82
Untreated	23	0	—	14	61	2	39	3	13
Three years									
Treated	24	5	21	11	46	8	33	23	96
Untreated	10	0	—	3	30	7	70	2	20

had more than one laser treatment. In bilateral cases, the poorer eye was treated whenever possible. Follow-up of the untreated group, having an average age of 59 years, averaged 2.6 years.

Visual acuity had improved at 1-year follow-up examination in 15% of treated eyes and had worsened in 16% (table). In none of the untreated eyes was acuity improved, and in 45% it became worse. At 3 years, acuity had improved in 21% of treated eyes and worsened in 33%, but none of 10 untreated eyes had improved and 70% had become worse. Macular edema resolved minimally after photocoagulation. Circinate deposits nearly always resolved in treated patients, but small deposits of exudates often remained in the fovea. The response to treatment could not be related to age or sex, but an initial acuity of 6/18 or better was predictive of a better outcome.

It is believed that photocoagulation to the center of the circinate ring improves the visual course of diabetics with circinate retinopathy for at least 3 years. Macular edema rarely is completely eliminated, apparently because of microaneurysmal leakage close to the fovea. Diabetic circinate retinopathy should be treated before irreversible structural damage takes place.

▶ [Macular edema, believed to be due to retinal capillary leakage, has been thought by some to have a submacular choroidal component. This might account for its relative resistance to parafoveal photocoagulation.] ◀

10–8 **Coagulation Therapy of Proliferative Diabetic Retinopathy in Juveniles** was investigated by E. Gerke and G. Meyer-Schwickerath (Univ. of Essen). Sixteen male and 35 female selected juvenile diabetics (diabetes before the age of 12 and proliferative retinopathy before the age of 25) were treated over a 3-year period. The median age at time of diagnosis was 6.9 ± 3.4 years (minimum 2 months, maximum 12 years) and median age at appearance of proliferative retinopathy was 22.6 ± 2.3 (minimum 16, maximum 25 years). The varied degrees of the disease were classified as follows: type I, only peripheral proliferation; type II, papillary proliferation; type III, peripheral proliferation with epiretinal or intravitreal hemorrhages; type IV, papillary proliferation with or without peripheral proliferation with epiretinal or intravitreal hemorrhages. Of the 81 eyes, 31 were type I, 20 type II, 9 type III, and 21 type IV. After 3 years, the eyes with traction ablatio were assigned to types III and IV. The coagulation therapy was performed with xenon photocoagulation in 77%, with the argon laser in 3%, with diathermy in 13%, and with cryocoagulation in 7% of the patients. Within the 3-year period, each eye received an average of 2.6 coagulation treatments, of which 2.2 were administered the first year, 0.3 the second, and 0.1 the third. Results of therapy on both fundus disease and visual acuity are highly dependent on the morphological aspect of the fundus at the beginning of coagulation. Eyes with peripheral neovascularizations alone have no more neovascularizations in 65% after 3 years and eyes with papillary neovascularizations, only 20%. Vitreous hemorrhage further reduces this percentage. Blindness after 3 years is rare in eyes with peripheral neovascularizations alone (3%), but 52% of eyes with papillary neovascularizations and vitreous hemorrhage are blind after 3 years.

Coagulation therapy should be considered at the first sign of proliferative retinopathy in juvenile diabetics. A one-time coagulation treatment is rarely enough to arrest the disease.

▶ [Optic disc neovascularization does imply a more serious general retinal problem than focal retinal areas of new blood vessels. Nonetheless,

---

(10–8) Klin. Monatsbl. Augenheilkd. 179:157–160, September 1981. (Ger.)

10-9 **Advances in Treating Cystoid Macular Edema** are discussed by Andrew K. Vine. In cystoid macular edema (CME), intercellular fluid accumulates in perifoveal cystic spaces, mainly in the outer molecular and inner nuclear layers. It is best diagnosed by contact lens biomicroscopy of the macula. Presence of CME has been demonstrated by fluorescein angiography in 54% of cases of uncomplicated cataract extraction. Usually it results from a localized perifoveal breakdown of the inner blood-retinal barrier. Breakdown of the outer blood-retinal barrier is responsible in a minority of cases where the retinal pigment epithelium is incompetent. The specific causes of CME are listed in the table. Diagnosis can be confirmed by fluorescein angiography, which shows dilated, leaking perifoveal capillaries and, later, intraretinal cystic accumulation of fluorescein. When the outer retinal barrier has broken down, increasing leakage of dye is seen from the choriocapillaris into and often beneath the retina.

Treatment is aimed at the primary disease. Vitrectomy

CAUSES OF CYSTOID MACULAR EDEMA	
General	Specific
Ophthalmic surgery	Cataract extraction (Irvine-Gass syndrome); retinal reattachment; penetrating keratoplasty; filtering procedures; vitrectomy; photocoagulation; cryotherapy
Retinal vascular diseases	Diabetic retinopathy; hypertensive retinopathy; central retinal vein occlusion; branch vein occlusion; papillophlebitis; retinal telangiectasis; subretinal neovascularization; retinal macroaneurysms; radiation retinopathy; syphilitic retinitis
Inflammation	Pars planitis; posterior uveitis; vitritis; chorioretinitis; papillitis
Drugs	Epinephrine; nicotinic acid; griseofulvin
Dystrophies	Retinitis pigmentosa; dominant cystoid macular edema
Ocular tumors	Melanoma; hemangioma; metastatic tumor; nevus
Others	Vitreoretinal traction; preretinal gliosis; hypotony

(10–9) Int. Ophthalmol. Clin. 21:157–165, Fall 1981.

has been suggested in eyes with persistent CME after cataract extraction and, when combined with membrane peeling, it can be effective in treating CME secondary to preretinal gliosis or vitreoretinal traction. Photocoagulation has been used chiefly in cases of CME secondary to retinal vascular disease. Focal argon laser therapy is being used to treat CME secondary to localized retinal vessel leakage in several conditions, including background diabetic retinopathy and subretinal neovascularization. Occasionally cryotherapy is used to treat peripheral chorioretinal causes of CME, and it can be used in place of photocoagulation to treat retinal telangiectasis. Steroids are useful in treating CME secondary to intraocular inflammation. Periocular steroids have been useful in treating CME in aphakic eyes, but the effect is usually only temporary. Indomethacin has been shown to reduce the incidence of CME after cataract surgery. Systemic pretreatment with 15-(S)-methyl-prostaglandin E_1 stabilizes the vascular endothelium and preserves interendothelial tight junctions in animals, and it may be effective in preventing breakdown of the blood-retinal barrier to circulating vasopermeability factors.

10–10 **A Fluorescein Angiographic Study of Cystoid Macular Edema.** Norman S. Jaffe, Susan M. Luscombe, Henry M. Clayman, and J. Donald Gass (Univ. of Miami) performed fluorescein angiography prospectively in 66 patients who had undergone uncomplicated extracapsular cataract extraction and implantation of a Shearing posterior chamber intraocular lens. Primary posterior capsulotomy was performed in all cases. Eight patients had phacoemulsification. Only two studies (3%) were positive for cystoid macular edema, showing dye leakage in the macula. One eye had an acuity of less than 6/12; this patient had nystagmus and congenital amblyopia. The angiographic studies were performed 11 to 23 months after operation.

The occurrence of cystoid macular edema in patients having various types of cataract surgery and lens implantation is shown in the table. With extracapsular extraction and implantation of a Shearing posterior chamber lens and

INCIDENCE OF CYSTOID MACULAR EDEMA PROVED BY FLUORESCEIN ANGIOGRAPHY

		Procedures*		
		Miami Study Group		Current Study
Clinical Data	ICCE-Binkhorst	ECCE-Binkhorst, Intact Capsule	ICCE, No Implant	ECCE-PCL, Capsulotomy
Time between surgery and examination (mos)				
Range	16–24	16–24	16–24	11–23
Mean	19.4	20.3	19.7	17.6
Age of patients (yrs)				
Range	67–94	67–89	67–91	61–95
Mean		73.36†		74.02	72.87
With cystoid macular edema				
No.	18/117	2/44	8/94	2/66
%	15.4	4.5	8.5	3.0

ICCE designates intracapsular cataract extraction; ECCE, extracapsular cataract extraction; PCL, posterior chamber intraocular lens.
†Combined mean age for both Binkhorst groups.

primary posterior capsulotomy, there was a low incidence of cystoid macular edema, compared with intracapsular extraction with or without a Binkhorst intraocular lens. The present rate of proved cystoid macular edema is similar to that in a previous series of extracapsular extractions in eyes with intact posterior capsules. A posterior chamber intraocular lens may provide greater stability and less pseudophakodonesis than a Binkhorst prepupillary intraocular lens, and this may be more important than the presence of an intact posterior capsule.

Pseudophakic Cystoid Maculopathy: Study of 50 Cases. Cystic macular edema (CME) is one of the most common complications of intracapsular lens implantation. Alan L. Stern, Daniel M. Taylor, Lewis A. Dalburg, and Robert T. Cosentino reviewed 50 cases of pseudophakic cystoid macular edema (PCME) in a series of 821 consecutive intracapsular cataract extractions and intraocular lens implantations. Patients were followed over 1–4½ years. All the lenses were iris fixated. Thirty-three patients had Platina clip lenses, 13 had Copeland implants, 3 had Medallion suture implants, and 1 had a Federov implant. Various factors possibly predisposing to PCME were identified in 12 cases.

(10–11) Ophthalmology (Rochester) 88:942–946, September 1981.

The clinical course of the patients is shown in the table. Only 1 patient had benign, nonrecurrent disease without corticosteroid therapy. Benign, nonrecurrent disease occurred in 22% of patients in association with corticosteroid therapy. Fifteen patients had recurrent PCME responsive to corticosteroid therapy and had a final acuity of 20/40 or

CLINICAL COURSE OF 50 PATIENTS

Patient	Age	Sex	Lens	Date	Best VA	Final VA	Onset of CME	VA with CME	Recurrences	Response to Therapy	Comments
1	66	F	Copeland	6/77	20/25	20/40	3 mos	20/60	0	−steroids	Did not use steroids
2	55	F	Copeland	10/77	20/25	20/30	11 mos	20/100	0	+steroids	
3	58	M	clip	6/78	20/20−	20/20−	3 mos	20/60	0	+steroids	Holding nicely
4	59	M	clip	5/78	20/40	20/40	5 mos	20/200	0	+steroids	Subluxated 1 wk post-op
5	59	F	clip	6/78	20/25	20/25	6 mos	20/60	0	+steroids	
6	60	M	clip	12/76	20/40	20/40	6 mos	20/60	0	+steroids	
7	64	F	clip	1/78	20/25	20/25	3 mos	20/80	0	+steroids	Hemorrhage in macula
8	66	M	clip	3/76	20/40	20/40	4 mos	20/80	0	+steroids	
9	68	M	clip	9/76	20/25	20/40	12 mos	20/80	0	+steroids	Hemorrhage in macula
10	75	M	clip	6/78	20/30	20/30	6 mos	20/50	0	+steroids	Other eye 20/20 Copeland
11	77	F	clip	12/76	20/25	20/30	6 mos	20/40	0	+steroids	
12	78	F	clip	6/78	20/40	20/40	8 mos	20/200	0	+steroids	
13	39	M	suture	4/78	20/25	20/25	3 mos	20/100	2	+steroids	
14	52	M	clip	9/77	20/30	20/20	3 mos	20/100	1	+steroids × 2	
15	53	M	clip	1/78	20/20	20/30	2½ mos	20/100	1	+steroids × 2	
16	57	F	clip	12/75	20/20−	20/20−	6 mos	20/60	1	+steroids × 2	
17	59	M	clip	6/76	20/25	20/40	6 mos	20/400	1	+steroids × 2	Subluxuated lens, poor follow-up
18	60	M	clip	10/76	20/20	20/20	8 mos	20/70	1	+steroids × 2	
19	60	M	clip	11/77	20/25	20/25	3 mos	20/70	3	+steroids × 3	
20	61	M	clip	12/77	20/30	20/30	3 mos	20/60	1	+steroids × 2	Same patient as above
21	68	F	Copeland	5/75	20/20	20/30	16 mos	20/80	1	+steroids × 2	
22	68	M	clip	1/78	20/20	20/25	8 mos	20/60	1	+steroids × 2	Corneal edema upper 1/6
23	68	M	clip	4/78	20/40	20/40	7 mos	20/70	1	+steroids × 2	Upper 1/6 corneal edema; fellow eye 20/20 w/IOL
24	69	F	Copeland	4/75	20/30	20/40	5 mos	20/80	w + w*	+steroids	Other eye 20/25 w/implant
25	69	F	clip	5/77	20/30	20/40	6 mos	20/100	3	+steroids × 3	Upper 1/8 corneal edema
26	72	M	clip	1/77	20/25	20/30	4 mos	20/80	1	+steroids	
27	73	M	clip	3/78	20/30	20/30	5 mos	20/200	1	+steroids	Same patient as above
28	75	M	Copeland	2/76	20/25	20/25	10 mos	20/100	w + w	+steroids	
29	50	M	clip	10/76	20/20−	20/70	2½ mos	20/70	w + w	+steroids × 2	Chronic iritis
30	50	F	clip	5/77	20/30	20/60	6 mos	20/100	w + w	+steroids	Corneal edema
31	54	M	clip	3/77	20/20	20/50	17 mos	20/70	1	+steroids × 1	Alcoholic; trauma 17 months
32	55	F	clip	6/78	20/25−	20/60	5 mos	20/100	w + w	+steroids +Indocin	Chronic course, lamellar hole + corneal edema + hemorrhage in macula
33	58	M	clip	8/77	20/20	20/60	8 mos	20/100	0	+steroids	Vitreous haze
34	61	M	clip	8/77	20/25	20/80	7 mos	CF	0	+steroids	Subluxated 4 mos postop
35	63	M	Copeland	3/76	20/25	20/60	8 mos	20/70	0	−steroids	+ Corneal edema
36	64	F	clip	3/76	20/30	20/60−	6 mos	20/100	w + w	+steroids	Cystic macular changes macula hemorrhage
37	66	M	Copeland	1/75	20/25	20/80	2 mos	20/80	0	−steroids	Hyphema 1 day postop + hemorrhage in macula
38	68	M	clip	8/78	20/30−	20/80	10 mos	20/100	0	−steroids	Poor follow-up, hyphema 1 day postop
39	71	F	clip	12/77	20/30	20/60	3 mos	20/80	1	−steroids	Hemorrhage in macula;? SMD also
40	74	F	clip	2/77	20/80	20/80	3 mos	20/200	0	+steroids	Probable SMD also
41	78	F	Copeland	6/78	20/25	20/60	10 mos	20/200	1	+steroids	Trauma 5 mos postop with Berlin's edema
42	79	F	Copeland	4/76	20/40	20/80	9 mos	CF	w + w	+steroids	Hemorrhage in macula
43	58	F	clip	8/77	20/25	20/200	6 mos	20/100	1	+steroids × 1	+ Hemorrhage in macula CF acuity 2nd time
44	59	F	Fyodorov	12/76	20/40	20/200	5 mos	20/200	w + w	−steroids	+ Corneal edema, graft
45	61	F	Copeland	10/75	20/20	20/100	10 mos	20/60	3	+steroids × 2	Cystic maculopathy
46	62	M	clip	4/77	20/40	20/100	6 mos	20/100	0	−steroids	Maculopathy, vitreous loss; other eye w/lens 20/25
47	64	M	suture	10/75	20/25	20/200	6 mos	20/200	0	−steroids	Vitreous hemorrhage 5 mos postop, macular cysts
48	73	M	suture	2/76	20/60	LP	3 mos	20/200	w + w	−steroids	Chronic iritis, vitreous hemorrhage
49	78	F	clip	5/77	20/25	20/300	5 mos	20/60	w + w	+steroids	Corneal edema; grafted + vitritis.
50	84	F	Copeland	4/75	20/60	20/200	18 mos	20/200	0	−steroids	SMD noted preop

*w + w: waxing and waning.

better, whereas 9 patients had a final acuity of 20/100 or worse despite such therapy. In 13 patients, PCME recurred at least three times, and only 5 of these had a final acuity of 20/40 or better. All but 9 of 49 patients given corticosteroid therapy responded at least once. Five nonresponders did not receive an adequate dosage.

Pseudophakic cystoid macular edema (Fig 10–3) appears to be an inflammatory condition. Nearly all patients in this study had evidence of chronic, low-grade inflammation, and the condition responds rapidly to anti-inflammatory agents. The risk of PCME is inversely related to age at operation. Presently, intracapsular surgery and lens implantation are reserved for patients aged 70 and older. Implant surgery in patients aged 60–70 years is done by an extracapsular technique. In contrast to CME, PCME is not benign. Patients are treated with 60 mg of prednisone for 4 days, followed by 40 mg daily for 6 days, and then lower doses over the next 3–4 weeks. If necessary, triamcinolone is injected by the sub-Tenon route.

▶ [The etiology of cystoid macular edema associated with cataract surgery is theorized to be due to such diverse problems as hypotony, in-

Fig 10–3.—Fluorophotograph of pseudophakic cystoid maculopathy with multiple macular hemorrhages. (Courtesy of Stern, A. L., et al.: Ophthalmology (Rochester) 88:942–946, September 1981.)

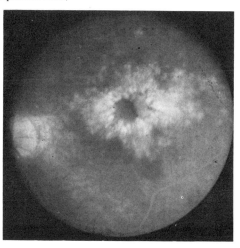

flammation, and loss of the vitreous support of the lens-iris diaphragm. Posterior chamber lenses appear to be associated with less cystoid macular edema, but there are differing reports about the effect of capsulotomy. Until we know more about the etiology and how best to treat the disease, it is difficult to make a final decision about which intraocular lens to use.] ◄

10–12 **The Histopathology of Cystoid Macular Edema.** Cystoid macular edema (CME) may follow intraocular surgery and compromise otherwise perfect results. Its cause remains unknown, and little is known of the histopathology of CME. J. Reimer Wolter (Univ. of Michigan) reviewed the findings in 10 cases.

Man, 75, had a chondroma removed from the right orbit and underwent re-resection 9 years later. Regrowth of the tumor 2 years later led to enucleation. Papilledema and spotty hemorrhages in the posterior retina were noted. A layer of vitreous exudate covered the retina posteriorly. Rubeosis iridis was observed, and there were early cataractous lens changes. The optic disc showed secondary atrophy. Advanced CME was observed in the foveal region (Fig 10–4). In addition to eosinophilic serous exudate on the pigment epithelium, there were pigment-filled macrophages and some fibrinous exudate. Large retinal cysts involved Henle's fiber layer, the nuclear layers, and the nerve fiber layer. Hemorrhages were noted in Henle's fiber layer and posteriorly over the outer aspect of the retina. The choroid was congested, with large blood-filled veins.

Early swelling of the foveal retina in CME occurs in Henle's fiber layer, the only layer of the central retina that allows for swelling without apparent destructive changes. Small cystoid spaces filled with plasmoid fluid then appear and enlarge, involving the neighboring nuclear layers, and degenerative changes are noted in foveal neurons and the glia. Eventually, the foveola is affected, and layer holes may develop. The central swelling is associated with petaloid folding of the inner retina. Exudates may accumulate in the cystoid spaces in the retina in the later stages, but these exudates are never very heavy.

Ocular hypotony is a leading concomitant of CME, especially when it occurs abruptly and in an irritated eye. Trauma and surgery are the chief causes of sudden hypotony. The separation of foveolar cones from the pigment ep-

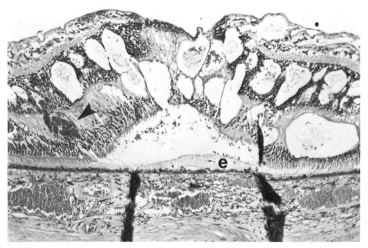

Fig 10–4.—Slightly parafoveolar horizontal paraffin section with many large cystoid spaces containing fibrinous exudate, deep retinal hemorrhage *(arrowhead)*, retinal fold of outer retina, central core degeneration, and shallow serous retrofoveal exudate *(e)*; choroid is congested. Hematoxylin-eosin, ×120. (Courtesy of Wolter, J. R.: Albrecht Von Graefes Arch. Klin. Exp. Ophthalmol. 216:85–101, April 1981; Berlin-Heidelberg-New York: Springer.)

ithelium that results from folding of the outer retinal layers explains central visual loss and leads to cone degeneration in the later stages. Changes in separation can explain clinically observed variations in vision in patients with CME.

Macular Edema and Cystoid Macular Edema. Cystoid macular edema is a retinal change seen in a variety of local ocular conditions and systemic diseases, consisting of cystlike spaces in the perifoveal region. Ben S. Fine (Armed Forces Inst. of Pathology) and Alexander J. Brucker (Univ. of Pennsylvania) performed microscopic studies on three eyes in which preenucleation fluorescein angiograms had shown the characteristic pattern of cystoid macular edema. Two patients, one a diabetic, had peripheral choroid melanomas; the third had diabetes only.

The tumor patients had minimal light microscopic evidence of retinal cystoid degeneration in the foveomacular region. Electron microscopic examination showed widespread swelling and degeneration of the Müller cell cytoplasm, particularly in the Henle fiber layer in the foveomacular region. Little or no widening of intercellular spaces was seen. The patient with diabetes only had characteristic findings of retinal cystoid macular degeneration. Some Müller cells in the inner retinal layers had degenerated. Degeneration of ganglion, bipolar, and photoreceptor cells was seen in all three cases. Degeneration of the outer segments of the foveolar photoreceptor cells was extensive in the eye from one of the tumor patients, who had a serous detachment of the foveomacula. Hypertrophy and occasional edema of capillary endothelial cells in the adjacent vasculature were observed, especially in the diabetics. The retinal capillary pericytes were altered in all cases.

The edematous process appears to begin with intracytoplasmic swelling of Müller cells, which is probably secondary to vascular abnormalities. Subsequently, there is progressive edema and liquefaction necrosis of Müller cells, besides neuronal degeneration, probably secondary to prolonged Müller cell dysfunction, liquefaction necrosis, or both, and increasingly large cystic spaces are formed. The edema of Müller cells may be a result of a faulty retinal vasculature or of an incompetent retinal pigment epithelium.

▶ [Both choroidal vascular occlusion and retinal vascular leakage have been implicated in the pathology of cystoid macular edema. There is a wide gamut of diseases that affect the ocular vasculature; therefore, the discovery of specific etiologies and treatment may be more difficult than heretofore imagined.] ◀

10–14 **Argon Laser Photocoagulation of Subretinal Neovascular Membranes.** Subretinal neovascular membranes, which are proliferative vessels that arise from the choriocapillaris and extend in the plane between Bruch's membrane and the retinal pigment epithelium, pose a significant threat of loss of central vision when present in the posterior pole of the eye. The most common causes are senile macular degeneration and the presumed ocular histoplasmosis syndrome. Hunter L. Little, Robert L. Jack, and Arthur Vassiliadis used photocoagulation to treat sub-

---

(10–14) Trans. Am. Ophthalmol. Soc. 78:167–189, 1980.

retinal neovascular membranes in eyes with senile choroidal macular degeneration and presumed ocular histoplasmosis. Treatment with the argon laser was indicated for serous or hemorrhagic detachment of the retina within the macula, and with evidence of a subretinal neovascular membrane without foveal involvement. An average of about 2½ sessions of argon laser therapy was administered, usually with a 200-μ spot size, 400–500 mW of power, and a 0.2-second exposure time. The technique is illustrated in Figure 10–5.

A total of 143 eyes with senile macular degeneration and 45 with presumed ocular histoplasmosis were treated and followed up for 6 months or longer. Of 59 eyes with senile macular degeneration that had initial acuities of 20/40 or better, 45% were stabilized at this level, and half of the 102 eyes with vision of 20/80 or better were stabilized. Women had worse initial acuities but better final acuities than men. The most favorable visual prognosis was for eyes with a

Fig 10–5.—Illustration showing pattern of argon laser photocoagulation lesions used for treatment of subretinal neovascular membrane. (Courtesy of Little, H. L., et al.: Trans. Am. Ophthalmol. Soc. 78:167–189, 1980.)

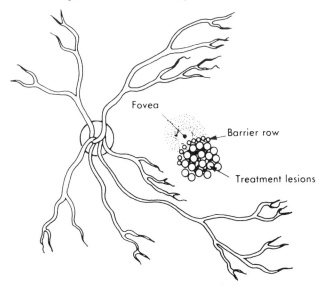

membrane more than 300 µ from the fovea, which was a far more important factor than the diameter of the membrane. Better visual results were obtained in eyes with presumed ocular histoplasmosis. Nearly 60% of eyes with initial acuities of 20/40 or better and more than 75% of those with acuities of 20/80 or better were stabilized. Women had a better response in this group as well, and the chief prognostic factor again was the distance from the membrane margin to the fovea.

Intense argon laser photocoagulation is helpful for patients with subretinal neovascular membranes caused by senile macular degeneration or presumed ocular histoplasmosis. Close follow-up is necessary, with repeated coagulation when evidence is obtained of residual subretinal neovascular membrane.

Argon Laser Photocoagulation of Choroidal Neovascular Membranes is discussed by Irvin L. Handelman, Michael L. Klein, and Richard G. Chenoweth. Choroidal neovascular membranes can develop in a variety of macular diseases that affect the retinal pigment epithelium, Bruch's membrane, and the choriocapillaris, and can lead to a significant, often permanent reduction of central vision. High-quality fluorescein angiography is necessary to photocoagulate neovascularization. Only lesions that are at least 125 µ from the foveal avascular zone (Fig 10–6) should be considered for treatment. Membranes between the disc and macula can be safely treated. Intense burns of long duration are placed to cover an area up to 100 µ beyond the borders of the lesion. Retrobulbar anesthesia is useful. After outlining the membrane with 100-µ burns for 0.1–0.2 second, the border is treated starting on the foveal side with 100- to 200-µ spots of 0.2 second duration. The center is then treated with 200- to 500-µ overlapping burns of 0.2- to 0.5-second duration.

The chief risk is inadvertent treatment of the foveal region. Retinal striae are common but usually have little visual significance. Subretinal hemorrhage is rare. Improved visual outcome has not yet been shown in treated eyes, but this question is currently under examination by the Mac-

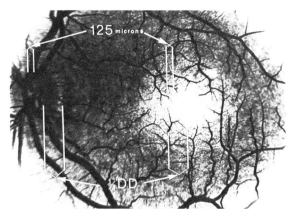

Fig 10–6.—Minimum distance for safe treatment of choroidal neovascular membrane to center of fovea is one-fourth disc diameter, or 125 μ from the avascular fovea. (Courtesy of Handelman, I. L., et al.: Int. Ophthalmol. Clin. 21:87–98, Fall 1981.)

ula Photocoagulation Study, which is a multicenter trial sponsored by the National Eye Institute. Patients with presumed ocular histoplasmosis, senile macular degeneration, and idiopathic choroidal neovascularization are included in the study. Destruction of choroidal neovascularization is technically feasible in some eyes by using intense burns of long duration that completely cover the membrane.

▶ [The treatment of subretinal neovascularization with laser has been advocated by many, but most series are small. A National Eye Institute-sponsored macular photocoagulation study is under way using the multicenter, prospective, randomized clinical trial mechanism, and in another year there should be some information available. Until then, the best course of action might be to enter one's patients in the study rather than make a decision whether to treat or not treat.] ◀

–16 **Treatment of Macular Subretinal Neovascularization With the Red-Light Krypton Laser in Presumed Ocular Histoplasmosis Syndrome.** Subretinal neovascularization in the presumed ocular histoplasmosis syndrome leads to visual impairment that does not respond well to medical management. Yuval Yassur, Emil Gilad, and Isaac Ben-Sira report the case of a patient with macular subre-

---

(10–16) Am. J. Ophthalmol. 91:172–176, February 1981.

266 / OPHTHALMOLOGY

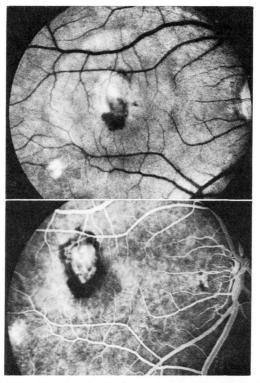

Fig 10–7 (top).—Posterior pole of right eye shows macular subretinal neovascular lesion. Retinal hemorrhage covers fovea. Second lesion is seen 2 disc diameters inferotemporal to macula.

Fig 10–8 (bottom).—Venous phase of fluorescein angiography shows early leakage of lesions and staining of fine peripapillary scars.

(Courtesy of Yassur, Y., et al.: Am. J. Ophthalmol. 91:172–176, February 1981.)

tinal neovascularization well suited to treatment by krypton-laser photocoagulation.

Woman, 50, had had an abrupt fall in acuity in the right eye a few months before the initial examination. Acuity was 6/120 on the right and 6/6 on the left, and an elevated grayish macular lesion was seen in the right fundus. The lower part of the hemorrhage extended into the fovea (Fig 10–7). A smaller subretinal lesion was present 2 disc diameters beneath and temporal to the fovea. A round atrophic choroidal scar was present in the upper temporal equatorial region. Two atrophic choroidal scars were present in the periphery of the left fundus. Fluorescein angiography of the macular lesion showed a choroidal neovascular membrane that leaked profusely (Figs 10–8 and 10–9). The areas of neovascularization were destroyed using the continuous red-light krypton laser (Fig 10–10). Atrophic chorioretinal scars were seen in the treated area within a few weeks, and the hemorrhage regressed and disappeared. Angiography confirmed complete de-

Fig 10–9 (top).—Fluorescein angiography at 2 minutes shows late leakage of membrane.
Fig 10–10 (bottom).—Immediate results of medium-intensity krypton laser photocoagulation of macular lesion and strong-intensity treatment of second lesion farther away from macula; krypton laser was applied only to lighter hemorrhage and did not extend into dark foveal hemorrhage.
(Courtesy of Yassur, Y., et al.: Am. J. Ophthalmol. 91:172–176, February 1981.)

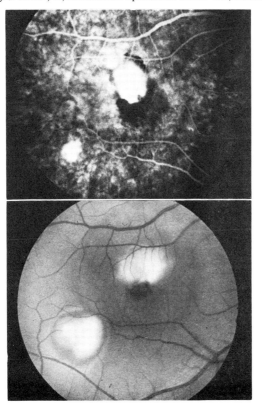

struction of the neovascular membrane. Acuity 6 months after treatment was 6/60. The patient was able to read J7 with a low-power lens. The fixation point was below the fovea.

This may be the first case of treatment of a histoplasmatic macular subretinal neovascular membrane with the red-light krypton laser. Less whitening of the retina was necessary and less energy was needed than is usual when such a lesion is destroyed by argon-laser therapy. Krypton-laser therapy might be indicated before acuity has deteriorated irreversibly when a macular subretinal neovascular membrane is present less than 0.25 disc diameter from the fovea.

▶ [The macular photocoagulation study has added krypton red as one of the treatment modalities tested. This laser can be used closer to the fovea than argon and in the presence of blood because it is little absorbed by xanthophyll or hemoglobin.] ◀

10–17 **Pathologic Myopia and Choroidal Neovascularization.** Pathologic myopia is the seventh leading cause of blindness in adults in the United States. It has been reported that choroidal neovascularization develops in as many as 10% of eyes with an axial length of more than 26.5 mm. Mary L. Hotchkiss and Stuart L. Fine (Johns Hopkins Med. Inst., Baltimore) reviewed the data on 81 patients with severe myopia, all but 3 of whom had a refractive error of -6 diopters or more. Thirty-three patients had a choroidal neovascular membrane at the posterior pole, 4 of them in both eyes. None of these patients had evidence of other degenerative disease of the posterior segment.

Lacquer cracks were more common in patients with choroidal neovascularization, and retinal hemorrhages occurred almost exclusively in this group. At follow-up, 3 of 14 eyes with neovascular membranes within the foveal avascular zone had improved two or more lines on the Snellen chart, while 7 eyes had lost this degree of vision. Of 5 eyes with neovascular membranes extending to the edge of the foveal avascular zone, 4 had lost two or more lines of vision at follow-up (Fig 10–11). Only 1 of 8 eyes with neovascular membranes outside the foveal avascular zone had improved on follow-up, 5 of these 8 eyes had been treated

---

(10–17) Am. J. Ophthalmol. 91:177–183, February 1981.

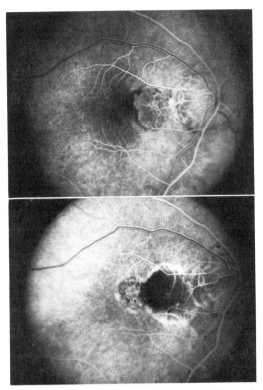

Fig 10–11.—View of right eye of 34-year-old man with 4-week history of decreased visual acuity (6/22.5) in that eye. **Top,** neovascular membrane extending to edge of avascular zone was treated with argon-laser photocoagulation. **Bottom,** angiogram taken 1 year after photocoagulation of membrane. Despite initially successful treatment, new vessels ultimately grew inside avascular zone; visual acuity, 6/48. (Courtesy of Hotchkiss, M. L., and Fine, S. L.: Am. J. Ophthalmol. 91:177–183, February 1981.)

by argon laser photocoagulation. Of 16 eyes without choroidal neovascularization, 3 had lost two or more lines of acuity at follow-up.

About half the eyes with choroidal neovascular membranes that were followed up became legally blind. Final acuity may be related to the position of the neovascular membrane within the posterior pole. Laser photocoagulation may be of use in treating neovascular membranes outside the foveal avascular zone or those extending to the edge of the perifoveal capillary network.

▶ [If photocoagulation is proved beneficial in presumed histoplasmosis syndrome or senile choroidal macular degeneration, or both, it might be reasonable to mount a prospective, randomized clinical trial of its efficacy in pathologic myopia.] ◀

▶ ↓ Retrolental fibroplasia is a disease we thought was in the past, but pediatricians are now able to save premature infants that previously would not have survived, and part of the treatment is oxygen. There are now new methods of monitoring oxygen with skin sensors as well as indwelling, self-calibrating catheter sensors and even ocular oxygen sensors; however, sometimes, to save an infant's life, retinal toxic doses must be administered. In the following four articles, treatment with both vitamin E and photocoagulation is discussed. ◀

10–18 **Retrolental Fibroplasia: Efficacy of Vitamin E in a Double-Blind Clinical Study of Preterm Infants.** Because the development of retrolental fibroplasia (RLF) is related to exposure to highly concentrated oxygen, the use of vitamin E, a naturally occurring antioxidant, for prophylaxis and also for treatment has been of interest. Helen Mintz Hittner, Louis B. Godio, Arnold J. Rudolph, James M. Adams, Joseph A. Garcia-Prats, Zvi Friedman, Judith A. Kautz, and William A. Monaco (Baylor College of Medicine, Houston) undertook a double-blind study of the efficacy of vitamin E in preventing severe RLF when given orally in pharmacologic doses to high-risk preterm infants. A total of 150 infants weighing 1,500 gm or less at birth who required supplemental oxygen for respiratory distress were entered into the study, and 101 who lived at least 4 weeks were evaluated. Fifty infants received 100 mg of vitamin E per kg daily from their first day; the other 51 received a control dose of 5 mg/kg.

No vitamin E toxicity was observed. The treatment and control groups were clinically comparable. Significant disease was reduced substantially in the study group, although there was no significant reduction in the overall occurrence of RLF. In control infants the best predictors of severity were gestational age, weighted oxygen score, intraventricular hemorrhage, sepsis, and birth weight. When these factors were used in a multivariate analysis of both

(10–18) N. Engl. J. Med. 305:1365–1371, Dec. 3, 1981.

groups, the high vitamin E dosage was found to reduce the severity of RLF significantly.

Treatment with 100 mg of vitamin E per kg daily significantly reduced the severity of RLF in preterm infants in this study. Vitamin E appears not to eliminate the occurrence of mild to moderate RLF. It may not be wise to withhold vitamin E until after oxygen has been administered and vitreous neovascularization has been identified. An increase in dosage may be indicated if several risk factors are present. No adverse effects have resulted from oral vitamin E administration, and the risk-benefit ratio strongly favors early, high-dose administration to high-risk preterm infants.

10–19 **Retrolental Fibroplasia: New Look at an Unsolved Problem.** Lois Johnson (Univ. of Pennsylvania) points out that, although uncommon, blindness from retrolental fibroplasia (RLF) still occurs as a complication of the increased survival of small premature infants. Retinal anoxia causes the abnormal neovascularization of RLF. The proliferative, vaso-obliterative changes result from hyperoxia. Most RLF that presently is diagnosed is mild in degree and resolves spontaneously, but blinding and lesser degrees of visual handicap still occur. The vessels of the immature retina are especially sensitive to changes in oxygen tension. Retinal changes identical to those seen in human infants with RLF have been produced in the kitten in the absence of hyperoxia by mechanical occlusion of the retinal arterioles. Marked individual variation in response to hyperoxia has been observed in infants.

Owens and Owens first evaluated a possible protective effect of vitamin E in infants exposed prematurely to an oxygen-rich atmosphere. The kitten studies of Phelps and Rosenbaum supported the use of megadose vitamin E therapy. The author, in 1972, began a series of clinical trials designed to evaluate high-dose vitamin E therapy. The dose of α-tocopherol used was much lower than that used in Phelps' kittens. When evaluated at 1–2 years, many control infants had significant visual morbidity, including am-

---

(10–19) Hosp. Pract. 16:109–121, May 1981.

blyopia, despite the apparent complete regression of active RLF after hospital discharge. The incidence of sequelae at age 1–2 years was lower in vitamin E-treated infants. Vitamin E treatment was associated with a significant reduction in the incidence and severity of RLF, after controlling for various known risk factors. A double-blind clinical trial of vitamin E treatment in infants is currently being carried out.

▶ [We look forward to the results of the prospective randomized clinical trial testing the efficacy of vitamin E in retrolental fibroplasia.] ◀

Acute Retinopathy in Premature Infants Following Oxygen Therapy. P. Ryzman, H. Hamard, H. Mondon, A. Lefrançois, J. P. Relier, A. Minkowski, G. Moriette, E. De Gamarra, Ch. Couturier, and G. Laguenie (Paris) report 5 cases of retinopathy of prematurity observed among 1,750 premature infants during a 4-year period. In all cases, arterial PaO_2 exceeded 100 mm Hg at least once, despite carefully administered and monitored oxygen therapy. In 4 eyes a laser photocoagulation was performed, resulting in two regressions, a stabilization with sequelae and a fibroplasia.

Since the first recognition of the pathogenetic effect of hyperoxygenation on the retina of the premature infant and the possibility of retrolenticular fibroplasia, assiduous control of oxygen therapy considerably lessened the frequency of these lesions that had affected some 30% of premature infants weighing less than 1,500 gm in 1942. The proposed treatment has curative as well as preventive elements. As in all ischemic retinopathy of proliferative neovascular origin, it is a matter of destroying the hypoxic zones secreting an angiogenic factor, resulting in atrophy of neovascular structures and fibroblastic tissue. Photocoagulation and cryocoagulation are used. In terms of prevention, oxygen therapy should be rigorously monitored with a view toward the danger of overdose immediately after birth. Moreover, indirect ophthalmoscopic surveillance must be systematically maintained for at least 3 months for possibly required photocoagulation in evolutive forms of retinopathy. Regular follow-up for several years will aid early recognition of eventual secondary lesions.

▶ [This is a small series, and the long-term effects of retinal ablation in an infant are completely unknown. Perhaps it is benign, but one wonders about vitreous retraction and peripheral vascular insufficiency over the decades after photocoagulation.] ◀

▶ ↓ The following two articles reach opposite conclusions about the relationship between blood transfusion and retrolental fibroplasia. ◀

Blood Transfusion: A Possible Risk Factor in Retrolental Fibroplasia. The occurrence of sustained hyperoxemia in premature infants without subsequent retrolental fibroplasia (RLF) and the development of cicatricial RLF in newborn infants without hyperoxemia suggest that other important factors may influence the interaction between oxygen and immature retinal vessels. Exchange transfusions may be associated with severe RLF. Christine Clark, Judith A. H. Gibbs, Robert Maniello, Eugene W. Outerbridge, and Jacob V. Aranda (McGill Univ., Montreal) evaluated this relationship in 58 infants weighing under 1,001 gm at birth who lived for at least 3 weeks; all but 2 infants required oxygen therapy for a mean of 28 days. Sixteen of these infants received exchange transfusions. Study also was made of 70 consecutive newborn infants with variable birth weights who received oxygen therapy. Nine received exchange transfusions.

Cicatricial RLF was significantly more frequent in the low birth weight infants who had exchange transfusions. No difference in mean peak PaO_2 or the duration or level of oxygen therapy was seen between the transfused and nontransfused groups. In the oxygen-treated group, there was a significant increase in active retinopathy in the transfused group. The transfused and nontransfused groups showed no difference in mean peak PaO_2 values or in the incidence of bag and mask ventilation with an inspired oxygen fraction of 1.0. Transfusion was associated with an increased rate of retinopathy only in "low-risk" infants. Retinopathy developed in 3 of the 5 twins in the oxygen-treated group, all of whom received transfusions. Gross indices of morbidity showed no significant differences between the transfused and nontransfused infants.

The reason for the relation between RLF and blood transfusion is not clear, but an increased availability of oxygen to tissues might lead to greater oxygen toxicity in the retinal vessels. Low birth weight infants given blood transfusions require ophthalmoscopic follow-up.

10-22 **Retrolental Fibroplasia and Blood Transfusion in Very Low Birth Weight Infants.** An association between multiple blood transfusions and exchange transfusion and retrolental fibroplasia (RLF) has been suggested. Linda M. Sacks, David B. Schaffer, Endla K. Anday, George J. Peckham, and Maria Delivoria-Papadopoulos (Univ. of Pennsylvania) examined the role of transfusion as a contributing factor in the development of RLF in 90 infants weighing 1,250 gm or less at birth, all of whom received oxygen therapy. The hematocrit reading was maintained at 40%–50% by replacement blood transfusions, and exchange transfusion was done when indicated for hyperbilirubinemia or hyaline membrane disease.

The mean birth weight was 1,050 gm, and the mean gestational age was 29.2 weeks. Forty-five infants received exchange transfusions. Acute proliferative RLF was seen in 54% of infants, but it had resolved totally at follow-up in 31 of 49 infants. Cicatricial RLF developed in 18 infants. Retrolental fibroplasia was significantly associated with the duration of oxygen therapy and of more than 40% oxygen therapy as well as multiple replacement transfusions, but not with birth weight, gestational age, or exchange transfusion. The incidence of RLF in infants given more than 130 ml of packed red blood cells per kilogram was 43%. The association of RLF with replacement transfusions remained significant after controlling for the duration of therapy with more than 40% oxygen, but not after controlling for the duration of oxygen therapy.

Exchange transfusion is not related to the development of RLF in very low birth weight infants, but an association with replacement blood transfusion is evident, though it is

(10–22) Pediatrics 68:770–774, December 1981.

not significant after controlling for the duration of oxygen therapy. Apparently, the adverse effect of oxygen on retinal vessels is more significant than the effect of transfusing adult hemoglobin. There is a need for further study of possible undesirable effects of multiple replacement transfusions, such as iron-loading, interference with biologic antioxidant effects of vitamin E, and microembolism to the retinal circulation.

10–23 **Prognosis for Central Vision and Anatomical Reattachment in Rhegmatogenous Retinal Detachment With Macula Detached.** Successful anatomical repair of retinal detachment is achieved in a high proportion of cases, but the final central visual acuity is often disappointing, especially if the macula was detached preoperatively. Paul Tani, Dennis M. Robertson, and Alice Langworthy (Mayo Clinic) reviewed the results of scleral buckling in 473 eyes treated for rhegmatogenous retinal detachment in which the macula was detached at the time of initial operation. The eyes were treated between 1969 and 1977.

Attachment was achieved in 90% of eyes (table). The functional result was favorable in 37% of 470 eyes, with a final acuity of 20/50 or better. These patients were significantly younger than the others, but the outcome could not be related to sex, trauma to the involved eye, or the presence or absence of vitreous hemorrhage, lattice degeneration, or aphakia. Three of 12 eyes without observed breaks did poorly. The visual results were related to the extent of retinal elevation. Severe cystoid macular edema tended to be associated with poorer functional results. The duration of detachment was related to the final visual outcome (Fig 10–12). Poorer functional results were associated with postoperative use of acetazolamide for increased intraocular pressure and with more than 50 cryopexy applications. Of 121 eyes with a significant preretinal membrane, 40% had a good functional result.

Only just over a third of these eyes with macular detachment did well functionally after scleral buckling, compared with 87% of cases in which the macula was spared. Both anatomical and functional success were positively related

Factors Significant to Anatomical Success and Good Postoperative Visual Acuity*

Factor	Anatomic Success No.	%	Good Visual Acuity (6/15 [20/50] or better) No.[†]	%
PREOPERATIVE FACTORS				
Visual acuity				
6/4.5 to 6/9 (20/15 to 20/30)	17 of 17	100	14 of 17	82
<6/9 to 6/15 (<20/30 to 20/50)	33 of 34	97	24 of 34	71
6/15 (20/50) or better	50 of 51	98	38 of 51	75
<6/15 to 6/30 (<20/50 to 20/100)	33 of 37	89	23 of 37	62
<6/30 to 6/60 (<20/100 to 20/200)	47 of 48	98	27 of 47[†]	57
6/60 (20/200) or better	130 of 136	96	88 of 135[†]	65
6/60 to 0.6/60 (<20/200 to 2/200)	69 of 71	97	26 of 71	37
Counting fingers or hand motions	215 of 248	87	60 of 246[†]	24
Light perception	14 of 19	74	0 of 19	0
Duration of detachment				
<1 mo	282 of 310	91	128 of 309[†]	41
>1 mo	143 of 161	89	45 of 159[†]	28
Intraocular pressure[‡]				
<5 mm Hg	2 of 7	29	0 of 7	0
5 to 20 mm Hg	390 of 425	92	164 of 422[†]	39
>20 mm Hg	20 of 23	87	5 of 23	22
Quadrants involved in detachment				
1	48 of 55	87	24 of 55	44
2	178 of 185	96	86 of 183[†]	47
3	96 of 104	92	45 of 103[†]	44
4 (not total)	42 of 45	93	11 of 45	24
4 (total)	60 of 81	74	6 of 81	7
Location of tear				
Anterior to or at equator	331 of 353	94	144 of 350[†]	41
Posterior to equator	85 of 104	82	28 of 104	27
Retinal folds fixed				
Yes	155 of 185	84	51 of 184[†]	28
No	273 of 389	94	123 of 287[†]	43
OPERATIVE FACTORS				
No. of cryoapplications[§]				
>50	36 of 48	75	6 of 47[†]	13
≤50	139 of 153	91	52 of 153	34
Subretinal fluid released				
No	84 of 87	97	41 of 87	47
Yes[∥]	342 of 385	89	133 of 382[†]	35
Extent of buckle				
<360 degrees	219 of 232	94	100 of 229[†]	44
360 degrees	208 of 241	86	73 of 241	30
Height of buckle				
Low or medium	331 of 355	93	150 of 353[†]	42
High	93 of 113	82	23 of 112	21

*Significant at $P < .05$.

[†]Final visual acuities were not available for 3 eyes. These eyes were therefore omitted from calculations.

[‡]Preoperative glaucoma was not significant in final visual acuity.

[§]Data were available for only 201 eyes, all treated recently.

[∥]Of 14 eyes that hemorrhaged from release site, 5 had final acuities of 6/15 (20/50) or better.

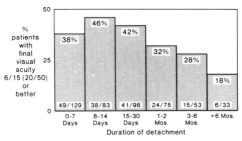

Fig 10–12.—Relation of duration of retinal detachment to postoperative visual acuity. Denominator of fraction in each bar identifies number of eyes in designated time interval, and numerator identifies number of eyes with final visual acuities of 6/15 (20/50) or better. (Courtesy of Tani, P., et al.: Am. J. Ophthalmol. 92:611–620, November 1981.)

to preoperative visual acuity. Functional recovery was strongly related to duration of detachment. It was also related to a shallowly detached macula, age younger than 60 years, and absence of postoperative choroidal detachment sufficient to cause glaucoma.

10–24 **Prognosis of Visual Acuity After Surgery For Detached Retina, With Special Reference to the Unaffected Eye.** Patients with a reattached retina sometimes report binocular diplopia, metamorphopsia, or anisometropia, and a substantial difference in acuity between the eyes may occur in such cases. Tsugio Amemiya, Hisatoshi Yano, Yuichiro Ogura, and Kenji Harayama (Kyoto Univ.) estimated postoperative visual acuity in patients with unilateral retinal detachments at intervals up to more than 5 years after successful reattachment. The study excluded patients with macular holes. A total of 600 cases were assessed.

Within 3 months after surgery, 14% of patients had acuity worse than 0.1 in the reattached eye and worse than 0.5 in the other eye; 36% had better than 1.0 acuity in the nondetached eye and worse than 0.3 in the reattached eye; and 20% had better than 1.0 acuity in the undetached retina and better than 0.8 in the reattached one. After 3–6 months, 24% of patients had 0.4–0.8 acuity in the reattached retina and better than 0.8 in the undetached one.

(10–24) Ophthalmologica 183:128–135, 1981.

After 1–2 years a small number of patients had better acuity in the reattached retina than in the nondetached one. After 2–5 years postoperatively, 13% of patients had better than 1.0 acuity in the nondetached retina and worse than 0.3 in the reattached one; 32% had better than 0.8 acuity in the nondetached retina and 0.4–0.8 in the reattached one; and 24% had better than 1.0 acuity in the nondetached retina and better than 0.8 in the reattached one. After more than 5 years there was almost no improvement in acuity; the average follow-up of this group was 6.7 years. About half the patients had a more than 0.6 difference in acuity between the two eyes more than 2 years postoperatively. Macular detachment was a poor prognostic factor in the 133 patients followed up for 3 years or longer.

Improvement in acuity in patients with reattached retinas may be expected for up to 2 years after surgery. Maximally recovered acuity tends to decline after more than 5 years postoperatively. A significant difference in acuity between the two eyes may be a cause of postoperative complaints.

▶ [Detachment of the macula, while repairable in a high percentage of cases, has a very poor visual prognosis.] ◀

10–25 **Retinal Dialysis: A Statistical and Genetic Study To Determine Pathogenic Factors.** A dialysis is a specific type of retinal tear that is oriented circumferentially and located adjacent to the ora serrata. Dialyses can be large with an elevated posterior edge, and thus may resemble giant tears that have not completely rolled over (Fig 10–13). William S. Hagler reports a prospective study of the pathogenesis of this type of retinal tear in patients who had retinal detachment surgery in 1960–1978. A total of 5,360 eyes were treated in 4,811 patients. A dialysis was observed in 9.8% of the eyes operated on.

Signs of trauma were present in 30% of cases with dialysis and in 4% of eyes in the comparison group. In two thirds of cases the dialysis was posterior to the ora; in most of the other cases there was an avulsion of the vitreous base. The average age of patients with dialysis was much lower than that of the comparison group. More men were

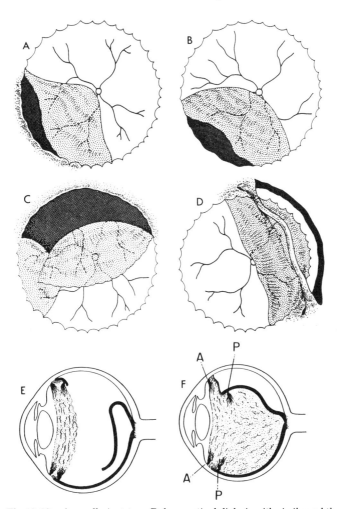

Fig 10–13.—**A,** small giant tear. **B,** large retinal dialysis with similar ophthalmoscopic appearance. **C,** large giant tear; retina typically rolls over and frequently ciliary epithelium is highly elevated. **D,** dialysis of ciliary epithelium; avulsed strip of ciliary epithelium may be intact *(above)* or occasionally torn. **E,** giant tear; vitreous base is always attached to anterior portion of retina and ciliary epithelium. **F,** dialysis showing posterior *(P)* attachment of vitreous base located posteriorly. Absence of vitreous detachment and bridging of dialysis by intact hyaloid prevent retina from rolling over. (Courtesy of Hagler, W. S.: Trans. Am. Ophthalmol. Soc. 78:686–733, 1980.)

REPORTED RATES OF DIALYSIS

Author	Year	Incidence of Dialysis
Shapland	1949	33% of 164 retinae detachments (RD)
Leffertstra	1950	14% of 1,428 RD
Tornquist	1963	17% of 672 RD
Tulloch	1965	10.9% of 442 RD
Donaldson	1967	15% of 667 RD
Hagler and North	1968	10% of 1,352 RD
Hilton and Richards	1970	69% of 26 RD
Chignell	1973	8% of 824 RD
Rodriguez	1972	19% of 1,103 RD
Chang	1979	20% of 502 RD
Hilton and Norton	1969	27% of RD < age 20
Hudson	1969	51% of RD < age 20
Gailloud et al	1969	19% of RD < age 20
Richardson	1969	25% of 118 RD < age 20
Chen and Dumas	1972	43% of RD < age 20
Winslow and Tasman	1978	40% of RD < age 16
Scharf and Zonis	1973	29% of RD < age 20

*Reproduced from Trans. Am. Ophthalmol. Soc. 78:686–733, 1980.

in the dialysis group. About 60% of patients with nontraumatic dialysis and about the same percentage of those with traumatic dialysis were free of symptoms, compared to only 22% of the nondialysis group. Eyes with dialysis were likelier to be hyperopic or emmetropic and less likely to be myopic or aphakic than the others. Only one quadrant was detached in about three fourths of the study cases, and in 19% of the eyes without dialysis. The duration of detachment was much greater in the study group. Intraretinal macrocysts occurred in one fourth of the eyes with nontraumatic dialysis. Concentric demarcation lines were present in 44% of this group, in 25% of eyes with traumatic dialysis, and in 10% of eyes without dialysis. Peripheral retinal degeneration was much more frequent in eyes without dialysis. Dialyses often involved the macula. Only 0.6% of eyes with nontraumatic dialysis and 4.1% of those with traumatic dialysis did not have successful reattachment, compared with 7.5% of the eyes without dialysis. Vision was improved in the majority in all groups when reattachment was achieved. Complications were comparable in the various groups.

Reported rates of dialysis are given in the table. Currently, a classification into anterior and posterior dialysis is appropriate, with further specification of contusion or penetrating trauma, contraction of vitreous membranes after chorioretinal inflammation or systemic vascular disease, and vitreous loss from intraocular surgery.

10–26 **Possible Relationship Between Lattice and Snail Track Degenerations of the Retina.** Lattice and snail track degenerations of the retina are common tractional lesions that may result in retinal breaks. They frequently occur in the same eye. Manoj Shukla and O. P. Ahuja (Aligarh Muslim Univ.) examined the relation between these conditions in 500 randomly selected patients, aged 8 to 66 years, 320 of them male. None had symptoms of retinal disease. Lattice degeneration was seen as isolated areas of retinal thinning oriented circumferentially in the periphery of the retina. Networks of white lines were seen within individual islands in advanced lesions. Snail track lesions appeared as elongated patches of retinal thinning with irregular borders.

Twelve of the 1,000 eyes examined contained both le-

Fig 10–14.—Lattice degeneration *(LD)* and snail track degeneration *(STD)* in same eye. (Courtesy of Shukla, M., and Ahuja, O. P.: Am. J. Ophthalmol. 92:482–485, October 1981.)

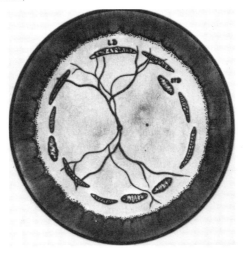

sions, although the lattice lesions predominated (Fig 10–14). Lattice degeneration was seen in 87 eyes of 62 subjects (12.4%); 25 had bilateral lesions. Snail track lesions were seen in 27 eyes of 17 subjects (3.4%), 10 of whom had bilateral lesions. Both lesions were most frequent in the second and third decades; neither increased with age. No sex associations were apparent. Both lesions affected myopic eyes, particularly those with myopia of more than 3 D. Fifteen subjects with lesions had relatives with the lesions. Both lesions showed a predilection for the temporal periphery of the retina, particularly the superotemporal quadrant. Vitreous attachments were seen at the margins of individual lattice and snail track lesions. The degenerative conditions were associated with 76 retinal breaks, most of them round. Breaks were present in 35% of subjects with lattice degeneration and in 29% of those with snail track lesions.

Striking similarities have been observed between lattice degeneration and snail track degeneration. The appearance of retinal breaks substantiates the close relation between the two tractional degenerative lesions. The association with round holes and the familial tendency suggest that these lesions represent local vascular changes.

▶ [This is a fine study, but the vascular hypothesis is difficult to prove. If one occludes the peripheral circulation in the experimental animal eye, neither lattice nor snail tract lesions are induced.] ◀

10–27 **Gyrate Atrophy of the Choroid and Retina: Biochemical Considerations and Experience With an Arginine-Restricted Diet.** Gyrate atrophy of the choroid and retina is associated with a deficiency of ornithine-δ-aminotransferase and accumulation of ornithine. Arginine, the precursor of ornithine, becomes an essential amino acid, because the deficiency not only blocks ornithine degradation but also prevents de novo synthesis of arginine (Fig 10–15). David Valle, MacKenzie Walser, Saul Brusilow, Muriel I. Kaiser-Kupfer, and Kirsti Takki treated 9 patients (7 females), aged 11 to 46 years, who had gyrate atrophy of the choroid and retina, with an arginine-restricted diet for 4 to 32 months. Eight patients had no significant change in plasma ornithine concentration when

---

(10–27) Ophthalmology (Rochester) 88:325–330, April 1981.

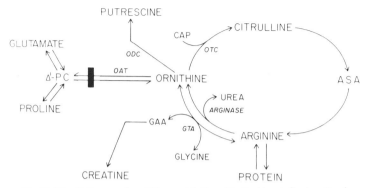

Fig 10–15.—Pathways of ornithine metabolism. Vertical bar indicates site of enzyme defect in gyrate atrophy of choroid and retina. *ASA,* argininosuccinic acid; *CAP,* carbamyl phosphate; *GAA,* guanidinoacetate; *GTA,* glycine transaminidase; *OAT,* ornithine-δ-aminotransferase; *ODC,* ornithine decarboxylase; *OTC,* ornithine transcarbamylase; Δ^1-*PC*, Δ^1-pyrroline-5-carboxylate. (Courtesy of Valle, D., et al.: Ophthalmology (Rochester) 88:325–330, April 1981.)

given pyridoxine for 2 weeks or longer. Protein intake was reduced, and patients received a mixture of essential amino acids, and α-amino isobutyric acid in a dose of 0.2 gm/kg daily for 1 day, followed by 0.1 gm/kg daily in the early stages.

The final reductions in plasma ornithine concentrations were twofold to sixfold (average, threefold). Patients tolerated the diet well, although 1 had persistent weight loss. Reduced concentrations of lysine, glutamate, glutamine, and ammonia returned toward normal when the plasma ornithine concentration was reduced. Three patients have maintained a long-term reduction in plasma ornithine concentration. No patient has had deterioration of vision or of other ophthalmologic functions while observing the diet.

An arginine-restricted diet results in a significant reduction in plasma ornithine concentration in patients with gyrate atrophy of the choroid and retina. No patient in this study had clinically significant hyperammonemia. Measured arginine or ornithine losses, or both, are considerably less than estimated arginine intake. Elucidation of this loss of ornithine could be of therapeutic benefit.

In an addendum, the senior author reports that 1 patient

Eclipse Retinopathy. S. P. Dhir, Amod Gupta, and I. S. Jain (Chandigarh, India) evaluated 30 patients who, despite warnings in the media, watched a partial solar eclipse in February 1980. All 10 affected patients were male; the mean age was 26.2 years. Most had gazed at the eclipse for 5 seconds or so. A total of 13 eyes had evidence of solar retinopathy. Two patients reported blurred vision, and 2 described positive scotomas, while 1 had only mild itching, and 5 had no complaints. Three patients had bilateral involvement.

Three eyes had an acuity of 6/6 or better at presentation, 6 had an acuity of 6/9, and 2 each had acuities of 6/12 and 6/18. None of the eyes had any significant refractive error. The fundus lesions were parafoveal in 4 eyes and perifoveal in 9. Severe lesions consisting of a gray-white patch indicative of severe retinal edema or acute retinal necrosis were present in 3 eyes. Moderate lesions, consisting of a red-brown granular area with a gray ring of retinal edema, were present in 5 eyes. Five eyes exhibited only a dark brown gran-

Fig 10–16.—Moderate eclipse retinopathy was present in both eyes. True lamellar macular hole developed at 3 weeks. Visual acuity in the left eye deteriorated from 6/9 to 6/18. (Courtesy of Dhir, S. P., et al.: Br. J. Ophthalmol. 65:42–45, January 1981.

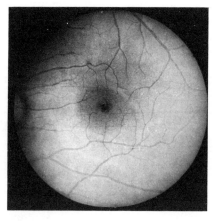

ular lesion at the macula without any retinal edema. Four patients had fluorescein angiographic abnormalities; 2 had microleaks in the parafoveal area.

Six of the 10 eyes followed up showed development of foveomacular holes. Four of these eyes showed visual improvement to 6/6 or better. In 1 case the macular hole disappeared in about 3 months. Follow-up fluorescein studies showed only faint window defects in 3 patients; no dye leakage was apparent.

The fovea appears to be spared in these cases by lack of foveal fixation. Visual acuity was not correlated with severity of lesions in the present cases. Most patients with moderate to severe burns develop a foveomacular hole surrounded by fine pigment clumps. True lamellar holes may develop if the inner retinal layers undergo necrosis (Fig 10–16). The final visual outcome in the present cases was excellent, in contrast to previously reported cases. Late visual deterioration developed in 1 patient who had a true lamellar macular hole.

10–29 **Fluorescence Fundus Photography by Retrobulbar Administration of the Dye, Photochemical Transillumination.** Kensaku Miyake and Kiyoshi Ohtsuki have found fluorescence fundus photography, performed after retrobulbar injection of fluorescein sodium, to be of value in diagnosis of several ocular conditions. A solution of 2 ml of 10% sodium fluorescein and 1 ml of lidocaine is injected with a 23-gauge needle, and gentle massage is performed. Photographs are taken from 30 seconds to 30 minutes after injection. Normally, small fluorescent spots appear within 3 minutes of dye injection in the posterior part of the fundus and fuse to form a geographic pattern within 7 minutes. At 7 to 10 minutes the entire posterior part of the fundus is fluorescent, and the retinal and choroidal vessels are seen in silhouette. Histochemical studies in 3 cases of glaucoma showed intense staining of the outer part of the sclera and retrobulbar tissue 5 minutes after retrobulbar dye injection. The choroidal stroma was stained uniformly at 25 minutes. At 90 minutes, dye was present in the posterior and anterior chambers.

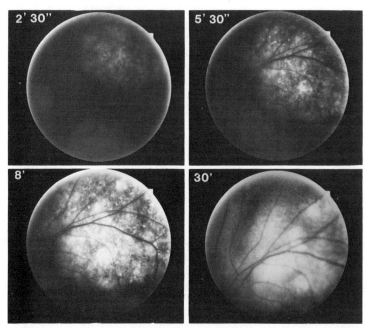

Fig 10–17.—Solitary choroid hemangioma. Fluorogram by photochemical transillumination. In phase I of photochemical transillumination there is faint, granular hyperfluorescence throughout entire area of tumor. The fluorescences join with one another and form mottled hyperfluorescence in phase II and become larger in phases III and IV. (Courtesy of Miyake, K., and Ohtsuki, K.: Jpn. J. Ophthalmol. 25:280–298, 1981; from Nakatsuka, K., and Takaku, I: Fluorescein fundus photographic findings in choroidal hemangioma by retrobulbar injection, Jpn. J. Clin. Ophthalmol. 34:885, 1980.)

Small choroidal tumors in rabbits were seen by photochemical transillumination but not clearly by standard fluorescein angiography. A malignant melanoma was detected more definitely by photochemical transillumination. The appearances of a solitary choroidal hemangioma are shown in Figure 10–17. Photochemical transillumination demonstrated choroid-stroma edema or separation in Harada's disease and showed fluorescein leakage in central serous retinochoroidopathy. Lesions of acute posterior multifocal placoid pigment epitheliopathy were larger on photochemical transillumination than the shadow defects seen on standard fluorescein angiography.

Photochemical transillumination provides intense staining of the posterior part of the choroid and sclera, which is useful in detecting such mass lesions as choroidal tumors. Further study is needed to determine the applicability of this approach to such choroidal disorders as Harada's disease and acute posterior multifocal placoid pigment epitheliopathy.

▶ [This is a more invasive technique than fluorescein angiography, but tumor staining is impressive. In standard late (1 hour or more) fluorescein angiograms, however, the sclera is routinely stained and, in fact, one can see the choroidal vessels as dark lines in front of and blocking the fluorescent sclera. Tumors also stain heavily at this late stage of angiography.] ◄

11. Neuro-ophthalmology

Blepharospasm

JONATHAN D. TROBE, M.D.

Department of Ophthalmology, University of Florida, Gainesville

The pathogenesis and treatment of essential blepharospasm have remained elusive. However, a review of the recent medical literature reveals some fresh insights and some encouraging, if preliminary, new modes of therapy.

The first step in managing blepharospasm is to recognize that it is not a single disease, but a sign that appears in many disease states. The clinician must first exclude:

1. *Trigeminal irritation* (keratitis, scleritis, uveitis, elevated intraocular pressure, meningitis)—which rarely produces sustained and completely uncontrolled eyelid closure.

2. *Difficulty with lid opening*—a supranuclear or bradykinetic disorder of upper lid elevation (not blepharospasm) seen in basal ganglia disorders.[1]

3. *Hemifacial spasm*—strictly unilateral, episodic facial contractions believed to be caused by extramedullary juxtapontine compression of the seventh nerve by an aberrant intracranial vessel. Separation of nerve and vessel by insertion of a sponge (Jannetta procedure) has been effective.[2-4]

4. *Spastic paretic facial contracture*—unilateral persistent facial contracture that may follow healed Bell's palsy. If accompanied by undulating contractions of the orbicularis oculi and no history of Bell's palsy, one should suspect intrinsic pontine disease, either glioma or multiple sclerosis.[5,6]

5. *Tonic blepharospasm*—delayed relaxation of the or-

bicularis oculi after forceful closure, occurring in muscle diseases such as myotonic dystrophy, tetany, hypothyroidism, and hyperkalemic periodic paralysis.[7]

6. *Reflex blepharospasm*—involuntary eyelid closure seen after tapping the forehead (globella) or touching the eyelids in premature infants and patients with extensive subcortical disease.[8, 9]

7. *Psychic blepharospasm*—intense and bilateral involuntary eyelid closure, which may be a hysterical manifestation in young females, usually responding to psychotherapy.

8. *Tics or habit spasms*—brief, patterned predictable episodes, usually involving the face. They usually occur in childhood and are rarely sustained enough to cause functional disability and mimic essential blepharospasm.[10] Persistent and evolving facial tics may be the first sign of Gilles de la Tourette's disease, an idiopathic basal ganglia disorder affecting boys in the first decade and responding to haloperidol, a dopamine antagonist.[11]

The large group of patients who do not fit clearly into any of these categories fall under the diagnostic rubric of "essential blepharospasm."[12-16] Not only has no inclusive pathogenesis been worked out for this "idiopathic" type, there is great controversy as to whether it represents fundamentally a psychopathologic or neuropathologic disturbance.

In support of the psychopathologic etiology is the frequent document of altered affect,[12, 13] especially depression, and the fact that blepharospasm resembles a facial tic and is sometimes relieved by placebos, tranquilizing medications, psychotherapy,[10, 17] behavior modification,[18, 19] and hypnosis.[20] As yet, there have been no comprehensive reports of the psychic disturbances in these patients, and results of successful psychotherapy are limited to isolated case reports.

In fact, the frustratingly low success rate of psychotherapy has reinforced the neuropathologic theory of the origin of blepharospasm. Further support for an "organic" basis for essential blepharospasm comes from the fact that it is often found in association with abnormal facial and head movements and postures that are similar to those seen in other neurologic conditions. The accompanying neurotic disturbances are believed to be reactions to the illness.

Patients who contract middle and lower facial muscles along with their lid closure are said to have the syndrome of "blepharospasm-oromandibular dystonia," first described by Meige in 1910.[21] The term *"dystonia"* implies a more *sustained* contraction than a spasm. Such sustained contractions lead to abnormal postures that change as different muscle groups become involved. Blepharospasm is often an isolated initial sign, with progression to include tonic and clonic contractions of muscle groups variously involving the eyelids, eyebrows, lips, tongue, jaw, larynx and pharynx, neck, and, rarely, the limbs.[22-24] Marsden[13] reported that of 30 cases of blepharospasm, 13 remained isolated while 17 showed dystonic features involving other facial and neck muscles.

Blepharospasm was also reported as a common feature of the dystonic facial grimacing found in patients in the early stages of Economo's encephalitis,[14] which appeared in the decade after the 1919 influenza epidemic and has not been described since. The blepharospasm and facial dystonia preceded the later development of the signs of postencephalitic Parkinson's disease. The coexistence of blepharospasm and Parkinson's disease is actually rare.[14]

Blepharospasm also has been described as a rare manifestation of "tardive dyskinesia," a movement disorder characterized by facial grimacing, intermittent jaw opening, lip smacking, and tongue protrusion.[25] Tardive dyskinesias are seen either spontaneously in the elderly, after levodopa treatment in Parkinson's disease, or, more commonly, after prolonged treatment of schizophrenics with neuroleptic medications, especially phenothiazines and butyrophenones.

Because the neurologic diseases that manifest blepharospasm are believed to be mediated by a wide variety of different neurotransmitter dysfunctions, the pharmacotherapy of blepharospasm has included virtually every drug known to influence these neurochemical agents. Based on the misimpression that blepharospasm was often linked to Parkinson's disease, there was great hope that the success of L-dopa in treating that disease might apply to blepharospasm. It has not helped.

The next approach was to consider blepharospasm part of a hyperkinetic disorder like Huntington's chorea, tardive dyskinesia, or Gilles de la Tourette's disease, which respond to dopaminergic antagonists such as haloperidol, reserpine, and tetrabenazine. Beneficial results have thus far been sparse or transient.[13, 25] Since an antagonism between dopamine and acetylcholine has been recognized in Parkinson's disease and Huntington's chorea, several investigators have attempted to manipulate the cholinergic system in blepharospastic patients. Unfortunately, the use of cholinomimetic agents such as physostigmine, choline chloride, and lecithin has met with only limited success.[26, 27]

However, there is exciting preliminary evidence that centrally acting *anticholinergic* agents may be more fruitful. Tanner et al.[28] applied a rigorous protocol involving acute sequential administration of centrally acting anticholinergic and cholinergic agents to 5 patients whose signs were evaluated by masked viewers of videotapes. In 4 of 5 patients, dystonic signs clearly improved acutely after anticholinergic administration and worsened with cholinergic treatment. The acute response reliably predicted the effect of chronic anticholinergic treatment in these patients.

These favorable results are consistent with those observed recently in anticholinergic treatment of other dystonic diseases such as dystonia musculorum deformans[29] and spasmodic torticollis in small numbers of patients.[30]

The anticholinergic used by Tanner et al.[28] in the acute trials was scopolamine; in the chronic trials, lasting up to 1 year, they used benztropine or trihexyphenidyl. Nine of the 12 patients tested had sustained relief of signs, but in 5 of these, therapeutic dosages could not be maintained because of either severe memory loss, sedation, or dry mouth.

Several investigators having some success in treating Meige syndrome patients with *baclofen,* a γ-aminobutyric acid (GABA) agonist;[31] GABA is a central neurotransmitter with inhibitory effects. Baclofen relieves spasticity and helps in some cases of tardive dyskinesia, but its value in the dystonias is yet unproved.

Likening blepharospasm to a myoclonic disorder has led

to the use of anticonvulsants. These generally have not helped, although 2 patients are reported to have responded to clonazepam (Clonopin), which has sedative properties.[32]

Until a drug with lasting benefit at nontoxic dosage levels is found, the mainstay of treatment of blepharospasm will be ablation of the seventh cranial nerve.[13–16, 33, 34] Alcohol injection at the junction of the seventh nerve branches and orbicularis oculi gives only temporary (3–6 months) relief; surgical section is effective if relatively proximal—either at the exit of seventh nerve from the stylomastoid foramen or in its intraparotid portion. More distal sectioning appears to be less effective, although Gillum and Anderson[35] recently described good results with extensive extirpation of the orbicularis oculi without neurectomy. Intracranial procedures are reserved for hemifacial spasm.

The most commonly performed operation for essential blepharospasm is differential extirpation of branches in the parotid gland, with relative preservation of those fibers destined for the lower part of the face. In a collective series of 100 cases, surgeons judged that blepharospasm was relieved in 69% of cases at 1 year after operation and 61% at 4 years.[34] Reoperations brought the success rate to a total of 75% at 4 years. In this series, the major complications were lower eyelid laxity (ectropion, 44%), paresis of the upper lip or drooping of the corner of the mouth (44%), and accentuation of upper eyelid dermatochalasis or brow droop (38%). About 50% of these complications were severe or persistent enough to require surgical correction, which was successful in all cases in averting permanent ocular complications.

Patients who have been debilitated by eyelid closure are so pleased they can now keep their eyes open that they usually are not disturbed by loss of facial expression or the usually mild problems with saliva control.

Among those who fail to obtain improvement with surgery in the early postoperative period are those in whom the orbicularis oculi remains functional (the innervating branches were inadequately or incompletely sectioned) and a perplexing group in whom the orbicularis is completely paralyzed and yet the eyelids remain closed! It appears that the levator palpebrae is not functioning—this is an upper lid opening problem rather than an accordian-like occlusion of the palpebral fissure. Patients in this group of nonresponders may sometimes be spotted before surgery by injection of a local anesthetic agent into the orbicularis oculi.[35] Those who are unable to open the eyes after evident paresis of this muscle should not have surgery; the only recourse in such patients is placebo, drug, or psychotherapy.

Blepharospasm remains an intriguing manifestation of a variety of pathologic states. The phenomenology of these states has become increasingly well-defined, and promising drug therapy may be available soon for properly selected patients. The interplay between psychologic and neuropathologic features, and the response to manipulation of central neurotransmitters, is reminiscent of Huntington's chorea, Parkinson's disease, Gilles de la Tourette's disease, and the dystonias. Based on the evidence so far, essential blepharospasm must be considered a forme fruste of an adult-onset idiopathic orofacial dystonia (Meige's syndrome) whose signs are, as with many other extrapyramidal diseases, exacerbated by emotionally trying circumstances. In its most flagrant state, it is a disabling affliction. Psychotherapy and drug therapy have not been effective enough in these patients, but may improve with greater understanding of the disease. Until that time, surgical ablation of the branches of the seventh nerve remains the treatment of choice, but should be reserved for the extremely debilitated because of some unpleasant side effects.

REFERENCES

1. Goldstein J.E., Cogan D.G.: Apraxia of lid opening. *Arch. Ophthalmol.* 73:155–159, 1965.
2. Ferguson J.H.: Hemifacial spasm and the facial nucleus. *Ann. Neurol.* 4:97–103, 1978.
3. Auger R.G.: Hemifacial spasm: Clinical and electrophysiologic observations. *Neurology (Minneap.)* 29:1261–1272, 1979.
4. Jennetta P.J., Abbasy M., Maroon J.C., et al.: Etiology and definitive microsurgical treatment of hemifacial spasm: Operative techniques and results in 47 patients. *J. Neurosurg.* 47:321–328, 1977.
5. Waybright E.A, Gutmann L., Chou S.M.: Facial myokymia: Pathologic features. *Arch. Neurol.* 36:244–245, 1979.

6. Boghen D., Filiatrault R., Descarries L.: Myokymia and facial contracture in brain stem tuberculoma. *Neurology (Minneap.)* 27:270–272, 1977.
7. Walsh F.B., Hoyt W.F.: *Clinical Neuro-ophthalmology*. Baltimore, Williams & Wilkins Co., 1969, vol. I, pp. 345–346.
8. Fisher C.M.: Reflex blepharospasm. *Neurology (Minneap.)* 13:77–82, 1963.
9. Irvine A.R., Daroff R.B., Sanders M.D., Hoyt W.F.: Familial reflex blepharospasm. *Am. J. Ophthalmol.* 65:889–890, 1968.
10. Langworthy O.R.: Emotional issues related to certain cases of blepharospasm and facial tics. *Arch. Neurol. Psychiatry* 68:620, 1952.
11. Shapiro A.K., Shapiro E., Wayne H.L.S.: The symptomatology and diagnosis of Gilles de la Tourette's syndrome. *J. Am. Acad. Child Psychiatry* 12:702–723, 1973.
12. Cavenar J.O., Brantley I.J., Braasch E.: Blepharospasm: Organic or functional? *Psychosomatics* 19:623–628, 1978.
13. Marsden C.D.: Blepharospasm-oromandibular dystonia syndrome (Brueghel's syndrome). A variant of adult-onset torsion dystonia? *J. Neurol. Neurosurg. Psychiatry* 39:1204–1209, 1976.
14. Henderson J.W.: Essential blepharospasm. *Trans. Am. Ophthalmol. Soc.* 54:453–520, 1956.
15. Bird A.C., McDonald W.I.: Essential blepharospasm. *Trans. Ophthalmol. Soc. U.K.* 95:250–253, 1975.
16. Coles W.H.: Essential blepharospasm. *South. Med. J.* 66:1407–1411, 1973.
17. Reckless J.B.: Hysterical blepharospasm treated by psychotherapy and conditioning procedures in a group setting. *Psychosomatics* 13:263–264, 1972.
18. Sharpe R.: Behavior therapy in a case of blepharospasm. *Br. J. Psychiatry* 124:603–604, 1974.
19. Hardar A., Clancy J.: Case report of successful treatment of a reflex trigeminal nerve blepharospasm. *Am. J. Ophthalmol.* 75:148–149, 1973.
20. Wickramasekera I.: Hypnosis and broad-spectrum behavior therapy for blepharospasm: A case study. *Int. J. Clin. Exp. Hypn.* 22:201–209, 1974.
21. Meige H.: Les convulsions de la face, une forme clinique de convulsion faciale, bilaterale et mediane. *Rev. Neurol. (Paris)* 10:437–443, 1910.
22. Tolosa E.S.: Clinical features of Meige's disease (idiopathic orofacial dystonia): A report of 17 cases. *Arch. Neurol.* 38:147–151, 1981.
23. Paulson G.W.: Meige's syndrome: Dyskinesia of the eyelids and facial muscles. *Geriatrics* 27:69–73, 1972.

24. Coles W.H.: Signs of essential blepharospasm. A motion-picture analysis. *Arch. Ophthalmol.* 95:1006–1007, 1977.
25. Crane G.E.: Persistent dyskinesia. *Br. J. Psychiatry* 122:395–397, 1973.
26. Casey D.E.: Pharmacology of blepharospasm-oromandibular dystonia syndrome. *Neurology (NY)* 30:690–695, 1980.
27. Tolosa E.S., Lai C.: Meige disease: Striatal dopaminergic preponderance. *Neurology (Minneap.)* 29:1126–1130, 1979.
28. Tanner C.M., Glantz R.H., Klawans H.C.: Meige disease: Acute and chronic cholinergic effects. *Neurology (NY)* [*Suppl.*] 31:78, 1981.
29. Fahn J.: The use of high-dose anticholinergics in dystonia. *Neurology (Minneap.)* 29:605, 1979.
30. Tanner C.M., Goetz C.G., Klawans H.C.: Cholinergic mechanisms in spasmodic torticollis. *Neurology (Minneap.)* 29:604, 1979.
31. Gollomp S., Ilson J., Burke R., et al.: Meige syndrome: A review of 31 cases. *Neurology (NY)* [*Suppl.*] 31:78, 1981.
32. Merikangas J.R., Reynolds C.F.: Blepharospasm: Successful treatment with clonazepam. *Ann. Neurol.* 5:401–402, 1979.
33. Reynolds D.H., Smith J.C., Walsh T.J.: Differential section of the facial nerve for blepharospasm. *Trans. Am. Acad. Ophthalmol. Otolaryngol.* 71:656–664, 1967.
34. Frueh B.R., Callahan A., Dortzbach R.K., et al.: The effects of differential section of the seventh nerve on patients with intractable blepharospasm. *Trans. Am. Acad. Ophthalmol. Otolaryngol.* 81:597–602, 1976.
35. Gillum W.N., Anderson R.L.: Blepharospasm surgery. *Arch. Ophthalmol.* 99:1056–1062, 1981.

11–1 **Screening Method for Chiasmal Visual Field Defects.** A distinction between chiasmal and prechiasmal lesions in patients with optic neuropathy is critical to the selection of appropriate management. Jonathan D. Trobe, Paulo C. Acosta, and Jeffrey P. Krischer (Univ. of Florida, Gainesville) evaluated a "selective" visual field procedure concentrating on a zone with borders 45 degrees to either side of the vertical meridian. Examination time is reduced from an average of 20 to 5 minutes per eye. Study was made of 28 eyes with hemianopic defects on conventional Goldmann perimetry, 17 with nerve fiber bundle defects, and 14 with no visual field defects. The hemianopic defects were in patients with proved chiasmal compressive lesions, usually

(11–1) Arch. Ophthalmol. 99:264–271, February 1981.

pituitary tumors. The patients with nerve fiber bundle defects had inactive ischemic or dysthyroid optic neuropathy and optic neuritis.

The selective procedure was completely sensitive and had a specificity of 84%. False positive results were obtained in five eyes with nonhemianopic nerve fiber bundle defects in reference fields whose borders fell within 15 degrees of the vertical meridian. All the hemianopic defects were identified by kinetic tests alone and all but one by static methods. Selective perimetry along the vertical meridian on the conventional and projected-stimulus tangent screen was slightly less sensitive than the same procedure done on the Goldmann perimeter, but it was equally specific.

The potential accuracy of office perimetry by the selective method remains to be determined, but it is a simple, concise, standardizable technique. A combination of kinetic and suprathreshold tests appears to be necessary. Static testing is especially helpful close to fixation, whereas kinetic testing across the hemianopic border would probably improve the specificity of the procedure.

▶ [There is no test more exhausting for the patient than visual field analysis. Automation may improve standardization and help the ophthalmologist, but studies like this make it possible to shorten the examination time, decrease the patient's difficulty, and furnish more reliable information.] ◀

11–2 **Pattern-Onset Visual Evoked Potentials in Suspected Multiple Sclerosis.** The averaged visual evoked potential (VEP) has been reported to be useful in diagnosis of multiple sclerosis and other disorders affecting the anterior visual pathways. Michael J. Aminoff and Alfred L. Ochs compared the VEP obtained by a standard checkerboard pattern-reversal stimulus with that obtained by pattern onset of the same checkerboard in 11 normal subjects and in 105 patients with possible multiple sclerosis referred for electrophysiologic evaluation.

In normal subjects, pattern-onset VEPs were generally larger, better defined, and less ambiguous than those elicited by pattern reversal, because of the biphasic wave form typically obtained with pattern-onset stimulation. The latency of the chief positive peak elicited by pattern-onset stimulation was significantly shorter than that elicited by pattern-reversal stimulation. Normal VEPs were recorded in 68 of the 105 patients with possible multiple sclerosis. In 9 others the records could not be adequately compared. In the other 28 patients, monocularly elicited potentials obtained by either technique or both were prolonged in latency to beyond 2.5 SD above the mean for normal subjects in at least one eye. Both methods showed a prolonged latency in 20 patients, in 6 of whom the abnormality was bilateral. In 7 patients the pattern-onset VEPs were delayed in both eyes, whereas the pattern-reversal VEPs were normal in both eyes. In 1 patient a prolonged-latency VEP was found on pattern-reversal stimulation, whereas the responses to pattern-onset stimulation were normal. Some patients had bilateral VEP abnormalities not indicated by the pattern-reversal technique. When abnormal VEPs were found with pattern-onset stimulation, both the principal positive and the principal negative waves generally were delayed. In all patients with abnormal VEPs, subsequent findings have so far been consistent with possible multiple sclerosis.

Pattern-onset VEP recording produces less ambiguous responses than pattern-reversal stimulation in normal subjects and reveals more abnormalities in patients with possible multiple sclerosis. When the visual system is adapted to the stimulating pattern, the pattern itself may become less effective in revealing abnormality within the visual pathways.

▶ [Visual evoked potential recording is essential in the diagnosis of multiple sclerosis. False positive results are rare and the authors' use of a new stimulus that appears to result in a more sensitive test is of considerable value. Pattern-reversal stimulation is more sensitive than flash stimulation, and now pattern-onset stimulation appears to be better than either one.] ◀

11-3 **Occipital Lobe Infarctions: Perimetry and Computed Tomography.** Robert H. Spector, Joel S. Glaser, Noble J. David, and Donald Q. Vining reevaluated standard views of striate cortex organization by performing computed tomography on 7 patients with varying patterns of homonymous visual loss caused by ischemic infarction of the occipital lobe. All patients had unilateral or bilateral occlusion of arteries supplying the visual cortex.

Woman, 35, had right homonymous visual loss preceding a migrainous headache. In contrast to previous episodes, the visual loss persisted. Perimetry done 22 days later showed complete right homonymous hemianopia (Fig 11–1, A). Acuity was normal bilaterally. Computed tomography showed a large infarction extending along the entire length of the left calcarine cortex (Fig 11–1, B).

Computed tomography is an effective means of demonstrating the anatomic extent of cerebral infarction in the occipital lobe for correlation with visual field findings. Ischemic necrosis of the posterolateral part of the striate cor-

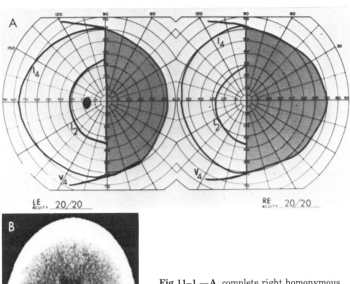

Fig 11–1.—**A,** complete right homonymous hemianopia. **B,** large left occipital infarction involves entire striate cortex *(arrows)*. (Courtesy of Spector, R. H., et al.: Neurology (NY) 31:1098–1106, September 1981.)

tex, where the "hemimacular" fibers project, correlated with homonymous field defects involving the central 5–10 degrees of vision in 4 of the 7 patients. Computed tomography provided data on the vertical disposition as well as the longitudinal extent of cerebral lesions.

The findings in patients with both unilateral and bilateral ischemic occipital lobe defects in this series are in accord with the clinicopathologic correlations proposed by Holmes and Lister in 1916. Their scheme of retinotopic organization appears to require no major alteration.

▶ [It seems amazing that a study like this can be done and computed tomography is only the beginning. Indeed, one of the problems is that the brain lesions are not visible during the immediate onset of the infarction, but this is not a problem for the techniques on the horizon. One of the new methods being developed is the use of nonradioactive xenon with computed tomography. Still more exciting is the use of nuclear magnetic resonance imaging using, instead of x-rays, entirely benign radio waves, to obtain detailed images of the brain.] ◀

11-4 **Gliomas of Intracranial Anterior Optic Pathways in Children: Role of Computed Tomography, Angiography, Pneumoencephalography, and Radionuclide Brain Scanning.** Mario Savoiardo, Derek C. Harwood-Nash, Rina Tadmor, Giuseppe Scotti, and Mark A. Musgrave (Hosp. for Sick Children, Toronto) compared the results of various diagnostic procedures in 22 children, seen since the introduction of computed tomography (CT) in 1975, with glioma of the optic nerves, chiasm, optic tracts, or more than one of these. In 16 patients the diagnosis was confirmed by operation and histologic study. The other 6 had excellent neuroradiologic evidence of tumor. Patients with evidence of a primary origin in other structures or without apparent intracranial extension were excluded.

All the patients who were operated on had low-grade astrocytomas. Four patients in the series had neurofibromatosis. The extent of the proved gliomas is shown in Figure 11–2. Ten patients had abnormalities on plain skull x-ray films, and tomography showed enlargement of one or both optic canals in all but 1 of 13 patients, sometimes accompanied by tunneling. Radionuclide brain scans were abnormal in 5 of 7 patients. Pneumoencephalography showed in-

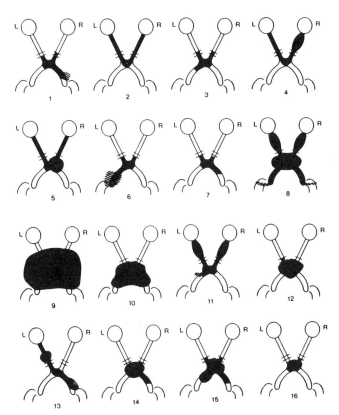

Fig 11–2.—Schematic drawings of gliomas of anterior optic pathways at operation in 16 patients. Tumor is indicated by solid areas; extension outside outline of optic pathways is indicated only when tumor reached considerable size, with nodular exophytic growth. Tumor contiguous to other structures in different planes, such as pulvinar, thalamus, or pineal region, is indicated by hatched areas. (Courtesy of Savoiardo, M., et al.: Radiology 138:601–610, March 1981.)

volvement of the chiasm in 10 of 14. Ten of 14 angiographic studies showed displacement and stretching of vessels indicative of a suprasellar mass. The entire extent of the tumors was best seen on CT. All but 5 tumors were enhanced to various degrees after contrast injection. Calcifications were seen in 3 patients, in 2 only on postirradiation CT scans. All patients but 1 had involvement of the optic chiasm. Spread to the optic tract was present in 13 patients, bilaterally in 5. Tumor reached the lateral geniculate body in 4 patients, bilaterally in 2. No tumor extended posteriorly to the optic radiations.

Computed tomography has become the single most useful means of evaluating gliomas of the anterior optic pathways, regardless of their extent. Air studies are more sensitive in showing minor changes in size of the optic chiasm and intracranial optic nerves. Only contrast-enhanced CT scans have demonstrated tumor spread along the optic tract, although in a few cases such extension was not apparent on CT studies.

11–5 **Reduced Contrast Sensitivity in Compressive Lesions of the Anterior Visual Pathway.** Patients with sellar masses frequently have visual abnormalities due to compression of the optic chiasm, optic nerve, or optic tract, but subtle deficits may not be detected by routine tests. Mark J. Kupersmith, Irwin M. Siegel, and Ronald E. Carr (New York Univ.) evaluated contrast sensitivity in 85 eyes of 46 patients in whom surgical or neuroradiologic observations suggested compression of the chiasm or optic nerve. Mean age was 47 years. Most patients had pituitary tumors. Pupillary abnormalities were present in 39 eyes and abnormal visual fields with use of a 2-mm red test object in 73 eyes. Color vision was abnormal in 59 eyes. Contrast testing was with the procedure of Arden and Jacobson, using a series of paper plates containing a bar pattern of fixed spatial frequency and varied contrast.

Eighty of the 84 evaluable eyes had cumulative contrast scores more than 2.5 SD above the control mean. Microadenoma patients with 20/20 acuity could hardly be distinguished from normal subjects. Several patients with unilateral lesions had normal contrast sensitivity in the uninvolved eye. As Snellen acuity worsened, contrast sensitivity at all spatial frequencies decreased. Contrast scores were lower after operation; the degree of improvement was predicted by the preoperative acuity. Postoperative patients, however, did not achieve sensitivities comparable with those of normal subjects. The residual losses were obvious to patients but were not revealed by Snellen acuity testing.

Contrast sensitivity appears to be a sensitive index of compressive lesions of the optic chiasm. Patients with little or no visual defect on routine testing may exhibit dramatic losses of contrast sensitivity. The procedure is useful in evaluating the immediate results of operation.

▶ [This study is convincing that contrast sensitivity is a sensitive index for chiasmal lesions. It is only fair to point out, however, that similar claims for the use of the test in other diseases such as glaucoma have been difficult to prove.] ◀

11-6 **Meningioma and the Ophthalmologist: Review of 80 Cases.** Duncan Anderson and Mourad Khalil (McGill Univ.) reviewed the records of 80 patients seen from 1960 to 1977 with proved meningiomas, all of whom had at least partial tumor removal. The 50 females and 30 males had a mean age of 57.4 years. The ophthalmologic symptoms are listed in Table 1 and the signs in Table 2. Ten patients had a third, fourth, or sixth cranial nerve palsy. About one third of patients had features related to the afferent visual system. Headache was reported by just under half the patients, and often had been present for some time before diagnosis. Twenty-six patients had an isolated seizure. The most common neurologic signs were hemiplegia and hemisensory loss. Ten patients were asymptomatic. Only 62% of skull x-ray films were abnormal. Three fourths of EEGs were abnormal, but the findings were often nonspecific. Four of 69 cerebral angiograms were normal.

Most meningiomas were in the frontal lobe and olfactory groove, followed by the parietal and parasagittal regions. Five of 35 patients with frontal lobe tumors had visual loss due to direct compression of the optic nerves. Five of 14 patients with parietal lobe tumors and 4 of 6 with occipital lobe tumors had field defects, usually homonymous. Six of 9 patients with sphenoid ridge meningiomas had loss of vision. On follow-up for 2 to 18 years after operation, 74% of patients were cured by one procedure and 11 others did well after two operations. Only 12% of patients died of tumor, mostly in the earlier years of the study. Nearly half the patients had no permanent disability after tumor removal. Fourteen patients had a visual or field deficit.

About one third of patients with meningioma in this se-

TABLE 1.—Ophthalmologic Symptoms in 80 Patients With Meningioma

Symptom	Number of Patients
Permanent visual loss	14
Transient visual loss	8
Symptomatic visual field loss	7
Diplopia	6
Proptosis	3
Orbital pain	3

TABLE 2.—Ophthalmologic Signs in 18 Patients With Meningioma

Sign	Number of Patients
Papilledema	16
Visual loss	14
Visual field defect	12
Third, fourth, or sixth nerve palsy	10
Nystagmus	9
Bony swelling	5
Exophthalmos	4

ries had ophthalmologic signs or symptoms. The brain scan was the most useful noninvasive study. All but 12% of patients were cured by operation. Eighteen percent of patients had a permanent visual or field deficit.

▶ [One third of patients with meningioma in this series had visual deficit, and it is disturbing that in almost one half of these patients the visual deficit was misdiagnosed initially.] ◀

11–7 **Management of Primary Optic Nerve Meningiomas: Current Status—Therapy in Controversy.** The management of primary optic nerve meningiomas is controversial. Melvin G. Alper (George Washington Univ.) reviewed experience with 55 patients. Orbital meningiomas may arise from the optic nerve meninges or invade the orbit from sites of origin within the cranial cavity. Theoretically, they also

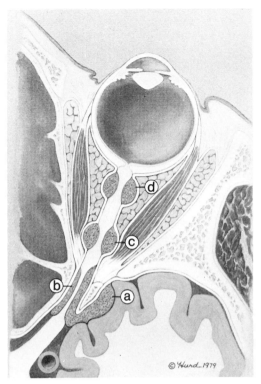

Fig 11–3.—The most common site of origin of an orbital meningioma is the cranial cavity *(A)* or, less often, the optic canal *(B)*. Other sites of origin include *(C)* the meninges of the optic nerve within the orbit, especially near the optic foramen and, less commonly, near the globe *(D)*, and the ectopic meningeal tissue in the orbit. (Courtesy of Alper, M. G.: J. Clin. Neuro-ophthalmol. 1:101–117, June 1981.)

may arise from ectopic meningeal tissue pinched off within the orbit during embryonic life (Fig 11–3). Meningiomas grow within the subdural space, up or down the dural sheath, invading the dura and obliterating the pial blood supply. They may encircle the optic nerve and compress it, causing atrophy with profound visual loss, or invade the nerve itself. Coronic compression of the optic nerve leads to the formation of retinociliary shunt veins. Computed tomography may show tubular or bulbous enlargement of the optic nerve, midorbital fusiform enlargement of the nerve, and enhancement after injection of contrast medium.

Of 12 patients under age 20 years who were followed up, 2 are alive without recurrence and 5 with recurrence. Four died with intracranial extension, and 1 died of Reye's disease. Seven of 12 patients aged 20–35 years are alive without disease and 4 with recurrence; 1 died of intracranial extension. Seven of 13 patients aged 35–50 years are alive without disease, and 2 with recurrent disease. Four died of other causes, but 3 of them had intracranial meningioma. Five of 6 patients older than age 50 years were alive without disease at follow-up; 1 died of associated causes. Sixteen patients required reoperation.

Younger patients who have lost vision should undergo removal of the optic nerve and the meningioma, followed by craniotomy with unroofing of the orbit and optic canal. Older patients with good vision are followed by computed tomography scanning every 6 months and visual field plotting every 3 months. If vision worsens and the apex of the orbit is spared, a Kroenlein approach may be tried; however, the author prefers to wait until vision is lost and then to remove the optic nerve totally along with the tumor. Recurrence in the orbital apex or intracranially calls for exenteration and craniotomy. Radiotherapy may be used as an alternative in adults.

11–8 **Paralysis of Cranial Nerves III, IV, and VI: Cause and Prognosis in 1,000 Cases.** James A. Rush and Brian R. Younge (Mayo Clinic) reviewed an unselected series of 1,000 cases of extraocular muscle dysfunction due to acquired lesions of the third, fourth, and sixth cranial nerves. Data were sought from 475 patients with paralysis from unknown, vascular, or traumatic causes, and 252 questionnaires were returned after an average interval of 5.7 years. The sex distribution of the large series was nearly equal. Three fourths of patients were older than age 35 years. The sixth nerve alone was affected in 419 cases, the third nerve in 290, and the fourth nerve in 172. There were 45 cases of paralysis of all 3 nerves, 35 of combined third and fourth

CAUSES OF PARALYSIS AND RECOVERY RATES OF AFFECTED CRANIAL NERVES*†

Cause	Cranial Nerves Affected							Total
	III	IV	VI	III and IV	III and VI	III, IV, and VI	IV and VI	
Undetermined	34/67	34/62	63/124	0/2	2/3	1/5	...	134/263
Trauma	17/47	24/55	27/70	1/6	3/6	7/13	...	79/197
Neoplasm	8/34	3/7	13/61	1/4	3/14	1/23	...	29/143
Vascular	44/60	24/32	51/74	...	2/5	1/1	...	122/172
Aneurysm†	15/40	1/3	10/15	3/6	1/2	2/4	1/1	33/71
Other	22/42	6/13	44/75	2/5	6/11	6/8	...	86/154
Total	140/290	92/172	208/419	7/23	17/41	18/54	1/1	483/1,000

*Numerator denotes number of patients known to have recovered partially or completely; denominator is total number of patients in each group; a few patients in each group were unavailable for follow-up and recovery is unknown.
†Includes 25 cases of subarachnoid hemorrhage.

nerve paralysis, and 19 of combined third and sixth nerve paralysis.

The cause of third nerve paralysis was undetermined in nearly one fourth of cases. The commonest identified causes were vascular factors and head trauma. Complete or partial recovery occurred in 48.3% of cases. More than one third of cases of fourth nerve paralysis were of undetermined cause. Head trauma was a factor in one third of these cases. Recovery was observed in 53.5% of cases. Paralysis of the sixth nerve was of undetermined cause in about 30% of cases. The leading specific causes were vascular disease, head trauma, and neoplasia. Recovery occurred in 49.6% of these cases. Infratentorial neoplasia was the commonest cause of multiple cranial nerve palsies. Multiple palsies remitted partially or completely in nearly 40% of cases.

This and other series of studies indicate a decline in the frequency of aneurysm-related cases of ocular paralysis. Recovery rates in cases of varying etiologies are shown in the table. More than two thirds of patients with palsies due to vascular disease recovered. The proportion of cases of undetermined cause remains high. Only 10 of 127 patients followed up who had no diagnosis made at the last examination reported that a cause had been identified.

11–9 **Epidemiology of Giant Cell Arteritis Including Temporal Arteritis and Polymyalgia Rheumatica: Incidences of Different Clinical Presentations and Eye Complications.** Giant cell arteritis is not rare in elderly persons. The most serious complication is blindness. Bengt-Åke Bengtsson and Bo-Eric Malmvall (Univ. of Göteborg) reviewed the findings in 126 patients in whom the diagnosis of giant cell arteritis was made between 1973 and 1975. Temporal artery biopsy provided histologic evidence of arteritis in 74 patients. The calculated annual incidence of giant cell arteritis was 9.3 per 100,000 persons, or 28.6 per 100,000 persons older than age 50 years. The respective figures for histologically proved giant cell arteritis were 5.5 and 16.8 per 100,000. Incidence rates are presented in the table.

Polymyalgia rheumatica was observed in 71% of all pa-

(11–9) Arthritis Rheum. 24:899–904, July 1981.

ANNUAL INCIDENCE OF GIANT CELL ARTERITIS IN GÖTEBORG, SWEDEN, 1973–1975 IN RELATION TO AGE AND SEX OF PATIENTS

	Men*		Women		Total	
	No. of patients	Incidence rate	No. of patients	Incidence rate	No. of patients	Incidence rate
All patients per 100,000 inhabitants	41 (28)	6.1 (4.2)	85 (46)	12.4 (6.7)	126 (74)	9.3 (5.5)
All patients per 100,000 inhabitants aged 50 years and over	41 (28)	20.4 (13.9)	85 (46)	35.3 (19.1)	126 (74)	28.6 (16.8)
Patients within each age group per 100,000 inhabitants in the same age group:						
50–59 years	6 (4)	6.8 (4.6)	6 (3)	6.4 (3.2)	12 (7)	6.6 (3.9)
60–69 years	13 (11)	19.8 (16.8)	27 (15)	34.3 (19.1)	40 (26)	27.7 (18.0)
70–79 years	14 (11)	40.4 (31.8)	39 (21)	78.6 (42.3)	53 (32)	62.9 (38.0)
80+ years	8 (2)	73.1 (18.3)	13 (7)	68.3 (36.8)	21 (9)	70.1 (30.0)

*Numbers in parentheses indicate biopsy-proved disease.

tients and in 79% of women. Signs or symptoms of temporal arteritis were present in 39% of patients. In 8% of patients only general symptoms were noted. Fifteen patients (12%) had ocular complications, including 9 with major complications resulting in permanently impaired acuity. Eight of these patients had anterior ischemic optic neuropathy, and 1 had retinal stroke. Four of these 9 patients had symptoms consistent with localized arteritis, and 5 had muscular or general symptoms only. Three had negative temporal artery biopsies. In 1 patient, acute blindness was the initial manifestation of giant cell arteritis. In the other 8, visual symptoms appeared 1–6 months after other manifestations of disease. The age of patients with major ocular complications was similar to that of the other patients.

Giant cell arteritis is not an uncommon condition, but it is rare in patients under age 50 years. Ocular complications may occur in patients with polymyalgia rheumatica who lack clinical evidence of temporal arteritis. Temporal artery biopsy is indicated in patients over age 50 with general symptoms, including fever of unknown origin and laboratory findings compatible with giant cell arteritis. Severe ocular complications can occur in any clinical form of giant cell arteritis. The most common complication is anterior ischemic optic neuropathy due to lesions in the ophthalmic artery or its branches. Steroids are indicated early in the course to prevent damage to the second eye; they usually fail to improve vision in already damaged eyes.

11–10 **The Tolosa-Hunt Syndrome: Further Clinical and Pathogenetic Considerations Based on the Study of Eight Cases.** The cause and pathogenesis in Tolosa-Hunt syndrome (THS) of remittent, sometimes recurrent episodes of painful ophthalmoplegia remain unclear. D. Inzitari, D. Sità, G. P. Marconi, and F. Barontini (Univ. of Florence) reviewed the findings in 8 patients, 3 men and 5 women aged 26–75 years. Three had recurrent attacks, 2 of them bilaterally. All patients had oculomotor nerve involvement, most often of the third and sixth nerves. Steroids relieved the pain but did not always reduce the duration of ophthalmoplegia. Three patients had a persistent deficit after a single episode. Steroid therapy, even in high dosage, did not influence the final outcome.

The pain is not vascular in nature, but rather resembles trigeminal or sympathetic pain. Pain preceded the onset of oculomotor weakness in all but 1 of the present cases. Vegetative symptoms were present in 3 patients. One patient had a clear family history of migraine. Cerebral angiograms have shown flattening and narrowing of the cavernous part of the internal carotid artery. Orbital phlebography has been reported to show complete or partial obliteration of the superior ophthalmic vein or the cavernous sinus, but the findings were normal in 4 of 5 cases in the present series. Elevated cerebrospinal fluid protein levels have been described and were observed in 2 of the present patients. Cranial and orbital computed tomography findings were normal in the 3 patients examined. The 3 patients with leukocytosis had an elevated sedimentation rate. No evidence of autoimmune disease was obtained. Visual evoked potentials were delayed in 3 of 4 cases, although the optic nerves were clinically normal.

These findings confirm the view that THS is a definite clinical entity, but its cause remains unknown. The occasional findings of carotidographic and venographic abnormalities and of systemic evidence of inflammation support Hunt's hypothesis of indolent inflammation of the cavernous sinus. Some clinical features may suggest a neuritis.

▶ [With the disease supposedly localized to the infraorbital fissure area, it is peculiar that the visual evoked response should be affected. The authors conclude that the Tolosa-Hunt syndrome may be an ocular polyneuritis, and it is fortunate that the disease responds well to corticosteroid therapy.] ◀

1-11 **Acephalgic Migraine: Fifteen Years' Experience.** Patrick S. O'Connor and Thomas J. Tredici (USAF School of Aerospace Medicine, Brooks AFB, Texas) report a study of 61 patients with acephalgic migraine seen from 1965 to 1979, the largest such series to be reported. Average age at onset (Table 1) was 31 years. Only one fourth of patients had a family history of migraine. Various scotomas were recorded (Table 2). The occurrence of other neurologic involvement was surprisingly frequent (Table 3). No persistent defects were observed. Most episodes lasted 5 to 30 minutes (Table 4). One patient was a heavy smoker, and 3

TABLE 1.—AGE AT ONSET

Age	No.	Percent
12–29	25/61	41%
30–35	20/61	33%
35–40	8/61	13%
Over 40	8/61	13%

TABLE 2.—SCOTOMAS

	No. Patients
Right homonymous	16/61
Left homonymous	16/61
Over both fields	2/61
Complete homonymous hemianopia	5/61
Monocular crescent	7/61
Altitudinal	4/61
Bitemporal	1/61
Bilateral central	7/61
Unilateral central	2/61
Tunnel vision	9/61
Amaurosis fugax	8/61

TABLE 3.—Other Neurologic Involvement

	No. Patients
Diplopia	7/61
Parasthesia	8/61
Dysphasia	4/61
Cloudy thinking	3/61
Dysarthria	2/61
Vertigo	1/61
Total	18/61 = 29.5%

TABLE 4.—Length of Spells

	No. Patients
50 to 60 seconds	2 (4)*
1 to 5 minutes	7
5 to 10 minutes	10
10 to 20 minutes	15
20 to 30 minutes	11
30 to 40 minutes	5
40 to 50 minutes	7
hours	4

*Whereas only 2 had spells lasting consistently less than 1 minute, 4 others with longer classic spells had many single episodes lasting less than 1 minute.

reported that exposure to flickering lights led to symptoms. Only 2 patients had a history of migraine headache.

The content and time course of attacks in these cases conformed to those of migrainous auras. The differential diagnosis includes recurrent microemboli and focal epilepsy. Only 1 patient in this study had a significant EEG dysrhythmia. The all-male nature of the group was the only nonrepresentative aspect. It may be concluded that acephalgic migraine is common, can occur at any age, and not infrequently occurs with other transient neurologic involvement. Acephalgic migraine should be considered in any patient with an acute, episodic neurologic disorder. It is most often seen by the ophthalmologist.

▶ [There is some debate about the use of the word "migraine" when the disease is free of headache. This seems primarily a semantic problem, made especially complex when it is realized that migraine means only "half-cranium." The important point is that most of these patients are seen by ophthalmologists.] ◀

Chapter 11–NEURO-OPHTHALMOLOGY / 313

11–12 **Ischemic Optic Neuropathy With Painful Ophthalmoplegia in Diabetes Mellitus.** Douglas A. Jabs, Neil R. Miller, and W. Richard Green (Johns Hopkins Med. Inst.) recently encountered 2 patients with adult-onset diabetes who simultaneously experienced unilateral painful ophthalmoplegia and severe ipsilateral retrobulbar optic neuropathy. The condition was relatively unresponsive to steroid therapy, but resolved spontaneously over 2–3 months. The patients were a woman aged 48 and a man aged 57 years. Acuity decreased rapidly in one eye in both patients. Histologic study of the optic nerve of the man following exploration, which showed the intracanalicular nerve to be erythematous and swollen, revealed ischemic necrosis with transitional zones between the necrotic and normal regions. Some peripheral areas of the infarcted zone were infiltrated by numerous histiocytes containing finely granular material. Some vessels showed lymphocytic infiltration of their walls, but none was occluded.

These patients both were middle-aged adults with mild diabetes. Acuity was lost over a week or less and reduced to no light perception, and multiple unilateral, painful cranial nerve palsies were present, involving the third and sixth nerves. The nerve palsies resolved totally. Steroid therapy did not relieve the pain. Histologic study in 1 case showed an optic nerve infarct. Both patients apparently experienced unilateral painful ophthalmoplegia and optic neuropathy from the microangiopathy associated with diabetes. This "orbital apex/cavernous sinus" syndrome should be considered in diabetics in whom other causes have been ruled out and who fail to respond well to steroid therapy. The differential diagnosis of painful ophthalmoplegia associated with ipsilateral optic neuropathy includes tumors, vascular lesions such as aneurysms and carotid-cavernous sinus fistulas, and inflammatory lesions such as the Tolosa-Hunt syndrome.

1–13 **Intracranial Pressure Following Optic Nerve Decompression for Benign Intracranial Hypertension: Case Report.** Optic nerve decompression has been shown

(11–12) Br. J. Ophthalmol. 65:673–678, October 1981.
(11–13) J. Neurosurg. 55:453–456, September 1981.

to reverse visual deterioration in patients with benign intracranial hypertension, but it is unclear whether this is due to a direct release of pressure on the optic nerve head or to a reduction in intracranial pressure from leakage of cerebrospinal fluid (CSF) through the windows cut in the dural sheath surrounding the optic nerve. Andrew H. Kaye, J. E. K. Galbraith, and John King (Melbourne) describe a patient with benign intracranial hypertension and visual failure in whom intracranial pressure was monitored before and after bilateral optic nerve sheath decompression.

Woman, 51, with constant headache for 14 months, was mildly hypertensive and had bilateral papilledema. Corrected acuities were 6/6 on the left and 6/12 on the right, with normal visual fields. A computed tomographic study of the brain yielded normal findings. The lumbar CSF pressure was 330 mm water. Optic disc swelling progressed over the next 6 months despite weight reduction and glycerol treatment, and transient visual obscurations developed. Bilateral optic nerve sheath decompression therefore was carried out, with creation of 3×5-mm windows in the dural sheath of the optic nerves. The baseline systolic intracranial pressure was about 30 mm Hg, and the amplitude of swings was 8 to 10 mm Hg. The b waves rose to a height of 45 mm Hg. The pressure did not change significantly after optic nerve sheath decompression. Papilledema subsided rapidly after operation, and the visual obscurations improved. Corrected acuity was 6/6 in both eyes 2 months postoperatively.

Visual acuity may be reduced in up to half of patients with benign intracranial hypertension. Elevated CSF pressure has a significant role in the development of papilledema. The exact mechanism of action of optic nerve decompression is unclear, but no fall in intracranial pressure was found in this patient after bilateral optic nerve sheath decompression. The improvement in papilledema appears to have been due to a local effect of decreased pressure on the optic nerve head.

▶ [Optic nerve sheath decompression is apparently effective in some cases, but indications for the procedure have not been clearly established. This patient evidently did not have periodic cerebrospinal fluid removal, nor was the possibility of a shunt considered.] ◀

12. Medical Ophthalmology and Drug Therapy

Opportunistic Infections

LEE M. JAMPOL, M.D.

Eye and Ear Infirmary, University of Illinois, Chicago

Many recent articles in the ophthalmic literature describe ocular infections caused by unusual opportunistic organisms.[1] These organisms rarely produce infections in healthy persons or healthy eyes; instead, they show a marked predisposition for immunodebilitated or immunosuppressed patients or tissues that have been damaged from other causes. Opportunistic pathogens may cause keratitis, scleritis, uveitis, retinitis, chorioretinitis, orbital cellulitis, or endophthalmitis. The increased rate of diagnosis of opportunistic infections is partly the result of improved diagnostic acumen. However, the incidence of these infections is undoubtedly increasing.

Among the factors most important in the increasing frequency of these infections is the use of corticosteroids. Topical corticosteroids predispose to viral or fungal keratitis. The use of high doses of systemic corticosteroids in patients with renal transplants, cancer, acquired diseases of connective tissue, and other conditions predisposes to the occurrence of systemic opportunistic infections; these infections may involve the eye. The use of other immunosuppressive drugs, such as azathioprine in organ transplant recipients or potent cytotoxic drugs in patients with malignancies, is similarly immunosuppressive. Other factors in the development of opportunistic infections include the use of potent antibiotics that destroy the normal bacterial flora and allow overgrowth of unusual organisms, indwelling intravenous cannulas and narcotic abuse that provide unsterile portals of entry for organisms, and longer survival of patients with malignancies, especially lymphoreticular tumors. Other factors that may also be important are listed in Table 1.

Some of the more common opportunists seen in ophthalmology are listed in Table 2. I will briefly describe the clinical appearance of three opportunists that may affect the retina, a virus (cytomegalovirus), a fungus *(Candida),* and a bacterium *(Nocardia).*

CYTOMEGALOVIRUS RETINITIS

The cytomegalovirus is a DNA virus that differs from herpes simplex in its tendency to induce abnormal large cells that give the infection its name. Intranuclear and intracytoplasmic inclusions often are present. Cytomegalovirus infection is usually benign, and up to 80% of the population shows evidence of previous infection by age 35. The infection may be entirely asymptomatic, although there may be upper respiratory or lower respiratory tract involvement, gastroenteritis, or infectious mononucleosis syndrome. Congenital infections and infections in immunodebilitated patients are more serious.

TABLE 1.—FACTORS PREDISPOSING TO OPPORTUNISTIC INFECTIONS

Corticosteroids
Other immunosuppressive drugs
Irradiation
Antibiotics
Intravenous cannulas
Narcotic abuse
Malignancies
Dysproteinemias, congenital immune deficiencies
Acquired diseases of connective tissue
Trauma, surgery
Diabetes mellitus, acidosis
Bacterial, viral infections
Alcoholism
Decreased or abnormal polymorphonuclear leukocytes
Burns
Uremia

TABLE 2.—OPPORTUNISTS IN
OPHTHALMOLOGY (PARTIAL LISTING)

FUNGI

Candida
Aspergillus
Fusarium
Cryptococcus
Histoplasma capsulatum
Coccidioides immitis
Phycomycetes (mucormycosis)
Nocardia asteroides*

VIRUSES

Herpes simplex
Herpes zoster
Cytomegalovirus
Measles virus

PROTOZOA

Toxoplasma gondii

BACTERIA

Mycobacterium tuberculosis
Listeria
Others

*A filamentous bacterium.

Congenital cytomegalic inclusion disease,[2] which results from intrauterine infection of the fetus, should be distinguished from neonatal infections caused by cytomegalovirus. It is estimated that about 1% of all newborns are infected by cytomegalovirus before birth, and perhaps one third of these have significant morbidity from the infection. The baby may be asymptomatic or may be premature and show skin rash, fever, failure to thrive, thrombocytopenia, anemia, pneumonitis, gastroenteritis, or hepatitis. Splenomegaly is common. Microcephaly and cerebral calcification may be present. About one third of these babies have evidence of retinitis. Other ocular manifestations can include conjunctivitis, cataract, and optic nerve hypoplasia and colobomas. The retinitis frequently involves the macular areas.

Adult cytomegalovirus retinitis is a very different disease. It is found almost exclusively in immunodebilitated patients.[3] Renal and cardiac transplant recipients are very susceptible, and patients with leukemia and lymphoma frequently also are involved. Patients with cytomegalovirus infections also seem to be more susceptible to other opportunists. Recently, an association of cytomegalovirus infection, other opportunistic infections (e.g., *Pneumocystis carinii*), and Kaposi's sarcoma increasingly has been noted, especially in the male homosexual population.[4] The reason for this clustering of diseases is uncertain.

The earliest lesions of cytomegalic retinitis are small whitish or yellowish exudates that appear in the retina or at the level of the pigment epithelium. The lesions become confluent, with large areas of white necrotic retina. Retinal vasculitis and vascular occlusions occur. There frequently are multiple hemorrhages, and a branch vein occlusion may be misdiagnosed. The retinal vessels may become totally nonperfused. If the lesions heal, the area of retinitis shows gradually increasing hyperpigmentation. During this stage, retinal tears or detachment may occur. In rare cases, cytomegalic infection also may cause nonrhegmatogenous retinal detachment. The diagnosis of cytomegalovirus infection is based on a characteristic picture in combination with positive viral cultures of the urine, buffy coat of the blood, and other sites. Examination of tissues for giant cells and inclusions is helpful. Serologic testing also may be important. In our laboratory, complement fixing and immunofluorescent techniques are used. Treatment of cytomegalovirus should include an attempt to decrease the administration of immunosuppressive drugs. Systemic antiviral agents such as adenine arabinoside or acyclovir recently have been tested, but their efficacy for the retinitis remains uncertain. The differential diagnosis of cytomegalovirus infection includes herpes simplex retinitis, the acute retinal necrosis syndrome, and other causes of opportunistic retinitis.

Candida RETINITIS

Candida species (especially *Candida albicans*) is presently a frequent cause of retinitis. White fluffy vitreal exudates overlying a small focus of retinitis are characteristic. A review of eyes with *Candida* endophthalmitis has shown that 59% had white fluffy exudates.[5] Some of the patients also demonstrated retinal hemorrhages and nonspecific findings such as Roth's spots, posterior uveitis, and anterior chamber reaction. Papillitis may be present. The isolation of *Candida* from the throat, urine, and other sites in an immunosuppressed patient is not proof of systemic candidiasis. The presence of the characteristic ocular lesions, however, proves systemic involvement and necessitates the institution of therapy. Because of this, ophthalmologic consultations frequently are obtained in patients in whom systemic candidiasis is suspected. If the characteristic lesions are seen, therapy includes intravenously administered amphotericin B. Fluorocytosine also has been used in recent years and appears to act synergistically with amphotericin B. Newer antifungal drugs, including the imidazoles, recently have been tested. Vitrectomy may play a role in clearing the ocular infection, as may intravitreal antifungal therapy.

Nocardia CHORIORETINITIS

Nocardia asteroides often is listed under fungal infections, although it is really a filamentous bacterium. With few exceptions, it is found in immunosuppressed patients. Although most *Nocardia* infections begin in the lungs or the skin, the eye is a secondary site in 3% of cases.[6] At the time *Nocardia* chorioretinitis is diagnosed, many patients will show signs of systemic nocardiosis. The classic ocular finding in nocardiosis is a chorioretinal abscess that may have a white or yellow coloration.[7] These lesions, which may be multiple and bilateral, gradually enlarge, with increasing vitreal reaction. The diagnosis can be made from systemic investigation or from vitreal aspiration or vitrectomy, or both, with histopathologic or cytologic examination of the vitreous fluid. Therapy of *Nocardia* chorioretinitis and systemic nocardiosis includes the use of sulfonamides and other antibiotics. Because these patients frequently are immunodebilitated, the outcome is often poor. Vitrectomy may play a therapeutic role in management of the ocular infection, if a prompt response to antibiotics is not seen.

SUMMARY

Many opportunistic viral, fungal, and bacterial infections may involve the eye. The ophthalmologist should think of these infections in the proper clinical setting, namely, a damaged eye or a immunosuppressed or immunodebilitated patient. In some situations, the clinical picture is virtually pathognomonic of the type of infection (e.g., cytomegalovirus). At other times, the clinical appearance may be suggestive (e.g., *Candida* retinitis). Appropriate tests can confirm the appropriate diagnosis and may allow preservation of both life and vision in many patients.

REFERENCES

1. Jampol L.M.: Opportunistic intraocular and orbital pathogens, in Peyman G.A., Sanders D.R., Goldberg M.F. (eds.): *Principles and Practice of Ophthalmology*. Philadelphia, W.B. Saunders Co., 1980, pp. 1654–1657.
2. Montgomery J.R., Mason E.O., Jr., Williamson A.P., et al.: Prospective study of congenital cytomegalovirus infection. *South Med. J.* 73:590–595, 1980.
3. Murray H.W., Knox D.R., Green W.R., et al.: Cytomegalovirus retinitis in adults: A manifestation of disseminated viral infection. *Am. J. Med.* 63:574–584, 1977.
4. Centers for Disease Control Task Force on Kaposi's Sarcoma and Opportunistic Infections: Epidemiologic aspects of the current outbreak of Kaposi's sarcoma and opportunistic infection. *N. Engl. J. Med.* 306:248–252, 1982.
5. Edwards J.E., Jr., Foos R.Y., Montgomerie J.Z., et al.: Ocular manifestations of *Candida septicemia:* Review of 76 cases of hematogenous endophthalmitis. *Medicine (Baltimore)* 53:47–75, 1974.
6. Palmer D.L., Harvey R.L., Wheeler J.K.: Diagnostic and therapeutic considerations in *Nocardia asteroides* infections. *Medicine (Baltimore)* 53:391–401, 1974.
7. Jampol L.M., Strauch B.S., Albert D.M.: Intraocular nocardiosis. *Am. J. Ophthalmol.* 76:568–573, 1973.

12–1 **Immunosuppressive Therapy of Behçet's Syndrome: Long-Term Follow-Up.** M. Bonnet (Lyons, France) reports data on 18 patients treated with chlorambucil. In ad-

(12–1) J. Fr. Ophtalmol. 4:455–464, 1981. (Fr.)

dition, 6 patients whose severe ocular symptoms threatened acute and permanent blindness received antilymphocyte globulins. Follow-up periods ranged from 1 to 12 years, with an average of 4.5 years. The daily dose of chlorambucil was 1–2 mg/10 kg body weight during the first 3–4 weeks, then was decreased to 0.5 mg/10 kg body weight (lesser amounts, tried in 2 patients, were followed by recurrence). Associated treatments included local application of corticoids and mydriatic agents 3 times daily in eyes presenting signs of inflammation of the anterior chamber, extraction of cataracted lens (6 eyes), and retinal photocoagulation in 4 eyes with retinal or optic disc neovascularization secondary to retinal venous occlusions.

Recovery from ocular inflammation was total in 14 patients and partial in 4. Improvement was quite rapid in patients given antilymphocyte globulins—clinically evident 1 week after initiation of treatment. In those treated with chlorambucil exclusively, inflammatory bouts recurred several times during the first 2 months of therapy, but did completely disappear after 3 months of treatment. Recurrence was observed in 3 patients at an interval of 7 months to 6 years after conclusion of treatment, seemingly without correlation to duration of therapy.

The results of this study confirm that while chlorambucil and antilymphocyte globulins have improved the prognosis of Behçet's disease dramatically, it is by no means the ultimate answer, particularly in view of the risk of severe hematotologic complications with long-term use of chlorambucil.

12–2 **Indomethacin** is discussed by Irving M. Katz (Hahnemann Med. School, Philadelphia). Indomethacin is a nonsteroidal anti-inflammatory agent with potent prostaglandin-inhibiting effects. When instilled conjunctivally in rabbits, it inhibits increased intraocular pressure after arachidonic acid administration. Indomethacin also has analgesic properties. It is well absorbed after oral administration, with peak plasma levels occurring at 30–120 minutes. The drug penetrates readily into the rabbit eye. Double-blind studies have shown variable results from indomethacin ophthalmic suspension on inflammation associated with various states. Indomethacin begun before surgery and continued postoperatively may help prevent pupillary constriction at surgery and may help reduce postoperative anterior-segment inflammation and prevent aphakic cystoid macular edema. Further controlled studies are needed to establish the role of indomethacin in ophthalmic treatment, but preliminary results have been encouraging.

Systemic indomethacin therapy is contraindicated in patients with nasal polyps associated with angioedema or a bronchospastic reaction to aspirin or other nonsteroidal antiinflammatory agents. Its safety in pregnancy has not been documented. Indomethacin may mask evidence of infection and must be used with caution in patients with existing controlled infection. The drug can inhibit platelet aggregation, and caution is needed in patients with coagulation defects. Other side effects are dose related and should be less frequent with ocular than with systemic administration. Concurrent administration of aspirin reduces plasma indomethacin levels. Levels are increased in patients receiving probenecid. Indomethacin can reduce the natriuretic and antihypertensive effects of furosemide in some patients and also blocks the furosemide-induced increase in plasma renin activity.

Prostaglandin Assay in Human Aqueous Humor After Intraocular Implantation: Effects of Indomethacin. G. Baikoff, B. Charbonnel and M. Kremer (Nantes, France). Aqueous humor from 26 patients was collected just before surgery and on the fifth postoperative day to establish the variation in prostaglandin levels as well as the presence of a prostaglandin synthetase inhibitor in patients treated with indomethacin.

The anti-inflammatory effect of indomethacin is subjectively evident when compared with the dosage of corticosteroids administered postoperatively. Subconjunctival injection of soluble corticosteroids was guided by severity of the inflammatory reaction. Among 13 patients who did not receive indomethacin, 7 received a total of 19 subconjunctival injections of corticosteroids; among 13 patients treated with

---

(12–3) J. Fr. Ophtalmol. 4:593–595, 1981. (Fr.)

indomethacin only 5 were given a total of 7 injections. Although based solely on clinical criteria, the anti-inflammatory effect of indomethacin is significant, permitting reduction of the amount of steroids required by half. Indomethacin significantly inhibits the liberation of prostaglandin E_2 in human aqueous humor. Prostaglandin E_2 levels increased without specific treatment, but with systematic administration of indomethacin no significant increase was observed. The angiographically demonstrated opening of the blood-aqueous barrier and the preventive effect of indomethacin in this regard appears most certainly mediated by ocular prostaglandin E_2.

▶ [Renewed interest in indomethacin probably has been generated by the possibility that it is beneficial in the treatment of cystoid macular edema associated with cataract extraction. It is curious that cystoid macular edema has become a major problem parallel with intraocular lens implantation. Two questions are of interest. First, is indomethacin efficacious in the treatment of cystoid macular edema, and, second, is there now more of the latter? It has been suggested that patients with extracapsulár cataract extractions have a lower incidence of the disease, an observation that evidently escaped notice 30 years ago when extracapsular cataract extraction began to be replaced by intracapsular surgery.] ◀

12-4 **Pharmacology of Ocular Drugs: 6. Oral Contraceptives.** Gissur J. Petursson, F. T. Fraunfelder, and S. Martha Meyer reviewed data in the National Registry of Drug-Induced Ocular Side Effects bearing on adverse ocular effects from the use of oral contraception. An association with systemic thromboembolic disease has been well documented, but retinal vascular occlusive states related to oral contraception are only suspected. Cases of retinal arteriolar and central retinal artery occlusion have been described, as have retinal vein occlusions, ocular hemorrhages, and macular edema. Visual field defects, optic neuritis, and retrobulbar neuritis have been reported. Acquired color vision deficiencies may develop after long-term oral contraception. Some believe that some women with retinitis pigmentosa have an accelerated loss of visual function during pregnancy. Difficulty in contact lens wear has been attributed to corneal edema, lid edema, and changes in tear composition.

Oral contraceptive use should be asked about in the course of ocular examination. Adverse ocular effects of the pill occur, but are rare. Patients with evidence of neovascularization, vasculitis, thromboembolic disorders, vascular occlusive disease, or macular disease should be discouraged from using oral contraceptives. Those with transient ischemic attacks probably should discontinue use of oral contraceptives, as should subjects with ocular symptoms caused by migraine that are aggravated by oral estrogens. Use of oral contraceptives also should be discontinued by patients with macular edema or recent disorders of color vision. Pseudotumor cerebri with secondary papilledema can occur after the use of oral contraceptives, and is an indication for discontinuing their use. Women taking estrogens should have periodic ocular evaluation including funduscopy.

▶ [The questions about oral contraceptives and ocular disease appear to continue, with very few hard data one way or the other. Nonetheless, the recommendations in this article are probably sound because the issue has so many other ramifications that, more than likely, we will never have definitive data nor be able to launch a controlled clinical trial.] ◀

12–5 **Acetazolamide and Symptomatic Metabolic Acidosis in Mild Renal Failure.** Acetazolamide, which can result in a bicarbonate diuresis, is used widely in the treatment of glaucoma because of a reduction in aqueous humor formation. D. N. Maisey and R. D. Brown (Cambridge, England) describe 2 patients in whom acetazolamide therapy for glaucoma induced symptomatic metabolic acidosis. Both patients were elderly and had mild renal impairment. They received acetazolamide in a dose of 250 mg, 2 or 3 times a day. Both patients presented with confusion and tachypnea. The patients improved rapidly after acetazolamide therapy was discontinued and, in 1 case, sodium bicarbonate was administered. In 1 patient with small kidneys suggestive of end-stage nephritis, the plasma creatinine level fell only slightly.

These elderly patients experienced acute confusion a week after the start of acetazolamide therapy for glaucoma and had biochemical evidence of metabolic acidosis. Evidence of preexisting renal failure was obtained in both cases. Excessive amounts of bicarbonate may be lost through the renal

---

(12–5) Br. Med. J. 283:1527–1528, Dec. 5, 1981.

tubules in some patients with renal failure, and acetazolamide would be expected to inhibit partial reabsorption of the bicarbonate. Many elderly patients have undiagnosed mild renal failure. Urea and electrolyte levels should be measured before acetazolamide therapy is instituted. If renal function is impaired, further estimations should be made and the bicarbonate level should be watched carefully. If it falls to 20 mM/L or below, oral sodium bicarbonate may be given or, preferably, acetazolamide therapy discontinued.

▶ [The carbonic anhydrase inhibitors are superb for short-term use, but they do have a large spectrum of side effects, including renal calculi, nausea, diarrhea, anorexia, confusion, depression, paresthesias, and others, which make long-term use difficult in some patients.] ◀

12-6 **Fetal Alcohol Syndrome** is a pattern of malformations observed in children of women with a history of alcohol abuse during pregnancy. Marilyn Miller, Jeannette Israel, and James Cuttone (Univ. of Illinois) point out that several ocular abnormalities have been described in affected infants and that short palpebral fissures are one of the more consistent features of the syndrome.

Girl, aged 3 years, presented with a constant esotropia and poor vision in the left eye. She had weighed 2,445 gm at birth. She had remained hospitalized for 2 months for possible viral infection and had received oxygen therapy. The mother had a history of alcohol abuse. Physical and mental development had been slow. At age 5, features noted were malar hypoplasia, a high palate, a short fifth finger in both hands with camptodactyly, and distally placed thumbs. Telecanthus, mild epicanthus, long eyelashes, and slight ptosis (Fig 12–1) also were noted. A Peters anomaly was observed, with a central corneal haze with pigmentation on the left. High myopia was documented. Motility study showed 0–8 degrees of left esotropia and 0–24 degrees of right esotropia with occasional spontaneously nystagmoid movements. The patient could fix spontaneously with the right eye, but preferred fixation with the left eye much of the time.

Abnormality of the palpebral fissure, usually shortness, is the most characteristic ocular finding in fetal alcohol syndrome. Strabismus was present in over half of the authors' 9 cases. No paralytic component was evident in any case. A high incidence of moderate to severe myopia also was noted. Corneal opacities have been rarely reported in

---

(12–6) J. Pediatr. Ophthalmol. Strabismus 18:6–15, July–Aug. 1981.

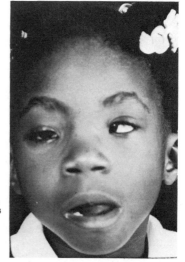

Fig 12–1.—Patient shows esotropia, mild ptosis OD, and telecanthus. Child also had a Peters anomaly of left cornea and high myopia. (Courtesy of Miller, M., et al.: J. Pediatr. Ophthalmol. Strabismus 18:6–15, July–Aug. 1981.)

fetal alcohol syndrome, but were present in 2 of the present patients.

Children with fetal alcohol syndrome are at considerable risk for a variety of ocular problems. The most prevalent ophthalmologic finding, a short horizontal palpebral fissure, appears to be due chiefly to a marked increase in intercanthal distances between the medial canthi, and to a lesser extent mild displacement of the lateral canthi.

▶ [The authors point out that the fact that maternal ingestion of alcohol may harm the fetus has been known for centuries. The risks for ocular problems are greater than heretofore recognized, with almost pathognomonic abnormalities of the palpebral fissure.] ◀

12–7 **Ocular Motor Signs in Some Metabolic Diseases** are reviewed by David G. Cogan, Fred C. Chu, Douglas Reingold, and John Barranger (Natl. Inst. of Health). Certain ocular motor disorders can be associated with specific metabolic defects as distinct syndromes. Some patients with Gaucher's disease have a progressive ophthalmoplegia for horizontal conjugate gaze. Four of about 50 patients evaluated had such a disorder, and 3 had findings simulating

---

(12–7) Arch. Ophthalmol. 99:1802–1808, October 1981.

those seen in congenital ocular motor apraxia. Vertical gaze palsy has been described in Neimann-Pick disease. The findings of downgaze paralysis, ataxia-athetosis, and foam cells may constitute a "DAF syndrome." An internuclear oththalmoplegia in which the adducting eye exhibits nystagmus on gaze to either side has been seen in abetalipoproteinemia.

Two of 6 patients with methylmalonohomocysteinuria had convulsive eye and lid movements. Slow eye movements have been observed in patients with olivopontospinocerebellar degeneration, besides an inability to initiate saccades. The combination of a form of ophthalmoplegia with pigmentary retinopathy also has been described. In ataxia-telangiectasia there may be inability to mobilize the eyes first for voluntary gaze and for the fast phase of vestibular nystagmus and later for pursuit movements. Eventually total ophthalmoplegia for these functions is present, whereas contraversive deviation of the eyes on rotation of the body is preserved. Horizontal and vertical movements are involved equally. Head thrusts are the rule.

12–8 **The Eye and Leprosy** are discussed by T. J. ffytche (St. Thomas' Hosp., London).

There may be between 500,000 and 750,000 persons in the world who are blind because of leprosy. A wide variety of ocular changes have long been recognized in this disease, but the underlying pathology and its consequences remain obscure. Facial nerve paralysis, a major cause of blindness, occurs in all forms of leprosy and may result in chronic exposure keratitis and subsequent corneal scarring and degeneration. The role of trigeminal neuropathy is less clear. All forms of leprosy can cause an acute iritis which, untreated, can lead to a profound and permanent loss of vision. In lepromatous leprosy the inflammation may be spontaneous and is believed to represent a reaction to the deposition of circulating immune complexes within the eye. True leproma of the cornea or iris is rare.

The so-called chronic iritis of lepromatous leprosy is responsible for the major visual impairment in the disease. It has the features of a basically degenerative process and de-

---

(12–8) Lepr. Rev. 52:111–119, June 1981.

velops quietly a few years after the onset of disease, causing no symptoms and very few signs at first. The iritis usually is bilateral. Iris pearls often are seen transiently in the early stages. Conventional mydriatics reportedly have little effect on the pupil, although synechiae are uncommon. A faint flare and fine atypical keratic precipitates, often pigmented, are noted in the anterior chamber. The condition may last for years and does not respond to local steroid therapy. Eventually there are signs of progressive iris atrophy and disintegration with increasing miosis. The relationship between leprosy and cataract remains unclear.

Pupillary testing may lead to the detection of systemic neurologic manifestations of leprosy. It may be possible to preserve the function of a failing dilator muscle by using direct sympathetic stimulants. The role of dopa and its breakdown products in relation to cataract formation and perhaps chronic iritis deserves further study. Long-term longitudinal studies and pathologic studies are needed to understand the natural history of the ocular manifestations of leprosy and the changes occurring in the iris nerves.

13. Surgery

Pars Plicata Surgery for Neonatal Anterior Segment Disease

MORTON F. GOLDBERG, M.D.

Eye and Ear Infirmary, University of Illinois, Chicago

Surgical indications for neonatal anterior segment diseases, including congenital cataracts, pupillary membranes, and persistent hyperplastic primary vitreous (PHPV), have been controversial. Invasive intervention traditionally has been viewed conservatively, particularly in unilaterally affected infants.[1] Surgical enthusiasm has been tempered by the technical difficulties of operative and postoperative care of neonatal and infantile eyes, especially when they are microphthalmic. Moreover, the difficulties of overcoming deprivation amblyopia, particularly after unilateral surgery, have been almost overwhelming. Contact lenses, spectacles, and patching regimens have constituted clinical mainstays for postoperative care, but have not been universally successful. Highly experimental approaches, including intraocular lenses[2] and epikeratophakic grafts,[3] also have severe limitations.

Despite these very real and distressing problems, two concurrent lines of development have occurred over the past few years, which suggest that a more optimistic viewpoint may now be in the offing. These events include quantitative methods of detection, measurement, and monitoring of amblyopia,[4] as well as better techniques of surgery for anterior segment diseases utilizing a transciliary body approach, specifically through the pars plicata.[1]

Amblyopia and Determination of Visual Acuity

First, with respect to the postoperative treatment of deprivation amblyopia, several reports indicate that even unilateral cataract (one of the most notoriously difficult rehabilitative problems) is compatible with normal or substantially improved acuity postoperatively, if a proper rehabilitative program is instituted quickly and pursued compulsively.[5-9] In a limited number of cases, this appears true even when some degree of microphthalmos exists,[5] but structural integrity of the optic nerve and macula is a necessary precondition. Thus, many cases of PHPV, which commonly have congenital anomalies of the optic nerve and macula, cannot be expected to achieve very useful vision, even with modern techniques of amblyopia management and technically uncomplicated microsurgery.

The development of three techniques of quantitative measurement of visual acuity has enabled the therapist to judge the evolution of postoperative visual acuity accurately and reproducibly. Thus, the use of different types of contact lenses and modifications of patching regimens has been enhanced considerably. These techniques involve measurement of the visual evoked potential, forced preferential looking, and optokinetic nystagmus. These quantitative measurements appear superior to traditional techniques of assessing the fixation pattern, nystagmus, and "visual behavior." Nonetheless, these clinical methods retain some utility, because they can be employed by any clinician without the need for specialized apparatuses or trained technical personnel.

Pars Plicata Surgery

The second major advance has been the availability of a series of innovative manual and automated vitrectomy instruments. Although developed for posterior segment disease, such as vitreous hemorrhage, they have proved to be extremely useful in removing opaque tissues from the anterior segment. Some anterior segment surgeons have utilized these vitrectomy instruments translimbally, relying on the traditional anterior segment entry site and avoiding, as much as possible, the vitreous itself. While sometimes effective, this approach has many disadvantages. Removal of a cataract with a vitrectomy instrument by a translimbal lensectomy approach can effectively eliminate the lenticular opacity, but is complicated by a high rate (23%)[10] of vitreous incarceration in the limbal wound and of cystoid macular edema.[5] A transciliary body approach minimizes these complications and has the following advantages[1]:

1. It is possible to remove opaque material in all axes through a single sclerotomy, utilizing a single, full-function vitrectomy instrument.
2. Both the anterior and posterior lens capsules can be removed completely and atraumatically to avoid subsequent problems with opacification.
3. It is possible to repair, if necessary, associated retinal pathology, such as breaks, detachments, or PHPV, during the same procedure.
4. It is also possible to utilize bimanual instrumentation, if necessary, such as intraocular diathermy or a chopping block technique, for cutting calcific or leathery tissue.
5. The vitreous can be removed atraumatically with the vitrectomy apparatus, and incarceration in a limbal wound is avoided.
6. It is possible (and desirable) to use an irrigated surgical contact lens in order to visualize the deep vitreous and fundus during the operative procedure. This permits removal of debris or abnormal tissue that falls into or is located within the preretinal space. Use of a limbal instrument precludes effective use of a surgical contact lens, and deep intravitreal manipulations are not possible.[1]

Bearing in mind the advantages of the transciliary body approach, attempts have been made[1, 11] to reduce those complications, such as entry-site dialysis of the retina, that are associated with a pars plana incision. We have been performing the transciliary body entry through the pars plicata for more than 5 years, and the procedure has had a remarkably low rate of complications when compared either to traditional limbal approaches (with manual or with vitrectomy instruments) or to the pars plana approach.[12, 13] For example, in a consecutive series of 32 such procedures for infantile and juvenile cataracts (with follow-up of 6 to 74 months), there were no entry-site dialyses, early or late retinal detachments (thus far), or postoperative pupillary block. There were no instances of hazy media requiring secondary surgery of any sort, although early complications included 3 cases of transient corneal edema, 1 of mild iris bleeding, and 1 with a 5-day period of hazy vitreous. Two eyes also had transient elevation of intraocular pressure, but no permanent sequelae resulted.[12] One patient had bilateral cystoid macular edema, although the true incidence may be found to be higher if routine fluorescein angioscopy is performed frequently in all neonatal eyes postoperatively.

Furthermore, after similar pars plicata surgery for 108 consecutive membranes that were followed up for an average of 3.8 years (range, 1 to 7 years), we detected no major operative complications.[1, 13] Vision improved in approximately 66% of the eyes. Vision in most of the others was approximately unchanged. About 4% of the eyes had worse postoperative visual acuity, which was attributable to preexisting glaucoma.[13]

Substantial growth of infants' eyes occurs to about 3 years of age. Thus, a major concern with transciliary body (including pars plicata) surgery and vitreous removal has been the potential for stunting growth of a neonatal eye, particularly when it is microphthalmic to begin with, or when it is infected with a growth-retarding virus such as rubella. In a limited number of cases followed carefully for these problems, such fears have proved to be unfounded.[1]

The pars plicata approach also has been advocated for the removal of PHPV. Here, the retina sometimes is pulled far anteriorly, and a transciliary body approach, especially through the pars plana, can be risky. The pars plicata approach can also result in retinal perforation.[14] In this disease, however, even translimbal entry has been complicated by inadvertent retinal biopsy.[1] Regardless of the technique to be used, other clinical judgments assume considerable importance. If, for example, the eye is only minimally deformed and the visual axis is clear, surgery usually is contraindicated, and the eye often can be treated adequately with pupillary dilatation or optical iridectomy and an antiamblyopia regimen. At the other end of the spectrum, if the eye is severely microphthalmic and if the vitreous, as demonstrated ultrasonically or by computed tomography, is filled with abnormal fetal tissue, there is little hope of salvaging the eye. The visual prognosis is equally bad if electroretinography shows no cone or rod responses. In these circumstances, a cosmetic scleral shell prosthesis (or possibly even enucleation) may be in the best interest of the patient rather than incurring the risks of sympathetic ophthalmia (or general anesthesia) by proceeding with operative intervention.

Between these two clinical extremes, decision-making for PHPV is extremely difficult. Depending on the findings from clinical inspection, ultrasonography, computed tomography, and electroretinography, the clinician may feel that removing the abnormal tissue, including the lens, may not only salvage the eye, but also may provide some improved vision. Surgery may seem indicated, for example, when there appears to be some useful vision and there is progressive, *documented* shallowing of the anterior chamber due to active centripetal contraction of the retrolental fibrovascular tissue and ciliary processes. The simple presence of centrally dragged ciliary processes, however, is not necessarily an indication for surgery, because such eyes can occasionally survive to adult life without intervention.[1, 15]

In any event, because of coexistent anatomical abnormalities as well as difficulties with amblyopia therapy, it is extremely unusual to have useful vision occur from even technically refined and uncomplicated modern surgery for PHPV,[1] and parents should be informed accordingly.

SUMMARY

In summary, the development of quantitative techniques for acuity measurements and amblyopia therapy has evolved pari passu with advances in microsurgical techniques using vitrectomy instruments. The pars plicata approach is a remarkably safe and effective technique for surgery of cataracts and of pupillary membranes in the childhood years.

Marked visual improvement can be anticipated with some confidence, assuming that surgery is uncomplicated and that the amblyopia regimen is instituted quickly and pursued compulsively. The proper method, if any, for management of many cases of PHPV has yet to be defined. Congenital anomalies of the optic nerve and macula often preclude useful vision, even when atraumatic, complication-free surgery is performed for this disorder.

REFERENCES

1. Goldberg M. F., Peyman G. A.: Pars plicata surgery in the child for pupillary membranes, persistent hyperplastic primary vitreous, and infantile cataracts, in *New Orleans Academy of Ophthalmology: Symposium on the Retina*. St. Louis, C. V. Mosby Co., in press.
2. Hiles D. A.: Indications, techniques, and complications associated with intraocular lens implantation in children, in Hiles D. M. (ed.): *Intraocular Lens Implants in Children*. New York, Grune & Stratton, 1979, p. 189.
3. Morgan K. S., Werblin T. P., Asbell P. A., Loupe D. N., Friedlander M. H., Kaufman H. E.: The use of epikeratophakia grafts in pediatric monocular aphakia. *J. Pediatr. Ophthalmol. Strabismus* 18:23–29, 1981.
4. Hoyt C. S., Nickel B. L., Billson F. A.: Review: Ophthalmological examination of the infant. *Surv. Ophthalmol.* 26:177–189, 1982.
5. Beller R., Hoyt C. S., Marg E., Odom J. V.: Good visual function after neonatal surgery for congenital monocular cataracts. *Am. J. Ophthalmol.* 91:559–565, 1981. (Article 13–12 in this YEAR BOOK.)
6. Pratt-Johnson J. A., Tillson G.: Visual results after removal of congenital cataracts before the age of 1 year. *Can. J. Ophthalmol.* 16:19–21, 1981.
7. Enoch J. M., Rabinowicz I. M., Campos E. C.: Postsurgical contact lens correction of infants with sensory deprivation amblyopia associated with unilateral congenital cataract. *J. Jpn. Contact Lens Soc.* 21:95–104, 1979.
8. Jacobson S. G., Mohindra I., Held R.: Development of visual acuity in infants with congenital cataracts. *Br. J. Ophthalmol.* 65:727–735, 1981.
9. Gelbart S. S., Hoyt C. S., Jastrebski G., Marg E.: Long-term visual results in bilateral congenital cataracts. *Am. J. Ophthalmol.*, in press.

10. Taylor D.: Choice of surgical technique in the management of congenital cataract. *Trans. Ophthalmol. Soc. U.K.* 101:114–117, 1981.
11. O'Malley C., Boyd B. F.: Closed-eye endomicrosurgery (Ab-interno microsurgery), in Boyd B. F. (ed.): *Highlights of Ophthalmology.* New York, Arcata Book Group, 1981, vol. 1, chap. 3.
12. Peyman G. A., Raichand M., Oesterle C., and Goldberg M. F.: Pars plicata lensectomy and vitrectomy in the management of congenital cataracts. *Ophthalmology (Rochester)* 88:437–439, 1981.
13. Juarez C. P., Peyman G. A., Raichand M., Goldberg M. F.: Secondary pupillary membranes treated by the pars plicata approach: Results of 108 cases. *Br. J. Ophthalmol.*, in press.
14. Federman J. L., Shields J. A., Altman B., et al.: The surgical and nonsurgical management of persistent hyperplastic primary vitreous. *Ophthalmology (Rochester)* 89:20–24, 1982.
15. Gieser D. K., Goldberg M. F., Apple D. J., et al.: Persistent hyperplastic primary vitreous in an adult: Case report with fluorescein angiographic findings. *J. Pediatr. Ophthalmol. Strabismus* 15:213–218, 1978.

13–1 **Cystoid Macular Edema After Aphakic Penetrating Keratoplasty.** Aphakic penetrating keratoplasty (APKP) and combined penetrating keratoplasty with lens extraction (CPKP) are highly successful procedures, but macular problems tend to develop or appear postoperatively, and visual acuity is disappointing, chiefly because of cystoid macular edema (CME) or preexisting macular degeneration. Steven G. Kramer (Univ. of California, San Francisco) has evaluated 132 eyes subjected to these procedures to determine whether vitreous manipulation altered the macular outcome. Eighty-four eyes had preexisting aphakia and underwent APKP with anterior vitrectomy (group 1); 48 underwent CPKP (group 2). Twenty-four of the 48 underwent anterior vitrectomy routinely immediately after lens extraction (group 2A); the other 24 did not (group 2B).

Overall rate of clear corneal grafts was 92%. Six months after operation CME was identified by fluorescein studies in 33% of cases. Only 2 of these eyes had a best corrected acuity of 20/70. The relation of CME to vitrectomy in eyes subjected to CPKP is shown in the table. The type of in-

---

(13–1) Ophthalmology (Rochester) 88:782–787, August 1981.

CYSTOID MACULAR EDEMA IN EYES SUBJECTED
TO COMBINED PENETRATING KERATOPLASTY
AND LENS EXTRACTION*

	With Vitrectomy (Group 2A)	Without Vitrectomy (Group 2B)
CME	8	1
No CME	16	23

*Difference between groups 2A and 2B is statistically significant ($P < .05$, $\chi^2 = 4.92$, Yates' correction applied).

strument used for vitrectomy (Kaufman Vitrector or O'Malley Ocutome) did not influence the occurrence of CME. The incidence of surgical complications such as adhesion between the iris and keratoplasty wound was 7%. Five of the 9 complications occurred in previously aphakic eyes.

Transpupillary vitreous excision should not be performed in association with CPKP unless it is unavoidable or strong indications are present. Iris wound adhesion may, however, be more likely when vitrectomy is not performed, and it may lead to compromised visual acuity through a graft rejection reaction or secondary glaucoma. Where vitreous excision is necessary because of vitreous prolapse or expected prolapse, nonpupillary routes for excising vitreous should be considered. Extracapsular cataract extraction may be considered in CPKP in the hope of maintaining an intact posterior capsular boundary and protecting the anterior vitreous face.

▶ [This is an important article because great enthusiasm for the partial anterior vitrectomy has developed in recent years, as it essentially eliminates anterior segment vitreous problems. It appears, however, that the procedure may be detrimental to the retina.] ◀

▶ ↓ The following three reports concern the use of sodium hyaluronate (Healon) in intraocular surgery. Advances in microsurgery have made many previously complicated intraocular manipulations a matter of routine. Sodium hyaluronate protects the corneal endothelium and maintains anatomical relationships during surgery. It is especially beneficial in a surgical training program. ◀

13–2 **Use of Sodium Hyaluronate (Healon) in Intracapsular Cataract Extraction With Insertion of Anterior Chamber Intraocular Lenses.** Sodium hyaluronate (Hea-

(13–2) Ophthalmic Surg. 12:646–649, September 1981.

lon) is a highly viscous disaccharide polymer useful in intraocular surgery. Its ability to facilitate penetrating keratoplasty and filtering procedures by separating tissue planes helps to prevent adhesions. G. William Lazenby and Geoffrey Broocker (Holiday, Fla.) evaluated the usefulness of Healon in intracapsular cataract extraction with insertion of an anterior chamber intraocular lens in a series of 40 eyes. Balanced salt solution or air was used to deepen the anterior chamber in 21 procedures and Healon in 19. In the latter group, Healon also was used to cover the anterior surface of the intraocular lens.

Endothelial cell loss was 13.5% in controls and 9.7% in patients given Healon treatment; however, the difference was not significant. No difference in corneal thickness was found between the two treatment groups. Intraocular pressure was significantly higher in the study group for 1–3 days after surgery, but pressure differences became insignificant after 1–2 weeks. This probably was a result of leaving excess Healon in the eye, interfering with aqueous flow. All but 3 of the operations done using Healon were considered easier than average and none was considered more difficult than average. Only 4 procedures done without Healon were considered easier, whereas 3 were considered more difficult than average.

Intraocular lens implantation was generally easier when Healon was used in this study. Movement of the lens during manipulation is dampened by Healon, reducing the risk of inadvertently damaging the cornea, angle structures, or vitreous face. Placement of the proximal feet or loop is facilitated by stabilization of the lens with Healon. When injecting Healon from above, the cannula should be advanced gradually in the direction of flow to prevent segmental deepening of the anterior chamber. Peripheral iridectomy should be done after the lens is in place. Only enough Healon to allow safe insertion of the lens should be used, and most should be washed out before closing the anterior chamber.

Sodium Hyaluronate (Healon) in Keratoplasty and IOL Implantation. Endothelial cells are lost during keratoplasty, leading to graft edema, but the loss may be prevented by coating the corneal endothelium with the viscoelastic substance sodium hyaluronate (Healon). Frank M. Polack, Thaddeus Demong, and Hamed Santaella (Univ. of Florida, Gainesville) evaluated Healon in 50 patients having penetrating keratoplasty for corneal edema, keratoconus, corneal scarring, or dystrophies. Ten of 20 aphakic patients with corneal edema received sodium hyaluronate at the time of surgery. Ten of 20 patients who had keratoplasty combined with extracapsular cataract extraction received sodium hyaluronate, while 10 received balanced saline solution. Eight other patients had bullous keratopathy and underwent cataract extraction and insertion of a posterior-chamber intraocular lens. Two patients had previous pseudophakos and corneal edema.

In aphakic keratoplasty, placement of sodium hyaluronate in the anterior chamber facilitated graft suturing and prevented lateral graft displacement. There was no evidence of iritis or unusual inflammation in hyaluronate-treated eyes. Intraocular pressures were lower in hyaluronate-treated than in control eyes on postoperative day 2 and subsequently. Similar observations were made in the patients having keratoplasty and cataract extraction. Corneal thickness and intraocular pressures were lower in hyaluronate-treated than in control eyes. Moderate iritis occurred in 2 patients in the group having intraocular lens insertion, and partial adhesions persisted for several weeks. Intraocular pressures were normal in all patients but 2, who received acetazolamide for 1 week after surgery. Specular microscopy indicated no significant difference in numbers of cells present in the study and control groups.

Sodium hyaluronate facilitates corneal transplantation in aphakic eyes and reduces endothelial trauma by decreasing the amount of graft manipulation necessary during suturing. Similar graft protection is observed in phakic eyes and in patients having grafting in conjunction with cataract surgery and intraocular lens implantation. It seems best to further refill the anterior chamber with balanced saline solution rather than sodium hyaluronate during and at the end of surgery. Excessive sodium hyaluronate can be removed and replaced by balanced saline solution.

▶ [Most would agree with the advantages of sodium hyaluronate use in intraocular lens insertion. Irrigating the material out of the eye, however, is difficult because of its viscosity and vitreous-like appearance. Perhaps a safer procedure is using a minimal amount and avoiding irrigation.] ◀

13-4 **The Use of Anterior Chamber Na-Hyaluronate in a Pseudophakic Patient Requiring Intravitreal Air During Retinal Reattachment Surgery.** Sodium hyaluronate (Healon) is a nontoxic material that is useful in maintaining the anterior chamber and the integrity of the corneal endothelium during several types of ocular surgery. Mano Swartz, Randall J. Olson, George C. Pingree, and Carolyn Sakauye (Univ. of Utah, Salt Lake City) successfully used sodium hyaluronate to maintain the anterior chamber in a patient with an intraocular lens during retinal reattachment surgery where intravitreal air was necessary.

Man, 50, with Parkinson's disease, had experienced a superotemporal field defect on the right. He had had bilateral intracapsular cataract extractions and implants of Worst Medallion lenses about 2 years earlier. A rhegmatogenous retinal detachment was found in the right fundus, associated with vision of finger-counting only. Reattachment surgery was carried out with the use of general anesthesia, cryotherapy, a silicone buckle, and a circumferential band. An air bubble was injected inferotemporally 4 mm posterior to the limbus because of retinal folds extending through the superior flap tears and communicating with the posterior part of the retina. The bubble flattened the anterior chamber and caused the intraocular lens to touch the corneal endothelium. Some air was released, and 0.4 ml of sodium hyaluronate was injected to deepen the anterior chamber. Keratopathy cleared within 5 days after surgery. The anterior chamber remained formed, and without flare or cells. The intraocular lens remained in place. The intravitreal air bubble resolved within 72 hours after surgery. Acuity was 20/30 by the second week after surgery.

Sodium hyaluronate provided a means of protecting the corneal endothelium in this patient when intravitreal air flattened the anterior chamber. Placement of Healon into the anterior chamber before intravitreal air or gas may be the best means of preventing touch of the corneal endothelium by an intraocular lens. Air-endothelial contact is avoided, and positive anterior chamber pressure is provided in the face of an open wound.

13–5 **Results With a Temporary Balloon Buckle for Repair of Retinal Detachment.** Harvey Lincoff (New York Hosp.-Cornell Med. Center) and Ingrid Kreissig (Univ. of Tübingen) evaluated an operation for retinal detachment in which a parabulbar space balloon is used as a temporary scleral buckle for 1 week. Cryopexy- or laser-induced adhesions are made around the break to obtain permanent attachment. A prospective study was conducted of 100 patients, with a mean age of 57 years, who had a single retinal break or group of breaks close together that did not subtend more than 6 mm. Only one quadrant was involved in 38 cases. The macula was completely detached preoperatively in 39 cases and partly detached in 11 others. Horseshoe tears were present in 74 cases.

The retinal break is located by transconjunctival cryopexy, and a siliconized latex balloon is inserted beneath the break and inflated with 0.75 to 2 ml of saline. The balloon closes the retinal break (Fig 13–1), and subretinal fluid

Fig 13–1.—Sagittal section of orbit showing balloon in Tenon's space after eye has been decompressed. Balloon has closed retinal break and retina has been reattached. (Courtesy of Lincoff, H., and Kreissig, I.: Am. J. Ophthalmol. 92:245–251, August 1981.)

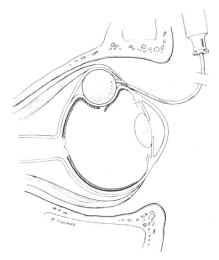

is absorbed. Generally only one or two localizing applications of cryopexy are necessary. The break is sealed with a laser after the retina comes into contact with the buckle.

Average follow-up was 21 months. The retinal break was closed successfully in 90 cases, and subretinal fluid was absorbed completely within a week in 82. Six retinas redetached after the balloon was removed. The macula was reattached promptly in 32 of the 39 cases with complete preoperative detachment. Complications included 2 cases of corneal erosion and single cases of iridocyclitis and choroidal detachment. Macular pucker occurred in 3 patients, 2 of whom had moderate iridocyclitis when the balloon was inserted.

Retinal breaks remained secure after temporary buckling and cryopexy or laser coagulation in 84 of 100 patients in this study. Complications were less frequent than with the sponge operation and other modern methods. Patients have been pleased with the absence of cosmetic defects. Air procedures are not indicated primarily except for treatment of large tears or other difficult detachment problems.

▶ [Other studies have shown that coagulation is not necessary for retinal adhesion, provided a buckle has closed the hole. This study shows that long-term buckles are not necessary as long as there is coagulation. It may be that in the former case, long-term buckles caused an inflammatory retinal adhesion.] ◀

13–6 **Fluid Silicon in Detachment Surgery.** R. Živojnović, D. A. E. Mertens, and G. S. Baarsma (Univ. of Rotterdam) discuss the indications, results, and complications in 90 consecutive cases of intravitreal silicon injection. These injections were performed according to the principles described by J. Scott. The patients, mostly with cases that were inoperable with standard techniques, underwent surgery in the period between the beginning of 1978 and the end of 1979. The follow-up period was between 5 months and 2 years. Before silicon injection, no patients could see more than hand motions and most could only perceive a gleam of light. In 18 patients, the operative eye was the only eye and in 8 patients the second eye had a 0.1 vision. In order to get an exact picture of the condition of the vitreous, all patients were examined with the binocular

(13–6) Klin. Monatsbl. Augenheilkd. 179:17–22, July 1981. (Ger.)

ophthalmoscope, the Goldmann-3 mirror-contact lens, and the panfunduscope. The procedure was done under intubation anesthetic and liquid silicon SF96 1,000 cSt was used for the injection.

Anatomical success was achieved in about 70% of the cases, including 9 patients with a three-fourths attached retina. Intraoperative complications were mostly hemorrhages, caused by preretinal tears, and were absorbed within several weeks. A choroidal hemorrhage may occur with the puncture and can be a very serious complication because increased intraocular pressure makes further silicon injection impossible. Extensive tears must be closed, and this is sometimes difficult. A new tear or the opening of an old one can be responsible for silicon getting under the retina, which presents a serious complication. However, sometimes the authors were successful in removing the subretinal silicon and closing the tear. Very few complications arose during the postoperative period.

The intravitreal silicon injection, carried out according to Scott's principles, makes it possible to help patients with massive periretinal proliferation (MPP), which until now was considered inoperable. With early surgery some complications can be prevented. Most of the late complications, such as cataract and glaucoma, can be treated surgically. At this time the question of silicon toxicity cannot be answered but the authors experienced no such complication.

▶ [Vitreous cavity silicon obviously facilitates complicated retinal detachment repair. Early, however, it was believed toxic to the retina. In the past few years, the question of its toxicity has been reexamined and, thus far, the results have been favorable.] ◀

13-7 **Effects on Corneal Endothelium of Anterior Chamber Reconstituents Instilled During Intracapsular Cataract Extraction.** Little attention has been given to possible effects of altering the composition of the aqueous during microsurgical procedures on the corneal endothelium. Most previous studies have been done in animals. R. M. Lang and D. T. R. Hassard (Univ. of Alberta) examined the effects of commonly used intraocular reconstituents in the living human eye. Studies were done in 77 patients un-

LOSS OF CORNEAL ENDOTHELIAL CELLS 6 AND 20 DAYS
AFTER INTRAOCULAR CATARACT EXTRACTION

Anterior chamber reconstituent	Loss (%), mean ± standard error	
	6 d	20 d
Miochol (M)	7.8 ± 2.7 (n = 6)	7.8 ± 2.3 (n = 6)
Air (A)	12.9 ± 6.0 (n = 7)	8.9 ± 5.0 (n = 10)
M + phenylephrine (P)	15.3 ± 7.8 (n = 17)	11.7 ± 4.3 (n = 21)
A + P	13.2 ± 8.6 (n = 6)	19.4 ± 4.8 (n = 10)
Balanced salt solution + P	19.2 ± 7.0 (n = 7)	13.3 ± 9.9 (n = 9)

dergoing intracapsular cataract extraction. Miochol (acetylcholine chloride in mannitol), air, 10% phenylephrine, or a balanced salt solution was introduced into the anterior chamber during operation. The central corneal endothelium was photographed before and 6 and 20 days after operation.

Corneal endothelial cell loss is shown in the table. Cell loss was greater when a combination of materials was used to reconstitute the anterior chamber. No significant change occurred between 6 and 20 days after operation in eyes reconstituted with Miochol. Cell recovery was observed in eyes reconstituted with air or with Miochol plus phenylephrine. In 7 of 8 patients with corneal endothelial cell losses exceeding 30%, phenylephrine was instilled at operation, and Miochol also was used in 6 of these. In the eighth patient the anterior chamber was irrigated with balanced salt solution after cataract extraction because of excessive dispersion of iris pigment during lens extraction.

Commonly used solutions introduced into the anterior chamber after lens extraction can have adverse effects on the corneal endothelium. Air may well have a short-lived deleterious effect on the endothelial cells. Endothelial cell function appears not to be altered by instillation of acetylcholine, but phenylephrine has an adverse effect on the corneal endothelium, and the combination of air and phenylephrine is particularly harmful. Anterior chamber reconstitution with Miochol appears to be indicated in cataract surgery. A broad iridectomy should be done if satisfactory dilation is not achieved, and corneal manipulation should be minimized.

▶ [It would be interesting to study the combination of sodium hyaluronate and acetylcholine chloride because these are now in general use by implant surgeons. The amount of corneal manipulation may be an important variable, especially the folding and distortion with opening of the anterior chamber during lens removal and implantation.] ◀

13–8 **Computerized Axial Tomography in Detection of Intraocular Foreign Bodies.** Computed tomographic (CT) scanning provides a rapid means of evaluating intraocular or intraorbital foreign bodies, or both, and can clearly demonstrate nonmetallic and multiple bodies and double perforations. Louis A. Lobes, Jr., M. Gilbert Grand, John Reece, and Ronald J. Penkrot (Univ. of Pittsburgh) used CT scanning to localize intraocular foreign bodies in 36 patients. Orbital-axial, coronal, and sagittal projections were used. All cuts were 7 mm thick.

Man, 20, sustained gunshot wounds of the face and had a laceration in the left eye 4 mm posterior to the limbus. Vitreous hemorrhage was present along the infratemporal arcade, and an impact site was seen with retinal edema. A CT scan showed a metallic-density foreign body along the infratemporal aspect of the scleral wall, apparently lying on the retina. A limbic incision was made in the area of the pars plana, but attempted extraction of the foreign body with a magnet failed. A vitrectomy was then performed, with removal of a lead foreign body. Final acuity was 20/50; a small macular pucker remained.

The CT scan is useful if lack of patient cooperation precludes traditional methods of localizing a foreign body. The CT study is safer than other methods, and the findings can be interpreted by nonspecialists. Small, anteriorly placed foreign bodies can be accurately localized by CT. Clear visualization of the posterior scleral wall is possible. It is reasonable to consider using CT as a primary means of localization in patients suspected of having intraocular or intraorbital foreign bodies.

13–9 **Transcranial Enucleation for Optic Nerve Tumor.** Conventional methods of enucleation do not permit exploration of the optic nerve or assure complete removal of tumor from the orbit, and they frequently require transection through tumor-containing tissue. Joel G. Sacks and James E. McLennan (Univ. of Cincinnati) performed transcranial enucleation in a patient, with enlargement of a proved benign astrocytoma of the optic nerve that threatened the chiasm and hypothalamus, who refused radiotherapy.

TECHNIQUE.—A unilateral frontal craniotomy is done, generally through a bicoronal scalp incision, and the orbital roof is exposed extradurally. The optic canal is unroofed by elevating the frontal lobe back to the sphenoid wing. The optic canal can be unroofed with a power-driven bur before the periorbita is incised axially, sparing the frontal nerve. Optimal exposure is obtained by entering the muscle cone at the lateral border of the superior rectus. If the tumor extends to the globe, the eye is mobilized with a 360-degree peritomy, and the globe is pushed posteriorly through the orbitotomy and the intermuscular incision. The ophthalmic artery is cauterized at the point of transection in or anterior to the optic canal (Fig 13–2). The intermuscular incision is closed before a prosthetic device is inserted through the peritomy. The

Fig 13–2.—Globe and contiguous optic nerve tumor are pulled superiorly through muscle cone, permitting mobilization of inferior portion of tumor and proper identification of its distal extent. (Courtesy of Sacks, J. G., and McLennan, J. E.: Neurosurgery 9:166–168, August 1981.)

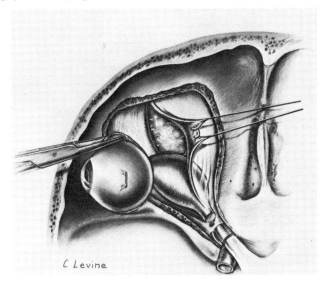

bony defect in the orbital roof is closed with tantalum mesh or alloplastic material.

This approach is indicated when a computed tomographic scan shows a large optic nerve tumor of undetermined nature. If the tumor is enlarging, the transcranial method permits direct inspection of the tumor, biopsy, and definitive treatment including en bloc enucleation, if necessary. If the optic foramen and canal must be unroofed because of posterior tumor extension, the muscle cone probably should be opened between the levator and the medial rectus muscles to avoid damaging the oculomotor nerve. If a normal segment of intervening optic nerve is not identified, it seems best to remove the tumor and globe together. Frozen sections are not generally reliable in showing the extent of tumor involvement, and if a meningioma is present, transection might lead to seeding of tumor cells within the orbit.

▶ [Computed tomography makes it possible to determine if there is intracranial extension necessitating transcranial surgery.] ◀

13–10 **Chest Pain in the Postoperative Ophthalmic Patient.** Surgical mortality has been reported to be 0.14 to 2.9 per 1,000 ophthalmic patients. Prevention of postoperative deaths requires the rapid and accurate assessment of the patient's condition after the onset of complications. Russell W. Neuhaus and Kenneth T. Meyer (Univ. of California, Los Angeles) reviewed the deaths that occurred among 17,632 patients seen in a 20-year period ending in 1974. Eleven patients (0.062%) died; all were postsurgical patients. Five deaths occurred after retinal detachment repair, and 3, after cataract extraction. Two patients had intraoperative cardiac arrest during local anesthesia and sedation, which necessitated cardiopulmonary resuscitation. Both these patients apparently died of diffuse cerebral anoxia. Three patients had confirmed myocardial infarctions. One cardiac arrest occurred 5 days after general anesthesia for retinal detachment repair. The 1 patient who had no postmortem examination had died after an unwitnessed cardiopulmonary arrest that occurred 8 hours after general

Differential Diagnosis of Chest Pain by Location	

Left neck and/or left arm
  Sensory nerve root compression
  Skeletal muscle strain
  Angina
Precordial
  Esophagitis
  Cardiac
    Pericarditis
    Angina
    Aortic dissection
	Pulmonary
	  Pleuritis
	  Pulmonary embolus
	  Pneumonia
	Epigastric
	  Pancreatitis
	  Peptic ulcer disease
	  Gallbladder disease
	  Angina

anesthesia. Six of the 9 patients who died postoperatively had had chest or epigastric pain after surgery.

Careful analysis of chest pain in ophthalmic surgery patients is necessary. The differential diagnosis is given in the table. Pulmonary embolism, myocardial infarction, congestive heart failure, and pneumonia all frequently can be managed successfully.

13–11 **Randomized Comparison of Four Incisions for Orbital Fractures.** Barbel Holtmann, R. Chris Wray, and A. Gerald Little (Washington Univ.) undertook a prospective comparison of 4 lower eyelid and orbital rim incisions for exposure of fractures of the orbital floor and infraorbital rim. Thirty-seven orbital rim and 36 lower lid incisions were made. There were 70 Le Fort II or zygomatic fractures, or both, involving the infraorbital rim and 3 blowout fractures of the orbital floor. The 43 male and 19 female patients were aged 16 to 72 years. The lower lid incision was made in a skin crease about half the distance between the lash margin and the orbital rim (Fig 13–3). The orbital rim incision was made directly over the rim (Fig 13–4). The conjunctival-lateral canthotomy incision is shown in Figure 13–5 and the subciliary incision in Figure 13–6.

Both the orbital rim and the lower lid incisions permitted adequate exposure of the infraorbital rim and orbital floor. No intraoperative complications were related to these incisions. One patient had a transient ectropion after a lower lid incision, and 2 had partial scar hypertrophy after lid

(13–11) Plast. Reconstr. Surg. 67:731–737, June 1981.

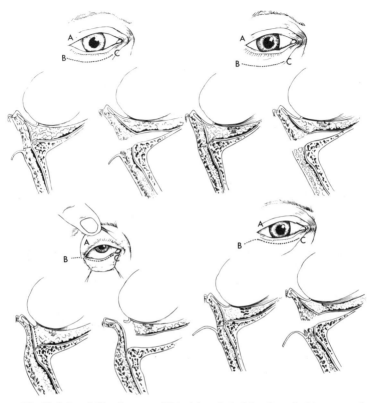

Fig 13–3 (top left).—Lower eyelid incision. *A*, incision through skin crease of lower eyelid. *B* and *C*, elevation of inferior skin flap and incision through orbicularis oculi muscle and periosteum over infraorbital rim.

Fig 13–4 (top right).—Orbital rim incision. *A*, incision through skin directly over infraorbital rim. *B* and *C*, orbicularis oculi and periosteum incised at same level as skin incision.

Fig 13–5 (bottom left).—Conjunctival-lateral canthotomy incision. *A*, incision through conjunctiva with lateral canthotomy extension. *B* and *C*, retroseptal approach with incision of periosteum over infraorbital rim.

Fig 13–6 (bottom right).—Subciliary incision. *A*, incision 2 mm below lid margin with lateral extension in skin crease. *B* and *C*, elevation of inferior skin flap and incision through orbicularis oculi and periosteum over infraorbital rim.

(Courtesy of Holtmann, B., et al.: Plast. Reconstr. Surg. 67:731–737, June 1981.)

incisions. The degrees of visibility of lower lid, orbital rim, and combined conjunctival-lateral canthotomy scars were comparable. Subciliary scars were slightly less visible than lower lid scars.

All these approaches provide adequate fracture exposure, but more rapid exposure is obtained with the more direct lower lid and orbital rim incisions. No morbidity followed orbital rim incisions in this series. The average scar after all the incisions is barely noticeable. The use of either lower eyelid or orbital rim incision for rapidly exposing orbital floor and infraorbital rim fractures is recommended.

13–12 **Good Visual Function After Neonatal Surgery for Congenital Monocular Cataracts.** Most workers have considered the monocular congenital cataract to be a nearly hopeless problem with little chance of successful visual rehabilitation. Richard Beller, Creig S. Hoyt (Univ. of California, San Francisco), Elwin Marg and J. Vernon Odom (Univ. of California, Berkeley) have obtained favorable long-term visual results in 8 infants who had removal of total monocular congenital cataracts in the neonatal period. Six children had standard lens aspiration, and 2 had combined lensectomy and vitrectomy. In the former group a constant infusion technique was used, and a complete posterior capsulotomy was done as part of the initial surgery. Fitting of contact lenses was begun within 4 days after surgery. When possible, the lens was removed only once a week for examination. Permanent corneal damage did not occur. Patching therapy was begun at the same time as contact lens fitting. The phakic eye tended to be patched for 4 to 8 hours a day, depending on visual-evoked potential measurements.

The results are given in the table. Five patients had improvement in acuity to 6/9 or better after a mean follow-up of 2.8 years. The 3 others improved to 6/24 or better; 1 was the oldest patient in the series, and the other 2 had serious contact lens problems and were without optical correction for at least 6 weeks. All 8 patients had clear heterotropia after patching therapy was begun. Four patients preferred fixation with the aphakic eye after good acuity was at-

CLINICAL DATA FOR EIGHT PATIENTS WITH MONOCULAR CONGENITAL CATARACTS
TREATED DURING THE NEONATAL PERIOD

Patient No.	Age At Surgery	Age Present (yrs)	Type of Surgery	Present Contact Lens	Final Visual Acuity in Aphakic Eye	Comments
1	6 days	3.3	Aspiration	Hydrocurve	6/9 (20/30)	Cornea 1.5 mm smaller in aphakic eye
2	3 days	3.1	Aspiration	Hydrocurve	6/7.5 (20/25)	Dense plaque on posterior lens capsule
3	20 days	3.1	Aspiration	Hydrocurve	6/24 (20/80)	Cornea 1 mm smaller in aphakic eye
4	41 days	3.0	Lensectomy, vitrectomy	Permalens	6/12 (20/40)	—
5	7 hrs	2.9	Aspiration	Hydrocurve	6/6 (20/20)	Cornea 1 mm smaller in aphakic eye
6	10 days	2.9	Lensectomy, vitrectomy	Bausch & Lomb	6/6 (20/20)	—
7	16 days	2.7	Aspiration	Hydrocurve	6/12 (20/40)	Cornea 2 mm smaller in aphakic eye
8	5 days	2.6	Aspiration	Permalens	6/9 (20/30)	—

tained. Six patients had surgery to correct the heterotropia, but none showed binocularity.

Surgery in the neonatal period probably is necessary for a successful visual outcome in infants with congenital monocular cataract. Alternative patching methods now are being studied to provide more binocular stimulation while maintaining good acuity in the aphakic eye. The lack of binocularity also may be related to the aniseikonia produced by the high-plus contact lenses. The use of a reverse Galilean telescopic correction may lead to better binocularity.

▶ [If the poor prognosis for monocular congenital cataracts is deprivation amblyopia during an early period, then operation and optical correction are essential before that period. The authors have obtained relatively good visual acuity but, thus far, no binocularity, so that some other factor or factors than monocular deprivation must affect this specialized visual function.] ◀

13-13 **Blepharospasm: Surgical Procedure for Therapy** is described by Arthur F. Battista (New York Univ.). Medical treatment usually is only temporarily helpful in severe and chronic cases of blepharospasm. The author has performed bilateral percutaneous fractional thermolytic destruction of facial nerve branches on 17 patients with bilateral blepharospasm. Local anesthesia is used to insert a no. 19 stimu-

---

(13–13) Ophthalmic Surg. 12:823–829, November 1981.

lating and heating needle subcutaneously to various facial nerve branches. Thermolytic lesions are made at 50–80 C as voluntary movements are monitored. From 8 to 35 lesions on each side are usually necessary to reduce or abolish involuntary lid spasms.

All patients operated on had had trials on various medications. The 13 women and 4 men had had symptoms for an average of 5½ years. Five patients had only one procedure. Six of 8 patients followed for more than 2 years after their last operation had 70%–80% improvement, and 1 had 50% improvement. Two of 6 patients followed for 1–2 years after their last operations had 60% improvement, whereas 4 had 70%–90% improvement. Significant complications were minimal. Several patients reported slight corneal irritation without sequelae. One patient had slow lid closure on one side after the thermolytic procedure.

The percutaneous thermolytic procedure for blepharospasm can be done with local anesthesia. Stepwise fractional destruction of facial nerve branches with the patient conscious permits assessment of the effects of the lesions and minimizes facial muscle weakness. Facial nerve function can be altered at any point from the small terminal branches to the main nerve trunk. Repeat procedures can readily be done to obtain further relief from muscle spasms. This procedure also has been used successfully in the treatment of hemifacial spasm.

13–14 **Ophthalmologic Use of Pulsed Neodymium Yag Lasers: Preoperative Aperture of Lenses Prior to Implant and of Secondary Cataracts Behind Implants.** D. Aron-Rosa, J.-C. Griesemann, and J.-J. Aron (Paris) introduce this new ultrarapid pulsing laser, permitting the finest microsurgery without opening of the eye. The basic principle is creation of a protective plasma (ionized gas created by volatilization of the medium) and augmentation of the mechanical effect of the laser wave impact without heating up the vitreous, cornea, iris, or retina. The importance of this technique is in the absence of heat, since any significant thermal increase in the anterior chamber may trigger uveal reactions or corneal edema, with endothelial

---

(13–14) J. Fr. Ophtalmol. 4:61–66, 1981. (Fr.)

dystrophy as an immediate or delayed side effect. All pigmented and nonpigmented ocular tissue may be cut without dangerous thermic effect. Temperature at the point of impact does not exceed 2×10^{-3} C. Moreover, the procedure does not require anesthesia and avoids introduction of foreign matter into the eye. The precision of impact of 50 μm virtually eliminates the risk of injury to the eye, or to an implant in surgical interventions that involve opening the capsule or softening the nucleus. Since 1978, more than 500 patients have been treated by this method for a variety of conditions, including rupture of the cyclitic membrane, iridectomy, secondary traumatic cataract, trabeculotomy, and goniotomy.

▶ [This instrument seems like it will be a valuable addition to our laser armamentarium. It is unfortunate that there are still no lasers that will do more than "soften" the lens when we need one that will vaporize it.] ◀

Management of Epithelial Cysts of the Anterior Chamber. Large epithelial cysts that cause reduced vision because of pupillary obstruction or cysts associated with uncontrolled glaucoma or iritis may require operation. William E. Bruner, Ronald G. Michels, Walter J. Stark, and A. Edward Maumenee (Johns Hopkins Univ.) use a closed-eye method in aphakic eyes to collapse the cyst and devitalize the epithelial cells by cryotherapy. In phakic eyes the cyst is dissected away from the cornea and partly excised by an open-sky approach, and transscleral cryotherapy then is applied to devitalize epithelial remnants.

TECHNIQUES.—A needle or cannula is placed through the limbus or pars plana in aphakic eyes to aspirate the cyst contents where the cyst is attached to the eye wall (Fig 13–7). A small vitrectomy probe then is used to excise the anterior part of the vitreous gel (Fig 13–8). Radial incisions in the iris can be made where necessary to collapse the cyst further. Air is injected through the infusion needle as fluid is evacuated through the vitrectomy probe. Transscleral cryotherapy is applied with a freeze-refreeze technique (Fig 13–9). Part of the air bubble then is removed and replaced with sterile physiologic solution.

Phakic eyes undergo cyst excision through an open-sky approach. The cyst contents are aspirated after a limbically based

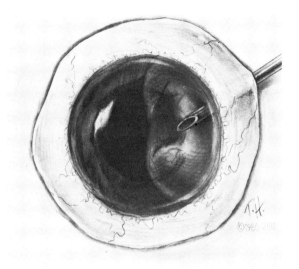

Fig 13–7.—Aspiration of epithelial cyst content through small-diameter needle introduced through limbus where cyst is attached to anterior chamber angle. (Courtesy of Bruner, W. E., et al.: Ophthalmic Surg. 12:279–285, April 1981.)

Fig 13–8 (left).—Excision of anterior vitreous gel with small-diameter probe to provide larger fluid-filled space for introduction of air bubble. Intraocular pressure is maintained by separate anterior chamber infusion needle (not shown).

Fig 13–9 (right).—Intraocular bubble filling anterior segment compresses cyst remnants against eye wall and provides thermal insulation during translimbic cryotherapy.

(Courtesy of Bruner, W. E., et al.: Ophthalmic Surg. 12:279–285, April 1981.)

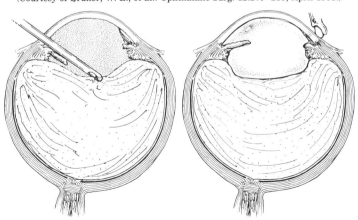

conjunctival flap is prepared. After air is injected into the anterior chamber, a spatula or small rod is used to break attachments between the cyst and the posterior part of the cornea. An incision is made throughout the limits of the cyst via the limbus, and the cyst is prolapsed into the incision and excised with scissors, with small pieces of adjacent iris. Transscleral cryotherapy is applied along the limbus after the limbic incision is closed and the anterior chamber is re-formed with air.

Seven eyes with epithelial cysts were managed by these methods, and successful anatomical results were obtained without recurrence of the cyst in each. One eye required further operation for epithelial ingrowth involving the central part of the cornea and had chronic corneal edema. Inadequate anterior vitreous was removed from this eye. Final acuity was 20/50 or better in three of the seven eyes. Two eyes had persistent cystoid macular edema, and one had amblyopia.

These methods are based on established principles of excision, or devitalization, or both of the epithelial tissue of cysts. The cause of cystoid macular edema after vitrectomy and cyst excision is unknown.

13–16 **The CT-Topography of Retrobulbar Anesthesia: Anatomic-Clinical Correlation of Complications and Suggestion of a Modified Technique.** R. Unsöld (Freiburg, West Germany), J. A. Stanley, and J. DeGroot (San Francisco) analyzed the anatomical relation of an injection needle, as traditionally placed in retrobulbar anesthesia, to the optic nerve, orbital vessels, and eye muscles, as shown on computed tomography (CT), in a human cadaver. The right eye was fixed in the traditional upward and inward position of gaze by sutures, and the injection was performed with a 25-gauge needle, 3.5 cm long and 0.5 mm wide, above the inferior orbital rim, about 0.5 cm medially to the lateral canthus. The needle was directed superiorly and medially toward the optic canal. In sequential inferior-superior sections, the different segments of the needle can be followed from the site of the puncture toward the tip of the needle within the orbital apex. Anatomical relationships were also studied with the use of an alternative technique. The left eye was fixed in a downward and outward position of gaze, and the site of puncture was the same, but the direction of the needle was lower, toward the inferior part of the superior orbital fissure. On CT study, the needle was shown to be remote from the optic nerve along its entire course and from the posterior segments of the superior ophthalmic vein and artery (Fig 13–10).

Numerous clinical complications following the traditional technique have been described. The most common complication is a retrobulbar venous hemorrhage, which is usually harmless and requires only postponement of surgery which otherwise would run a higher risk of vitreous complications. In some patients, occlusion of the central retinal artery has been reported after increased retrobulbar pressure caused by a retrobulbar hematoma. Transient visual loss or blindness, followed by a complete restitution of visual function, is thought to be a rather common phenomenon caused by a conduction block by the anesthetic agent. Permanent visual loss or blindness is a serious complication. Arterial hemorrhage with a sudden massive increase of retrobulbar pressure and subsequent ischemia is a rare but dangerous event requiring immediate surgical intervention. Perforation of the globe has been reported, particularly in patients with high myopia or colobomas of the optic nerve. Analysis of the topographic relationships of the main orbital structures and traditionally placed injection needle by CT study shows the needle to be in close proximity to the optic nerve, ophthalmic artery and its major branches, the superior ophthalmic vein, and the inferior oblique muscle.

Although most of the serious complications of retrobulbar anesthesia are rare, it seems desirable to modify the injection technique, with a resultant reduction in the risk of damaging the optic nerve, the ophthalmic artery and its branches, as well as the superior orbital vein. This can be achieved by having the patient look downward and outward, and directing the needle slightly lower toward the inferior portion of the superior orbital fissure. Preliminary trials with the alternate technique in about 50 patients have

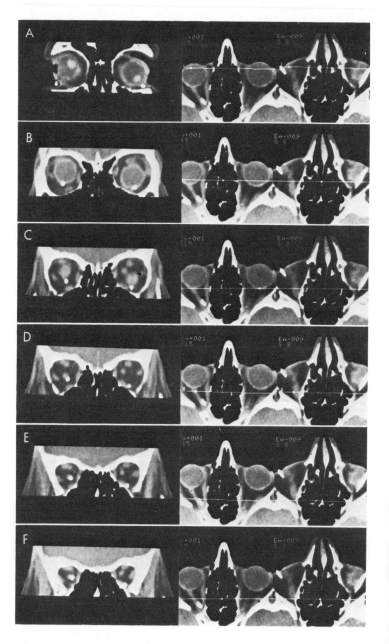

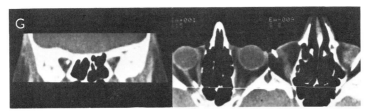

Fig 13–10.—Sequential anteroposterior computer reformations through both orbits. *Right,* coronal computer reformation; *left,* plane of coronal reformation on axial CT section. The position of gaze is demonstrated by the position of the lens. **A,** the site of the injection is symmetric on either side. Note closeness of the needle to the optic nerve shadow within the right orbit. Within the left orbit, the needle is remote from the nerve along its entire orbital course (**E–G**). The tip of the needle is demonstrated in the right orbit in front of the optic canal, in the left orbit in front of the lower portion of the superior orbital fissure (**F** and **G**). (Courtesy of Unsöld, R., et al.: Albrecht Von Graefes Arch. Klin. Exp. Ophthalmol. 217:125–136, August 1981.)

been promising, but more experience must be gained before definite recommendations can be made.

▶ [This new technique is apparently somewhat safer than the standard method of retrobulbar anesthetic injection. The nerves to the extraocular muscles do enter on their inner surfaces, and the ciliary ganglion is also between optic nerve and muscle. Thus, an injection some distance from the optic nerve and directed to the apex of the orbit might not be as effective as the usual muscle cone injection.] ◀

14. Basic Sciences, Injuries, and Miscellaneous

Giants of Visual Science

J. TERRY ERNEST, M.D.

University of Illinois, Chicago

The 1981 Nobel Prize for Physiology or Medicine was shared by David H. Hubel and Torsten N. Wiesel with Roger W. Sperry. Hubel and Wiesel received half the award for their spectacular work and insights into how the visual system works.

There are many giants of visual science; the first in modern times, perhaps, is Helmholtz, who invented the ophthalmoscope in 1851.[1] In addition to the ophthalmoscope, his work on vision and optics laid the foundation for all subsequent studies. Nobel Prizes were not awarded in those days, but Helmholtz surely would have received the honor.

Nobel Prizes have been awarded annually in physiology or medicine, physics, chemistry, literature, and peace since 1901 (a sixth prize, for economics, was added in 1969 by the National Bank of Sweden). The first vision scientist (and only ophthalmologist) to receive the award was Allvar Gullstrand. He was given the 1911 Nobel Prize for his work in physiologic optics.[2] That same year, Gullstrand invented the slit-lamp illumination system for the biomicroscope, which continues to be indispensable to our practices.[3] It is important to note that both Helmholtz and Gullstrand not only made fundamental discoveries in visual science, but also made revolutionary contributions to the clinical practice of ophthalmology.

More giants were to come. In 1967, Haldan Hartline, George Wald, and Ragnar Granit received the Nobel Prize for their studies of the chemical and physiologic visual processes of the eye. Although we remain a distance from the treatment of medical defects of the retina, these men gave us the first step toward the ultimate elimination of devastating retinal dystrophies and degeneration.

Hubel and Wiesel, in the tradition of Nobel laureates, have given us basic insights into how the visual system works, and they have helped us clinically. Their studies show that the newborn visual cortex responds to binocular images and that a loss of form vision by one eye results in a functional blindness at the level of the cerebral cortex. Therefore, it is necessary to treat eyes of strabismic children before the critical period when irreversible brain connections form.

We can all be proud to be ophthalmologists in this day and time, for we stand on the shoulders of giants and bring to our patients the finest visual science and ophthalmic care the world has known.

REFERENCES

1. Helmholtz H.: Beschreibung emir Augen-Spiegels. Berlin, A. Forstner'sce Verlagsbunchhandlung, 1851. Also in Shastid T. H. (trans.): Description of an Ophthalmoscope. Chicago, Cleveland Press, 1916.
2. Gullstrand A.: Einfuhrung in die Methoden der Dioptrik des Auges der Menschen, Leipzig, S. Hirzel, 1911.
3. Gullstrand A.: Demonstration der Nernstspaltlampe. *Ber. Versammlung Ophthalmol. Ges.* 37:374–376, 1911.

14-1 **Epinephrine Distribution After Topical Administration to Phakic and Aphakic Eyes.** Steven G. Kramer has examined the distribution of epinephrine after topical application in doses comparable to those used in the management of open-angle glaucoma. Epinephrine labeled with ^{14}C was topically administered to one eye of experimental ani-

---

(14–1) Trans. Am. Ophthalmol. Soc. 78:947–982, 1980.

mals, and, subsequently, labeled epinephrine was sought in the tissues of both eyes and in other tissues. A dose of 50 μl of 2% ^{14}C-epinephrine was applied to the center of the cornea every 5 minutes for a total of 6 doses, and the eyes were removed 2 hours after the first dose. Lens extraction was performed in about half the studies. Epinephrine also was infused into the carotid artery on one side, as were labeled dopamine and norepinephrine.

Phakic eyes showed significant intraocular uptake and storage of ^{14}C-epinephrine in the iris, ciliary body, and choroid after topical administration. When both eyes were aphakic, substantially more epinephrine was present on the treated side. Choroidal concentration when the treated eye was aphakic was about 2½ times greater than when the treated eye was phakic. No such difference was found for the untreated eyes.

Substantial uptake and storage of epinephrine were noted in the iris, ciliary body, and choroid after ipsilateral carotid artery infusion of epinephrine. Retinal storage was significantly greater on the side with the infusion. There was less uveal uptake and storage of epinephrine when superior cervical ganglionectomy was done on the same side as the subsequent infusion. The procedure did not affect retinal uptake, however. Low amounts of label were found in nonuveal tissues or nonocular tissues after topical epinephrine administration. Significant iris, ciliary body, and choroidal uptake and storage also were noted after intravenous infusion of epinephrine. Nonuveal ocular tissues had substantially lower uptake and storage. The retina had about twice the levels of uptake and storage as the optic nerve. Nonocular tissues with a rich sympathetic innervation showed significant uptake and storage of epinephrine after intravenous infusion.

Epinephrine must be used very cautiously in aphakic eyes, with special care when it is administered in only one eye, in the lowest effective concentration. It should not be used unless a therapeutic effect occurs. The use of commercial preparations of pilocarpine and epinephrine in combination may be dangerous, because they usually are given 4 times daily, twice as often as epinephrine is required.

▶ [Aphakic epinephrine maculopathy is a well-recognized entity. It is disturbing that the drug, while found in relatively high concentration at the posterior pole of the aphakic eye, is also found in the choroid, retina, and optic nerve of both treated and fellow eyes even when they are phakic.] ◀

14–2 **Pigment Epithelial Cells in Culture: Metabolic Pathways Required for Phagocytosis.** The effect of phagocytosis on the metabolic abilities of pigmented epithelial cells and the possible energy needs of these cells in initiating or sustaining phagocytosis are unknown. Eileen Masterson and Gerald J. Chader (Natl. Eye Inst., Bethesda) examined the role of the major glucose degradative pathways in the phagocytic process in cultured chick pigmented epithelial cells. Phagocytosis of bovine rod outer segments was assessed by the uptake of ^{3}H-labeled outer segments in cultures of embryonic chick pigmented epithelial cells. The participation of glycolysis, the tricarboxylic acid cycle (TCA) and cytochrome system, and the hexose monophosphate (HMP) shunt was evaluated.

Prolonged glucose deprivation substantially suppressed the uptake of labeled rod outer segments by cultured pigmented epithelial cells. Glucose transport into the pigmented epithelial cells was not increased by phagocytosis. Lactic acid production was increased in phagocytizing pigmented epithelial cells. Production of 1-^{14}CO$_2$ from 1-^{14}C-glucose was significantly decreased by phagocytosis, but 1-^{14}C-glucose uptake/utilization was unaffected. The findings indicated probable routing of glucose metabolism away from the HMP shunt during phagocytosis. Phenazine methosulfate stimulated the HMP shunt and dramatically reduced the uptake of rod outer segments. Cells incubated in 2,4-dinitrophenol (DNP) had reduced CO$_2$ production and glucose uptake/utilization; also, DNP significantly decreased phagocytosis. Ouabain and quinine retained some suppressive effects in the presence of glucose, whereas DNP and phenazine methosulfate had a vigorously suppressive effect.

Inhibitors of the TCA cycle and a lack of glucose markedly inhibit the phagocytosis of bovine rod outer segments by cultured chick pigmented epithelial cells. The TCA cycle

▶ [Retinal pigment epithelial cells phagocytize rod and cone outer segments. This is an important process that may be disrupted in aging and by disease. Whereas extrapolations from in vitro to in vivo are always difficult, the authors' pigment epithelium culture seems to be a superb system for studying the phagocytosis process.] ◀

14-3 **Increased Blood Pressure Following Pupillary Dilation With 2.5% Phenylephrine Hydrochloride in Preterm Infants.** Early ophthalmologic examinations now are done with pupillary dilating agents to detect retrolental fibroplasia in preterm infants, but the cardiovascular effects of these drugs have not been thoroughly examined. Bonnie J. Lees and Luis A. Cabal examined the cardiovascular effects of 0.5% tropicamide and 2.5% phenylephrine HCl in 7 distressed preterm infants on the first day of life. Birth weights ranged from 910 to 2,060 gm, and gestational ages ranged from 26 to 36 weeks. One drop of the medications was instilled in each eye, and cardiovascular status was monitored for 75 minutes. Full pupillary dilatation was achieved within 15–20 minutes.

The heart rate was increased at 6 minutes and decreased at 8 minutes, followed by a gradual return to baseline. The changes were not significant. All patients experienced a rise in arterial pressure after instillation of the drops. Peak increases in systolic, diastolic, and mean pressures of 25%, 23%, and 24%, respectively, were observed by 8 minutes. Significant elevations persisted for 30 minutes.

A significant increase in arterial pressure follows instillation of 0.5% tropicamide and 2.5% phenylephrine drops in preterm infants who are ill. It is possible that this effect has a role in the genesis of intraventricular hemorrhage, although the relation between arterial pressure and cerebral blood flow in the asphyxiated premature infant is unclear. The benefits of accurate gestational age assessment and funduscopy in ill premature infants must be weighed against the possible risks from increased arterial pressure.

Arterial pressure should be monitored when using mydriatic agents in this setting.

▶ [Ophthalmologists examining infants usually use small amounts of drug in an oil vehicle along with manual occlusion of the lacrimal sacs to minimize systemic absorption. Nonetheless, blood pressure effects occur and, as these authors point out, may be dangerous.] ◀

14–4 **The Symptom of Ocular Pain** is discussed by R. A. Hitchings (London). Pain in or around the eye is a common presentation to ophthalmologists. Patient descriptions of pain and their responses to ocular lesions that cause pain are infinitely varied. Ocular causes of pain in the eye are listed in the table. Pain may arise from direct stimulation of pain nerve endings or from excessive stimulation of other types of sensory terminals. Both the cornea and sclera are innervated by the ophthalmic division of the fifth cranial nerve. The uveal tract has shown minimal evidence of sensory innervation.

Mechanical stimulation after loss or disease of the corneal epithelium can produce pain directly. Pain can be prevented through more rapid healing, use of analgesics to reduce stimulation of pain fibers, and treatment of coincidental iritis. There is little direct sensory innervation of the posterior sclera; pain from posterior scleritis may be due to involvement of the short posterior ciliary nerves or inflammation of adjacent extraocular muscles and orbital structures. Kinins and prostaglandins released in the iris with breakdown of the blood-aqueous barrier can stimulate

Causes of Ocular Pain	
Site	*Disease*
Cornea	Erosion, foreign body, ulcer, bullous keratopathy
Sclera	Scleritis
Iris	Iritis, miotics, iridectomy, Argon laser, anterior segment ischaemia, thrombotic and acute angle-closure glaucoma
Ciliary body	Argon laser
Retina and choroid	Krypton laser. Glare and photophobia

(14–4) Trans. Ophthalmol. Soc. U.K. 100(Pt. 2):257–259, July 1980.

chemoreceptors in the nerve plexus of the ciliary body. Manipulation of the iris during iridectomy can cause pain from tugging at the iris root. The pain seen in glaucoma may be due to concurrent inflammation. Pain from iris inflammation can be managed with steroids to counter the release of tissue kinins and prostaglandin E_1 or with antiprostaglandins. Pain from iris miosis can be reversed by atropine. Pain from photocoagulation of the iris root can be minimized by ensuring that burns are of short duration.

Short-duration photocoagulation of the retina and choroid with the argon laser is painless, but use of the krypton laser may cause pain. Patients who cannot regulate the amount of light entering the eye may suffer from glare, and dark glasses may be of benefit. Photophobia may be viewed as undue sensitivity to light of normal luminosity. It classically occurs with ocular inflammation from either corneal disease or iritis. When photophobia is associated with miosis and is possibly due to spasm of the ciliary muscles, it is relieved by cycloplegics.

14–5 **Human Electroretinogram After Argon Laser Photocoagulation of Different Retinal Areas.** Photocoagulation is now an accepted treatment of diabetic retinopathy, although its beneficial effects remain unclear. Destruction of hypoxic regions may eliminate production of a vasoproliferative substance, and coagulation of large areas of the retina may leave the rest in better metabolic condition. Magnus Gjötterberg and Sven Blomdahl (Karolinska Inst., Stockholm) evaluated the results of photocoagulation in 20 diabetic patients aged 22–72 years, of whom most had early proliferative retinopathy. Initially 300 argon laser burns were applied during each of three occasions, with a spot size of 500 µm and an exposure time of 0.1 second. Moderately severe lesions were produced. In 10 eyes the treatment began in the posterior pole 15–40 degrees from the fovea, excluding the papillomacular zone, whereas in 10 other eyes the treatment began in the superior peripheral area. The third session in both groups included treatment of the inferior peripheral area.

Repeated treatments resulted in a substantial reduction

in all electroretinographic components. Central treatments tended to reduce the amplitudes more. Amplitude reductions were considerably greater than expected from the fraction of the total retinal area destroyed. The a-wave appeared to be the most diminished. Electroretinograms recorded immediately after the three treatment sessions resembled those recorded later.

Electroretinographic changes are related to photocoagulation of particular areas in eyes with proliferative diabetic retinopathy. Coagulation of a central region appears to reduce the electroretinogram more than if destruction of a peripheral area has occurred, probably because of different receptor concentrations. Argon laser coagulation appears to reduce the electroretinographic a-wave more than the b-wave. A small electroretinogram should not be considered a contraindication to vitrectomy in a photocoagulated patient.

▶ [There was tremendous variation in electroretinographic response. That may mean there are other factors besides the extent of photocoagulation that must be considered, such as the effects of the diabetes itself on the response.] ◀

14–6 **Laser-Induced Endovascular Thrombosis as a Possibility of Selective Vessel Closure.** Absorption of argon laser light by hemoglobin makes this modality suitable for the selective coagulation of neovascularizations. The small beam divergence of the laser permits small vessels to be treated without damaging surrounding tissues. K.-P. Boergen, R. Birngruber, and F. Hillenkamp attempted to occlude small vessels selectively in the rat mesentery while leaving the vessel wall intact. The circulation of the ileal mesentery was assessed by large-field microscopy while argon laser irradiation was applied, using a spot size of 70 μm and an exposure time of 23 msec. Studies were done during both undisturbed blood flow and when blood flow was reduced by pulling on the mesentery.

Endovascular thrombosis was achieved with energy levels less than 5 millijoules at reduced blood flow rates. The endothelium of the vessel wall on the opposite side maintained its continuity. Energy levels of more than 10 milli-

---
(14–6) Ophthalmic Res. 13:139–150, 1981.

joules were necessary for endovascular change at normal flow velocity. Short-term luminal occlusion was often observed, with interruption of blood flow. Disruption of the internal elastic lamina was noted at the site of laser application. Marked thrombocyte agglutination was present at the free end, and at the opposite wall the endothelium was completely removed. Fibrin formation was not observed. Repeated exposures led to complete vessel occlusion lasting several hours. The lumen was largely occluded by amorphous masses of clumped erythrocytes.

Specific vascular occlusion through the production of endovascular thrombosis with the argon laser apparently is feasible. The coagulation variables necessary for optimal vascular coagulation are not, however, available with current clinical lasers.

▶ [Although the retinal circulation autoregulates, at intraocular pressures above approximately 40 mm Hg the retinal blood flow is slowed. Perhaps focal treatment of abnormal blood vessels would be augmented by induced ocular hypertension.] ◀

14-7 **Prevention of Eye Injuries** was discussed by Tom Pashby (Hosp. for Sick Children, Toronto). In Canada, 30,000 people are registered as being blind; in one third of these, blindness might have been avoided. Prevention is the key to reducing the number of eye injuries and blind eyes.

Homes are filled with hazards, especially to children. Household items with sharp points or edges and caustic substances (especially those in spray cans) can cause severe visual injuries and should be kept out of the reach of children. Parents also must be alert to the dangers of children's toys. The kitchen, garage, and workshop are potentially dangerous areas. Pets and stray dogs are responsible for many lid lacerations. Other injuries have been caused by overheated carbonated drink bottles that have been shaken vigorously. Lighted cigarettes are responsible for eye burns, especially to babies. Adults making repairs in the home or on the car should use protective eye wear and familiarize themselves with the proper method of the work at hand.

Sports are responsible for many eye injuries. Many hockey

(14-7) Can. Fam. Physician 27:464-469, March 1981.

careers have ended because of blinding injuries. Changes in rules and the development of effective face protectors are reducing the number of eye injuries in organized hockey. A change of philosophy from "winning is everything" to playing for pleasure also has reduced injuries in amateur players. The growing popularity of squash and racket ball has increased the frequency of eye injuries. A Canadian Standards Association (CSA) has been formed to write a racket sports eye protector standard. Until CSA certification, it is recommended that all racket sports players wear an eye protector of the closed type with either plano or prescription plastic lenses. Eyes are vulnerable to injury in other sports as well (table). Again, depending on the sport, adequate masks or polycarbonate shields or goggles must be worn. Because amblyopia has a prevalence of 2%–4% in the general population, it is recommended that visual acuity be recorded for each eye before participation in sports.

A great number of eye injuries occur at work. The benefit of safety glasses, goggles, or shields cannot be overestimated. In the United States, 85,000 eyes (more than 2,000 per year) as well as $10 million in compensation payments have been saved. The Canadian Conference on Personal Protective Equipment in 1978 (COPE '78) stressed the need to assess the visual acuity of the workman to determine his suitability for the job, the need for sufficient lighting, and appropriate eye protectors.

The importance of prevention of eye injuries is gaining prominence. However, doctors are so involved in treating patients that they often neglect their potential role as stim-

COS Athletic Eye Injuries in Six Seasons

Sport	1972-73 No. of Injuries	1972-73 No. of Blind Eyes	1974-75 No. of Injuries	1974-75 No. of Blind Eyes	1976-77 No. of Injuries	1976-77 No. of Blind Eyes	1977-78 No. of Injuries	1977-78 No. of Blind Eyes	1978-79 No. of Injuries	1978-79 No. of Blind Eyes	1979-80 No. of Injuries	1979-80 No. of Blind Eyes	Total No. of Injuries	Total No. of Blind Eyes
Ice hockey	287	20	258	42	90	12	52	8	43	13	85	21	815	116
Ball hockey					24	3	8		9	2	16	1	57	6
Racket sports					48	3	12	1	28	1	58	1	146	6
Baseball					19	2	2		2		24	1	47	3
Football					11	1	2		3		2	1	18	2
Volleyball					1	1					7		8	1
Golf					5	1			1		1		7	1
Lacrosse					2		1		1				4	
Broomball					2	2					2		4	2
Skiing					1	1	1		3	2	1		6	3
Snowmobiling					2	1					1	1	3	2
Total	287	20	258	42	205	27	78	9	90	18	197	26	1115	142

ulators of prevention. Physicians also must take more responsibility for providing the media with *accurate* information on prevention and health care.

14-8 **Sports Eye Injuries: A Preventable Disease.** Paul F. Vinger (Harvard Med. School) points out that more than 100,000 school-age children in a year are expected to incur sports-related eye injuries and that 25% will have serious complications. Sixty percent of unprotected hockey players have eye or facial injury by high school. The average eye injury in hockey costs more than $1,200 in direct medical expenses alone. Certified face protectors greatly reduce eye and face injuries. Estimates of eye injuries in various sports are given in the table. Football faceguards have reduced facial injuries by more than 80%. Protection in racket sports can be obtained with a polycarbonate protector, either plano or a prescription lens. Contact lenses offer no ocular protection from impact.

Greater input from large ophthalmologic centers is needed in the area of eye protection in sports activities. More basic research is needed on the mechanisms of eye injuries from sports. Better public education also is essential. The public should know that 23% of emergency trauma admissions to

ESTIMATED EYE INJURIES IN VARIOUS SPORTS*

Sport	Emergency Rooms 1979	Emergency Rooms First Quarter 1980	Emergency Rooms and Private Practice 1979
Baseball	6,139	1,084	
Racket sports	4,259	1,439	9,184
Tennis, badminton	2,271	212	
Squash, racquetball, paddleball	1,988	1,227	
Basketball	5,362	2,712	
Football	2,024	244	
Bicycling	2,793	208	
Soccer	658	134	
Volleyball	710	212	
Hockey (all kinds)	481*	252*	
Gas-, Air-, Spring- Operated guns	1,273	508	

*Low numbers result from wearing protective masks.

(14–8) Ophthalmology (Rochester) 88:108–113, February 1981.

the Massachusetts Eye and Ear Infirmary were for sports injuries and that 20% were for intraocular foreign bodies. Manufacturers should be encouraged to make safer products, and regressive legislation such as the liberalization of air weapons or fireworks laws should be opposed.

14–9 **Pharmacokinetics of Fluorescein in the Vitreous.** Vitreous fluorophotometry has been used to investigate ocular abnormalities in diabetes and other diseases such as retinitis pigmentosa. A. G. Palestine and R. F. Brubaker (Mayo Clinic) compared the kinetics of orally and intravenously administered fluorescein in the blood and the vitreous. An optical device was developed that permits the same region of vitreous to be analyzed on successive occasions in a given person. Six young, normal subjects were studied. Sodium fluorescein 10% was injected intravenously over 4 minutes or given orally in 350 ml of a carbonated citrus beverage. The subjects were fasting at the time of administration. All but 1 received a dose of 7 mg of fluorescein per kg. The oral and intravenous studies were done at least a week apart. Vitreous and blood fluorescein concentrations were determined over 8 hours by fluorophotometry and fluorescence polarization.

The free fraction of fluorescein ranged from 0.10 to 0.14. The intravenous blood concentration fell rapidly, whereas the vitreous concentration rose rapidly. Oral fluorescein administration produced lower peak blood concentrations and lower vitreous concentrations than did intravenous administration. Peak blood concentrations of orally administered fluorescein usually occurred at 30 minutes. After 4 hours the oral and intravenous pharmacokinetic curves were similar. The average vitreous concentration after intravenous injection peaked at 2 hours and remained constant for several hours. After oral administration, the vitreous concentration rose and fell more slowly and lacked a distinct plateau phase. Calculations indicated that increasing retinal permeability has results identical with those of decreasing the active transport pump.

Fluorescein is most easily administered orally, and the risk of a serious reaction probably is lower than from intravenous injection. Variability in absorption, however, introduces uncertainties unless systemic concentrations are measured. The active transport and plasma binding of fluorescein, and retinal permeability, should be taken into account in interpreting fluorophotometry data.

14–10 **Vitreous Fluorophotometry: Identification of Sources of Variability.** Slit-lamp vitreous fluorophotometry (VF) is a noninvasive means of measurement of fluorescein in various ocular compartments and has been used to show early breakdown of the blood-ocular barrier. Elevated vitreous fluorescein levels have been reported in diabetic patients even when no retinal pathologic conditions were found by angiography or ophthalmoscopy. Thomas C. Prager, David J. Wilson, Graham D. Avery, James H. Merritt, Charles A. Garcia, Gary Hopen, and Robert E. Anderson (Houston) have identified several variables that directly influence VF readings. Studies were performed in normal human subjects and in an artificial eye. Subjects received 7 mg of 25% fluorescein sodium per kg intravenously and were examined an hour later.

Ocular pigmentation was a significant factor in VF readings. Fluorescein in the choroidal circulation significantly influenced VF readings taken at the retinal surface and in the posterior vitreous. Heavy pigmentation in dark-eyed subjects screened out choroidal fluorescence more effectively than the light pigmentation of blue-eyed subjects. Vitreous readings taken near the retina closely followed the decline in plasma fluorescein levels. The amount of measured fluorescein was influenced by the slit width of the exciting light; the effect was less evident at narrow slit widths.

These variables must be taken into account when quantitative VF is performed. Ocular pigmentation can be partly controlled by determining relative reflectance, or its contribution can be reduced by using a narrow slit width and taking measurements beyond the main choroidal sphere of influence. All VF measurements should be made at the same time, particularly if posterior vitreous values are needed.

▶ [The authors of this article and the preceding one have demonstrated

---

(14–10) Invest. Ophthalmol. Vis. Sci. 21:854–864, December 1981.

that there are many more factors affecting vitreous fluorescein measurements than heretofore recognized. Indeed, it may be that there are still more variables to be discovered. The conclusion is that, for the time being, fluorophotometry data must be analyzed extensively and extreme care must be taken in the interpretation of its meaning.] ◀

14–11 **Efficiency of Ordinary Sunglasses as Protection From Ultraviolet Radiation.** Anderson and Gebel reported that ultraviolet transmittance by commercial sunglasses may be a cause for concern. G. Segrè, R. Reccia, B. Pignalosa, and G. Pappalardo (Naples, Italy) attempted to verify this finding because of the marked increase in the use of such spectacles by persons of all ages. Fifty pairs of sunglasses obtained from various commercial sources were evaluated. The optical transmission spectrum was measured with a spectrophotometer. Although sunglass wearers may be exposed longer to sunlight, this is not a quantifiable factor. Pupillary adaptation depends on light flux, and the consequent radiation damage depends on radiant intensity and wavelength. In the ultraviolet range, there was a crossing over of the curve of some lenses with that representing the specific solar radiance. Such lenses offer no protection from ultraviolet radiation.

Although Anderson and Gebel may have exaggerated in stating that the dose received with spectacles is twice as great as that received by the naked eye, in many cases the use of sunglasses may result in a considerable risk. Better information will help the public in selecting sunglasses; the most expensive glasses are certainly not always the best. Such information should be made compulsory by law and should be presented in a clear, easily understandable manner.

▶ [Defective sunglasses may increase eye exposure because individuals think they are protected and remain in bright sunlight and pupils may dilate. The transmission should be flat in the visible with U.V. and I.R. blocking but this is seldom the case with most commercially available sunglasses.] ◀

14–12 **Damage to Monkey Retina by Broad-Spectrum Fluorescent Light.** In a variety of animals, structural retinal damage follows excessive exposure to visible light. Stephen M. Sykes, W. Gerald Robison, Jr., Morris Waxler, and To-

---

(14–11) Ophthalmic Res. 13:180–187, 1981.
(14–12) Invest. Ophthalmol. Vis. Sci. 20:425–434, April 1981.

ichiro Kuwabara attempted to determine thresholds for morphological change after fluorescent light exposure in the retinas of 10 adult rhesus and pigtail monkeys aged 5–15 years. Light intensities of 5,900–24,700 lux were delivered from daylight fluorescent bulbs. The eyes were removed for microscopic study 15 hours after the end of exposure.

Exposure to 24,700 lux resulted in marked disruption of photoreceptor outer segments, which appeared poorly aligned and abnormally twisted. Nearly all receptors in the macula were affected to some degree. No such changes were seen in the patched eye. The ultrastructural appearances are shown in Figure 14–1. The primary site of rod damage was the distal end of the outer segment, where swelling and

Fig 14–1.—Retinal pigment epithelium *(PE)* and distal portions of photoreceptor outer segments *(OS)* of macula in retina. **A**, patched eye. **B**, eye exposed to 24,700 lux. Only rod outer segments are shown. Vacuoles *(V)* associated with membrane lamellae in the pigment epithelium were distributed irregularly in both exposed and unexposed retinas; original magnification ×7100. (Courtesy of Sykes, S. M., et al.: Invest. Ophthalmol. Vis. Sci. 20:425–434, April 1981.)

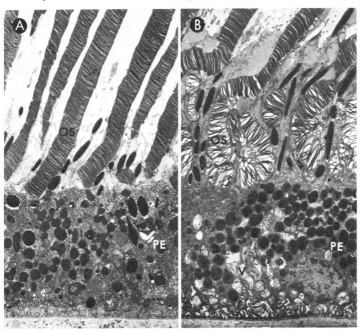

disk membrane separation were evident. Cone damage was of the proximal type, with vesicle and vacuole formation and membrane reorganization. Less misalignment of the outer segment was seen at 19,400 lux. At 10,800 lux, damage essentially was restricted to the proximal regions of the outer segments of photoreceptor cells that appeared to be cones. Damage at lower exposure levels was marginal. At 5,900 lux, fewer than 5% of photoreceptors in the macula were affected, and damage was of the proximal type only.

The primate retina can be damaged at levels of illumination that potentially may be encountered. The findings may not be applicable to laser therapy, because the thermal lesions produced by brief laser exposures differ substantially from the photochemical lesions due to broad-spectrum light exposures. The lesser amount of ocular pigment present in human beings may make them more susceptible than monkeys to photochemical retinal damage.

▶ [Work continues in this important area and, whereas this particular study emphasizes the normal environment, the use of direct and indirect ophthalmoscopes would also seem to be of some concern.] ◀

14–13 **Onchocerciasis.** B. O. L. Duke (Geneva) describes onchocerciasis as a disease of the eye and skin that follows infection with the filarial worm *Onchocerca volvulus*. It is transmitted by female black flies of the genus *Simulium*. An estimated 20 to 40 million persons are infected with *O. volvulus*. Intense infections tend to build up from repeated inoculations of infective larvae. Blindness rates as high as 15% may be found in villages in the African savanna region. The microfilariae, appearing some 9–18 months after a bite, live in the human host for some 1–2 years. Ocular lesions include sclerosing keratitis, iridocyclitis, chorioretinal lesions, and optic atrophy. Patients seen in Great Britain usually have light infection, acquired during brief exposure in an endemic area, with itching and perhaps a reddish, papular rash and occasionally a few microfilariae in the eye. There may be a mild punctate keratitis, which responds well to treatment. Such patients rarely develop severe ocular lesions.

(14–13) Br. Med. J. 283:961–962, Oct. 10, 1981.

Currently treatment is with diethylcarbamazine citrate (DEC-C) to kill the microfilariae, and an attempt is made to dampen the often violent local and systemic reactions due to death of the parasite. A course of suramin injections then is given to kill the adult forms, followed by more DEC-C to kill residual microfilariae. Treatment may last 2–3 months. No chemoprophylaxis is available. Visitors to endemic areas must try to avoid places where *Simulium* are biting and wear protective clothing. *Simulium* are controllable by organic chemical larvicides, and it is hoped that the parasite eventually will die out of the human population and that the disease will disappear. A nontoxic drug for use in treatment of onchocerciasis is needed badly. An agent should have a convenient dosage schedule and should kill or permanently sterilize the adult worms of *O. volvulus* without producing a microfilaricidal reaction.

▶ [The author states that the pharmaceutical industry is not much interested in developing drugs against tropical parasitic diseases because of the poor possibility of profit.] ◀

14–14 **Prevalence of Ocular Manifestations of Leprosy in Port Moresby, Papua New Guinea.** Roger Dethlefs reviewed the ocular abnormalities in 109 leprosy patients seen at Port Moresby General Hospital in a 4-month period in 1978. The findings are shown in the table. Fifty-two percent of the patients had ocular complications, and 12% had sight-threatening lesions, including lagophthalmos and anterior uveitis. Five of 7 patients with uveitis had lepromatous leprosy. No potentially sight-threatening lesions were found in patients with tuberculoid leprosy. Mean patient age was 26.3 years, and mean estimated duration of disease was 7.2 years. A total of 777 leprosy outpatients currently being seen at the hospital had a mean age of 28.3 years and a mean duration of disease of 6.5 years.

The prevalence of ocular complications and serious lesions was lower in this series than in other reported studies. As in other series, uveitis was most frequent in patients with lepromatous leprosy. Only 4 patients had acuity less than 6/9 in one eye, and 3 of them had had trauma to the affected eye; 1 patient had superficial punctate kerati-

---

(14–14) Br. J. Ophthalmol. 65:223–225, April 1981.

PREVALENCE OF OCULAR LESIONS ACCORDING TO LEPROSY TYPE

	Tuberculoid	Borderline	Lepromatous
Madarosis	—	22	27
Lid infiltration	—	6	8
Epibulbar lesions	—	—	—
Superficial keratitis	—	10	10
Corneal hypoaesthesia	—	7	7
Band keratopathy	—	—	—
Flare	—	1	3
Cells	—	1	4
Posterior synechiae	—	—	1
Keratic precipitates	—	2	4
Iris pearls	—	—	3
Choroidal lesions	—	—	—
Interstitial keratitis	—	—	1
Leprous pannus	—	—	—
Lagophthalmos	—	6	—
Total	9	70	30

tis. There was 1 case of interstitial keratitis that affected the peripheral cornea only and 1 case of nonvascularized superficial keratitis with "chalk flake" opacities in the upper cornea near the limbus. The other cases of keratitis were superficial and related to either lagophthalmos and exposure, or a trigeminal nerve deficit.

▶ ["Madarosis" (table) is from the Greek word for "bald," and it means "loss of the eyelashes or eyebrows."] ◀

14-15 **Evolution of Ophthalmic Sutures** is reviewed by Wendell L. Hughes, Ramon Castroviejo, J. Elliott Blaydes, Samuel D. McPherson, Jr., Charles T. Riall, William L. Himsel, and Richard L. Kronenthal. Various suture components and fabrication methods have been investigated in parallel with the development of needles for use in

(14–15) Ann. Plast. Surg. 6:48–65, January 1981.

ophthalmic surgery. Progressively smaller sutures down to size 11-0 have been developed, permitting successful work on the most delicate ocular tissues. Silicone, Teflon, and other coatings have been used on both the suture and the needle to attain smoothness. Both permanent and absorbable synthetic sutures are available in a variety of forms. Dyes are used to enhance the visibility of fine sutures. Various metals also have been used as suture materials. Microsurgical instruments have been devised to manipulate tiny needles and sutures in work on delicate intraocular tissues.

The ideal suture provides apposition of the wound long enough for adequate healing to occur and then leaves the wound. The PDS material developed by Ethicon is a long-term absorbable suture with many interesting possibilities. Over 300 different needle-suture combinations are now available to the ophthalmologist.

Continued improvements in needles, sutures, and packaging technology will be necessary as new ophthalmic procedures are developed. A means of joining strands of suture with a tissue-compatible cement or solvent, or heat, to eliminate the bulk and occasional uncertainty of a knot would be a real advantage, particularly for continuous mattress sutures. Sutures then could be made practically friction free to reduce tissue drag and tissue entrapment. Another possibility is replacement of the needle by treating or tempering the end of the suture so that it could be molded and sharpened to a point.

▶ [These fine surgeons have written a delightful article mostly from an historic point of view. It is difficult to keep from wondering, however, if the future is not going to be microstaples and tissue glue rather than needles with microfilaments.] ◀

Beware Recessive Genes. Calbert I. Phillips and Marjorie S. Newton (Edinburgh) have learned to consider recessive genes as a possible cause of any unusual bilaterally symmetric ocular disease. Five families with two blind children have been encountered, in which the birth of the second child might have been prevented if autosomal recessive genes had been suspected as the cause of blindness in the first child. The diagnoses included bilateral macular

---

(14–16) Lancet 2:293–297, Aug. 8, 1981.

"coloboma," bilateral nonattachment of the retina, asphyxiating thoracic dystrophy (Jeune's disease) and retinitis pigmentosa, congenital retinal aplasia (Leber's congenital amaurosis), and retinitis pigmentosa, metaphyseal chondrodysplasia, and brachydactyly. In two sibships with affected males only, X-linked transmission was a consideration. The diagnoses were bilateral macular "coloboma" and retinal aplasia, and bilateral nonattachment of the retina.

Autosomal recessive disease typically appears in only one generation. Consanguinity increases the risk that children will be affected by diseases due to autosomal recessive genes. If only males are affected, the possibility of X-linked disease must be considered even if previous generations have not been affected. In some families with dominant disease, one person may have only one affected eye, whereas others are bilaterally affected. There is a danger of invoking recessive genes too often to explain difficult clinical problems. Intrauterine infection and drug toxicity must also be considered. In small families, which are common today, the chance that recessive disease will appear even once is small. Recessive disease should be considered when any unusual condition is seen, especially if it is bilaterally symmetric.

14–17 **Genetic Counseling for Parents of Children With Impaired Vision** is discussed by J. François (Univ. of Gent). Genetic counseling at the university clinic is conducted for retinoblastoma (37%), uveacoloboma (15%), tapetoretinal degeneration (11%), congenital glaucoma (11%), and various eye diseases (26%). Consanguinity of parents is also a reason for counseling. A complete obstetric, personal, and familial case history should be established to discover a teratogenic and not a genetic cause of the disease. The three large groups of genetic diseases are: (1) chromosomal diseases, (2) monogenetic diseases, and (3) polygenetic (or multifactorial) diseases, which depend on several pathologic genes and possibly are affected by environmental factors.

The empirical risk of children being born with a disease or malformation is reported. In healthy families with normal parents, the probability is 2% to 4%; when healthy parents are first cousins, the risk is 5%. Of course, the risk is greater in affected families. When the mother or father is affected and there is no consanguinity, the risk is 20%, but when the parents are first cousins, it is 32.5%. When both parents are affected it is 100%. When the parents are normal but one child is affected, the risk for the other children is 25%. When the mother or father is affected and there is already one child affected, the risk for the other children is 50%. When a grandparent is affected, the risk for the grandchildren is 10%. When an aunt or an uncle is affected, the risk for the nephews and nieces is 7%.

In genetic counseling, the parents must understand that no physician can guarantee a normal child. Parents also must understand that the mendelian risks are the same for each pregnancy. Finally, parents must be aware of a 2% to 4% risk of a major congenital anomaly for each child. From the human and psychologic point of view, the counselor must convince the parents that they are not responsible for their child's disease and that both the husband and the wife may carry pathologic genes (every individual carries 2 to 10 pathologically recessive genes). Finally, it is not the counselor's responsibility to impose a decision. Only the parents can decide whether they want more children.

▶ [The authors of this article and the preceding one emphasize the importance of genetic counseling. The issues may be both difficult to understand and in some cases painful for the parents. A team consisting of the physician, a social worker or family counselor, and the minister might be the most helpful.] ◀

14–18 **Coping With Sudden Blindness.** Rudolf Hoehn-Saric, Elizabeth Frank, Lawrence W. Hirst, and Charlotte G. Seltser (Johns Hopkins Univ.) describe a patient who was instantly blinded without other disability or disfigurement, and who illustrates the response of a well-functioning person to sudden disaster.

Man, 20, a college student from a middle-class family with strong religious beliefs and rural traditions, had been an active, outgoing person with good social skills and strong leadership ability. A bullet from the gun of a person outside his house pierced the wall and entered the patient's lateral canthal area, destroying both globes but not the brain or face. The only result other than total blindness was temporary impairment of the sense of smell. Bilateral enucleation was carried out. Although extremely upset and frightened, the patient began talking about rehabilitation on the night of operation and recalled having "bargained with the Lord" to accept blindness if there were no other disabilities. He was optimistic from the outset, obtained full family support, and was able to obtain expensive learning materials and equipment and to finance his rehabilitation. The patient remained realistic and goal directed, always expressing optimism. He continued to be able to visualize his surroundings. The most disturbing aspect of his condition were vivid dreams, which eventually became less intense. The patient was little interested in the outcome of the trial of his assailant, feeling that if anyone were going to ruin his life it would be himself, not the assailant.

This patient's rapid rehabilitation and lack of major affective disturbance can be attributed to good hospital care, active family support, a healthy personality, and an optimistic outlook on life. His ability to recognize meaning in life without losing sight of his actual limitations assured his speedy rehabilitation and an inner satisfaction that could not be gained from intellectual questioning.

14–19 **Ramble in Chinese Ophthalmology, Past and Present.** Chen Yaozhen reviewed early descriptions of various ocular diseases in China. One of the earliest records of glaucoma is that of a disciple of Confucius who lived at about 500 B.C. Another description is available from the eighth century A.D. The overall prevalence of glaucoma in China today is about 0.5%. Cases of treatment of cataract are available from the ninth century A.D. Senile cataract is found in up to 7% of rural populations in China today. The origin of trachoma has been said to be in the nomadic races of Mongolia, from where it spread westward with the Mongol invasions and eastward to the American continent. The first distinct records of trachoma in China are from the sixth century A.D. Trachoma is found today in about two thirds of a rural population in the north of China and in about one third of rural subjects in the south.

▶ [Glaucoma has been documented to have blinded people 500 years before Christ, and no doubt before that, just as the disease often does today despite our best efforts.] ◀

14–20 **Manpower Studies for the United States: II. Demand for Eye Care: A Public Opinion Poll Based on a Gallup Poll Survey.** Robert D. Reinecke and Theodore Steinberg analyzed data from a survey of the general public involving 3,067 interviews of adults in 1979 regarding the provision of eye care. The goal was to obtain an approximation of the civilian population of the United States aged 18 and older.

About half of the subjects reported knowing the difference between an ophthalmologist and optometrist, and more than three fourths of these preferred to receive eye care from an ophthalmologist. Most of those who did not know the difference also selected an ophthalmologist. Forty percent of the subjects knew a specific ophthalmologist whom they saw regularly or would see if the need arose. About three-fourths believed that healthy adults should have an eye examination every 2 years, but only about half reported having examinations this often. About one-fifth reported having had a medical eye emergency requiring ophthalmologic care. About 40% of subjects receiving third-party payments had been examined by an ophthalmologist; 45% by an optometrist. About 60% of the sample reported having seen advertisements concerning eye care.

Fewer than half of the adults in this survey had a regular ophthalmologist. A large majority of subjects felt that, if there were a national health care program, it should cover the cost of routine eye examinations. Just more than one third of the sample believed the current number of ophthalmologists to be correct, while just more than half believed that the current number of optometrists is correct.

(14–20) Ophthalmology (Rochester) 88:34A–47A, April 1981.

Subject Index

A

Acephalgic migraine: experience with, 311
Acetazolamide: and renal failure, 324
Acidosis: metabolic, and acetazolamide, 324
Age: and normal visual acuity, 67
Air: intravitreal, during retinal reattachment, 339
Alcohol syndrome: fetal, 325
Aldose reductase: in diabetic cataract, 185
Allergic conjunctivitis: clobetasone butyrate and sodium cromoglycate in, 82
Allograft reactions: after keratoplasty, 111
Amblyopia, 48
 anisometropic
  myopic, contact lenses in, 50
  therapy of, 48
 CAM treatment of, evaluation, 52
 stimulus deprivation, 49
 strabismic, contact lenses in, 51
 vergence eye movements in, dynamic, 61
Anesthesia
 corneal, during timolol, 64
 retrobulbar, CT in topography of, 341
Angiography
 fluorescein, in macular edema, 256
 of glioma of intracranial optic pathway, in children, 300
Anomalies: of facial contour, prefabricated sculptured implants in, 26
Anterior chamber
 angle in intraocular pressure increase, argon laser in, 135
 cysts, epithelial, 352
Aphakic
 correction, extended-wear contact lenses for, 74
 eye, epinephrine distribution in, 360
 keratopathy, keratoplasty in, 109
 keratoplasty, penetrating, macular edema after, 335
Aqueous
 -blood barrier breakdown, and cyclocryotherapy, 158
 humor
  after implant, intraocular, 322
  timolol penetration into, 146
 -venous shunt for glaucoma, 169
Arginine-restricted diet: in atrophy of choroid and retina, 282
Argon (see Laser, argon)
Arteritis
 giant cell, eye complications in, 308
 temporal, eye complications in, 308
Atopic
 dermatitis (see Dermatitis, atopic)
 keratoconjunctivitis, sodium cromoglycate in, 81
Atrophy: of choroid and retina, arginine-restricted diet in, 282

Autoimmunity: iridocyclitis and HLA B8 in black patients, 205

B

Balloon buckle: in retinal detachment repair, 340
Behçet's syndrome:
immunosuppressive therapy of, 320
Birth weight: very low, retrolental fibroplasia and transfusion, 247
Blepharospasm: surgical procedure for, 350
Blindness: sudden, coping with, 379
Blood
-aqueous barrier breakdown, and cyclocryotherapy, 158
pressure increase after pupillary dilation, in prematurity, 363
transfusion in retrolental fibroplasia, 273 ff.
Brain scanning: of glioma of intracranial optic pathway, in children, 300
Bronchoconstrictive effect: of timolol and obstructive lung disease, 154
Bronchospasm: after timolol, 153
Bullous keratopathy: keratoplasty in, 109

C

CAM treatment: of amblyopia, evaluation, 52
Cancer: of eye, metastatic, complication of, 205
Carcinoma, 15 ff.
of eye adnexa, incompletely excised, 15
lid, basal cell, 15
Care: of eye, survey of demand for, 381
Cataract, 179 ff., 185 ff., 190 ff. congenital
good visual function after surgery, in newborn, 349
visual acuity after surgery before 6 months, 196
in dermatitis, atopic, 193
diabetic, aldose reductase in, 185
extraction, 186 ff.
extracapsular, pseudophakos implant and (in primate), 190
intracapsular, reconstituents and corneal endothelium, 342
intracapsular, sodium hyaluronate in, 336
intraocular lens implant after, 187
length of hospital stay for, 186
formation, effect of diabetes on, 180
glaucoma and, 194
in G6PD deficiency, 192
with lens extraction, visual disturbances due to glasses or lenses, 71
secondary behind implant, pulsed neodymium laser in, 351
senile, diabetes and salicylate in, 183
surgery, 179 ff.
effectiveness of, 180
indications for, change in, 179
ultraviolet risk factor and, 193
Cell(s)
epithelial, pigment, and phagocytosis, 362
-mediated event in retinal traction, 234
Cellulitis: orbital, in children, 39
Chest pain: in postoperative ophthalmic patients, 346
Chiasmal visual field defects: screening for, 296
Children
cellulitis, orbital, 39
glioma of intracranial optic pathway, 300

infant, fitting of contact lenses
      for, 72
  melanoma of, uveal, 210
  newborn, good visual function
      after cataract surgery in,
      349
  palsy of, VI nerve, 59
  refractive errors in, high,
      screening for, 46
  retinopathy of, diabetic,
      coagulation in, 254
  strabismus, photographic
      screening for, 46
Chinese ophthalmology: review of,
    380
Choriocapillary occlusion: in
    Moschowitz's disease, 227
Chorioretinitis: vitiliginous, 225
Choroid
  atrophy, arginine-restricted diet
      in, 282
  detachment, discussion of, 223
  melanoma (*see* Melanoma,
      choroid)
  neovascular membranes,
      photocoagulation of, 264
  neovascularization, and myopia,
      268
  tumors, nerve, 219
Clobetasone butyrate: in allergic
    conjunctivitis, 82
Coagulation: in diabetic
    retinopathy, 254
Computed tomography: in
    melanoma of choroid, 214
Conjunctiva
  in dyscrasia, immunoglobulin-
      producing, 90
  erythroplasia of Queyrat of, 88
  melanoma, prognostic factors, 85
  melanosis of, precancerous,
      cryotherapy for, 87
Conjunctivitis
  allergic, clobetasone butyrate
      and sodium cromoglycate in,
      82
  inclusion, adult, 80
Contact lenses, 50 ff., 71 ff.
  in amblyopia, myopic
      anisometropic, 50
  extended-wear, 73 ff.
    for aphakic correction, 74
    for myopic correction, 73
    soft, in strabismic amblyopia,
        51
  hard, fitting, in infant, 72
  meibomian glands and, 29
  visual disturbances due to, in
      cataract with lens
      extraction, 71
Contraceptives: oral, and eye, 323
Convergence insufficiency: surgery
    of, 55
Cooper permalens: experience
    with, 74
Cornea
  anesthesia during timolol, 152
  changes in conjunctivitis, adult
      inclusion, 80
  endothelium, 123 ff.
    in diabetes, 123
    after lens implant,
        intraocular, 124
    after reconstituents in
        cataract extraction, 342
    replacement of, 116
  laceration, keratoplasty in, 114
  preservation, prolonged donor,
      110
  thickness in diabetes, 123
  transplant (*see* Transplantation,
      cornea)
  ulcer, herpes keratitis after, 120
Corticosteroids: in Graves'
    ophthalmopathy, 37
Cranial
  intracranial (*see* Intracranial)
  nerves III, IV and VI, paralysis
      of, 306
Cromoglycate (*see* Sodium,
    cromoglycate)
Cryosurgery, 17 ff.
  complications of, 19
  lamella, in distichiasis, 17
Cryotherapy
  cyclocryotherapy and blood-
      aqueous barrier breakdown,
      23

in precancerous melanosis of conjunctiva, 87
CT (*see* Tomography, computed)
Cyclocryotherapy: and blood-aqueous barrier breakdown, 158
Cyst: epithelial, of anterior chamber, 352
Cystoid
 macular edema (*see* Macula, edema, cystoid)
 maculopathy, pseudophakic, 257
Cytology: of conjunctiva in dyscrasia, 90

D

Dermatitis, atopic
 cataract in, 193
 infraorbital fold in, 40
Diabetes mellitus, 181 ff.
 in cataract
  aldose reductase in, 185
  senile, 183
 corneal thickness and endothelium in, 123
 effect on cataract formation, 180
 lens changes and, senile, 181
 optic neuropathy and ophthalmoplegia in, 313
 retinopathy of (*see* Retinopathy, diabetic)
Dialysis: retinal, pathogenic factors in, 278
Diet: arginine-restricted, atrophy of choroid and retina in, 282
Disc (*see* Optic, disc)
Distichiasis: lid splitting and cryosurgery in, 17
Double elevator palsy, 60
Dry eye: the questionably, 28
Dyscrasia: immunoglobulin-producing, of conjunctiva, 90
Dysthyroidism: optic nerve in, 38

E

Eclipse retinopathy, 284
Edema (*see* Macula, edema)

Electroretinography: after photocoagulation of retina, 365
Elevator palsy: double, 60
Endocrine ophthalmopathy, 31
Endothelium (*see* Cornea, endothelium)
Epikeratophakia: surgical correction, 103
Epinephrine
 distribution in phakic and aphakic eyes, 360
 in intraocular pressure lowering, 147
Epiphora: congenital, natural history, 28
Epithelial
 cells, pigment, and phagocytosis, 362
 cysts of anterior chamber, 352
 disease, herpes ocular, 117
Erythroplasia of Queyrat: of conjunctiva, 88
Esotropia: congenital, monofixation syndrome in, 46
Exotropia, intermittent, 53 ff.
 surgery in, necessity of, 54
 surgical results, 53
Eye
 cancer metastatic, complication of, 220
 carcinoma of adnexa, incompletely excised, 15
 care, survey of demand for, 381
 complications in giant cell arteritis, 308
 contraceptives and, oral, 323
 dry, the questionably, 28
 foreign body detection with CAT, 344
 herpes epithelial disease, 117
 histoplasmosis syndrome, laser for neovascularization in, 265
 hypertension (*see* Hypertension, ocular)
 immunology, review of, 203
 injuries, 367

SUBJECT INDEX / 387

prevention of, 367
  sports, prevention of, 369
  intraocular (see Intraocular)
  lens implant, corneal
    endothelium after, 124
  leprosy and, 327
  manifestations of leprosy,
    prevalence in New Guinea,
    375
  melanoma, rates of, 207
  melanosis, and lid pigmented
    lesion, 86
  motor signs in metabolic
    diseases, 326
  movements, dynamic vergence,
    in strabismus and
    amblyopia, 61
  pain, symptom of, 375
  pemphigoid, cicatricial, 89
  refraction (see Refraction)
  tissue, ^{32}P uptake by, in
    melanoma, 222
  torsion and retinal meridians, 63
Eyelid (see Lid)

F

Facial contour deformities:
    prefabricated sculptured
    implants in, 26
Fascia lata: use and fate of, in
    surgery, 24
Fetus: alcohol syndrome, 325
Fibroplasia (see Retrolental
    fibroplasia)
Fluorescein
  angiography in macular edema,
    256
  in vitreous, pharmacokinetics of,
    370
Fluorescence photography:
    retrobulbar administration
    of dye, 285
Fluorescent light: damaging retina
    (in monkey), 372
Fluorophotometry: vitreous, and
    variability, 371
Foreign bodies: intraocular,
    detection with CAT, 344

Fracture: of orbit, four incisions
    for, 347
Frisby test: for screening, 69

G

Genes: recessive, beware of, 377
Genetic counseling: for parents of
    children with impaired
    vision, 378
Giant cell arteritis: eye
    complications in, 308
Glasses: causing visual
    disturbances in cataract
    with lens extraction, 71
Glaucoma, 131 ff., 156 ff., 166 ff.
  angle-closure, complications of
    iridectomy in, 143
  cataract and, 194
  chronic simple, optic disc
    hemorrhage in, 160
  congenital, goniotomy in, 167
  low-tension, timolol and
    intraocular pressure in, 149
  neovascular, after central retinal
    vein obstruction, 156
  open-angle
    clinicopathology of, 166
    laser in, 136
    laser in, argon, 132 ff.
    uncontrolled phakic, argon
      laser trabecular surgery in,
      133
  secondary, and iris
    neovascularization, 157
  shunt in, aqueous-venous, 169
  surgery, lens injury during,
    168
  timolol in, 145
    with other drugs, 146
Glioma: of intracranial optic
    pathway, in children, 300
Glucose-6-phosphate
    dehydrogenase deficiency:
    cataract in, 192
Goniotomy: in congenital
    glaucoma, 167
Graft: allograft reactions after
    keratoplasty, 111

Graves'
  disease, orbital, 32
  ophthalmopathy, corticosteroids in, 37

H

Hamartoma: iris, and von Recklinghausen's neurofibromatosis, 217
Healon (*see* Sodium hyaluronate)
Hemorrhage
  optic disc, 160 ff.
    in glaucoma, 160
    in hypertension, ocular, 160 ff.
  vitreous, pseudo, 236
Herpes
  keratitis (*see* Keratitis, herpes)
  ocular epithelial disease, 117
Histoplasmosis syndrome: ocular, laser for neovascularization in, 265
HLA B8: and iridocyclitis in black patients, 205
Hyaluronate
  Na-hyaluronate and retinal reattachment, 339
  sodium (*see* Sodium, hyaluronate)
Hyperplasia: of conjunctiva, melanocytic, 87
Hypertension
  intracranial, optic nerve decompression in, 313
  ocular
    optic disc hemorrhage in, 160 ff.
    prophylactic therapy of, 164

I

Immunity: systemic, in herpes keratitis, 121
Immunoglobulin-producing dyscrasia: of conjunctiva, 90
Immunology
  corticosteroids in Graves' ophthalmopathy and, 37
  of eye, review of, 203
  of keratoplasty, penetrating, 112

Immunosuppressive therapy: of Behçet's syndrome, 320
Implant
  intraocular, aqueous humor after, 322
  lens
    intraocular, after cataract extraction, 187
    intraocular, corneal endothelium after, 124
    intraocular, sodium hyaluronate and, 337
    laser in, pulsed neodymium, 351
  prefabricated sculptured, in facial contour deformities, 26
  pseudophakos, and cataract extraction (in primate), 190
Indomethacin, 321 ff.
  discussion of, 321
  intraocular implant and, 322
Infant: contact lens fitting for, 72
Infarctions: occipital lobe, 298
Infraorbital fold: in atopic dermatitis, 40
Intracranial
  hypertension, optic nerve decompression in, 313
  optic pathway, glioma of, in children, 300
Intraocular
  implant (*see under* Implant)
  lens (*see* Lens, intraocular)
  pressure, 147 ff.
    argon laser of anterior chamber angle in, 135
    in glaucoma, low-tension, 149
    lowering with timolol and epinephrine, 147
Iridectomy, peripheral, 142 ff.
  case review, 142
  in glaucoma, complications of, 143
Iridocyclitis: and HLA B8 in black patients, 205
Iridotomy: laser, technique and safety, 144
Iris, 215 ff.
  hamartoma and von

Recklinghausen's
neurofibromatosis, 217
"melanoma," as nevus, 215
neovascularization, and
secondary glaucoma, 157
Ischemic optic neuropathy: in
diabetes, 313

K

Keratitis, 119 ff.
herpes, 119 ff.
bilateral, 119
after corneal ulcer, prognosis,
120
immunity in, systemic, 121
Thygeson's superficial punctate,
122
Keratoconjunctivitis
atopic, sodium cromoglycate in,
81
phlyctenular, tetracycline for, 83
Keratomileusis: pathologic
features of, 102
Keratopathy: aphakic bullous,
keratoplasty in, 109
Keratophakia, 100 ff.
epikeratophakia, surgical
correction, 103
evaluation of, 100
pathologic features of, 102
update on, 100
Keratoplasty
(*See also* Transplantation,
cornea)
penetrating, 106 ff.
allograft reactions after, 111
aphakic, macular edema after,
335
immunology of, 112
in keratomileusis, 102
in keratopathy, aphakic
bullous, 109
in keratophakia, 102
after laceration of cornea, 114
selecting patients for, 106
visual results after, 108
sodium hyaluronate in, 337
Keratotomy, radial, 96 ff.
experience with, 98

UCLA clinical trial of, 96
Kidney failure: and acetazolamide,
324
Krypton laser: in macular
subretinal
neovascularization, 265

L

Laser, 365 ff.
argon, 131 ff.
of anterior chamber angle in
intraocular pressure
increase, 135
in glaucoma, open-angle, 132
in glaucoma with trabecular
tightening, 131
photocoagulation (*see*
Photocoagulation, argon
laser)
in glaucoma, open-angle, 136
-induced endovascular
thrombosis, and vessel
closure, 366
iridotomy, technique and safety,
144
neodymium, pulsed,
ophthalmologic use of, 351
red-light krypton, in macular
subretinal
neovascularization, 265
Lens
contact (*see* Contact lenses)
extraction for cataract, visual
disturbances due to glasses
or lenses in, 71
implant (*see* Implant, lens)
injury during glaucoma surgery,
168
intraocular, 187 ff.
Shearing, position of, 189
sodium hyaluronate and,
336
senile changes, and diabetes,
181
Leprosy
eye in, 327
eye manifestations of,
prevalence in New Guinea,
375

Levator recession: in thyroid-related lid retraction, 33
Lid, 20 ff.
　carcinoma, basal cell, 15
　pigmented lesion, and ocular melanosis, 86
　retraction, secondary to thryoid ophthalmopathy, 27
　splitting in distichiasis, 17
　surgery, discussion of, 22
　tumors of sweat gland origin, 16
　upper
　　eversion of, congenital total, 20
　retraction, thyroid-related, 33
Light: fluorescent, damaging retina (in monkey), 372
Lung disease: obstructive, and bronchoconstrictive effect of timolol, 154

M

Macula
　detachment, 275
　edema, 261
　edema, cystoid, 255 ff., 260 ff.
　　angiography of, fluorescein, 256
　　histopathology of, 260
　　after keratoplasty, penetrating, 335
　　treatment advances, 255
　　in vitreoretinal traction, 232
　neovascularization, laser in, 265
　pucker, vitreous surgery for, 235
Maculopathy: pseudophakic cystoid, 257
Manpower studies: for eye care, in U.S., 381
Meibomian glands: and contact lens wear, 29
Melanocytic hyperplasia: of conjunctiva, 87
Melanoma, 207 ff.
　choroid, 211 ff.
　　extraocular extension of, 213
　　metastatic, prognosis in, 211
　　tomography in, computed, 214
　conjunctival, prognostic factors, 85
　of eye, rates of, 207
　of iris, as nevus, 215
　^{32}P uptake in ocular tissue, 222
　uvea, 208 ff.
　　in children, 210
　　metastases from, 208
Melanosis, 86 ff.
　of conjunctiva, precancerous, cryotherapy for, 87
　ocular, and lid pigmented lesion, 86
Meningioma, 303 ff.
　ophthalmologist and, 303
　optic nerve, management, 304
Metabolic diseases: ocular motor signs in, 326
Metastases
　of choroidal melanoma, 211
　in eye cancer, complication of, 220
　from uveal melanoma, 208
Migraine: acephalgic, experience with, 311
Monofixation syndrome: in congenital esotropia, 46
Monolayer: corneal endothelial, formation, 116
Moschowitz's disease: choriocapillary occlusion in, 227
Motor signs: ocular, in metabolic diseases, 326
Müller's muscle excision: in thyroid-related lid retraction, 33
Multiple sclerosis: visual evoked potentials in, 297
Muscle
　Müller's muscle excision in thyroid-related lid retraction, 33
　"slipped muscle," discussion of, 64
Myopathy: thyroid, diagnosis and treatment, 36
Myopia: pathology of, and choroidal neovascularization, 268

Myopic
  amblyopia, contact lenses in, 50
  correction, extended-wear contact lenses for, 73

N

Na-hyaluronate: and retinal reattachment, 339
Nail pigmentation: after timolol, 132
Neodymium laser: pulsed, ophthalmologic use of, 351
Neovascular
  glaucoma after central retinal vein obstruction, 156
  membranes (see Photocoagulation, argon laser, of neovascular membranes)
Neovascularization, 265 ff.
  choroidal, and myopia, 268
  of iris and secondary glaucoma, 157
  macular retinal, laser in, 265
  optic disc, correlation with rubeosis iridis, 251
Nerve(s), 304 ff.
  cranial, III, IV and VI, paralysis of, 306
  optic (see Optic, nerve)
  retinal, fiber defects in ocular hypertension, 160
  VI, palsy, benign recurrent, in children, 59
  tumor of choroid, 219
Neurofibromatosis: von Recklinghausen's, and iris hamartoma, 217
Neuropathy: optic, ischemic, in diabetes, 131
Nevi: iris "melanomas" as, 215
Newborn: cataract surgery in, good visual function after, 349

O

Oblique
  inferior, anterior transposition of, 57
  paresis, masked bilateral superior, 60
Occipital lobe infarctions, 298
Ocular (see Eye)
Onchocerciasis: discussion of, 363
Ophthalmic
  plastic surgery, fascia lata and sclera in, 24
  postoperative patients, chest pain in, 346
  sutures, evolution of, 376
Ophthalmologist: and meningioma, 303
Ophthalmology: Chinese, review of, 380
Ophthalmopathy
  endocrine, 31
  Graves', corticosteroids in, 57
  thyroid, lid retraction after, 27
Ophthalmoplegia: painful, in diabetes, 313
Optic
  disc
    hemorrhage (see Hemorrhage, optic disc)
    neovascularization, correlation with rubeosis iridis, 251
  nerve
    decompression in hypertension, 313
    in dysthyroidism, 38
    meningioma, management, 304
    tumor, transcranial enucleation in, 344
  neuropathy, ischemic, in diabetes, 313
  pathway, intracranial, glioma of, in children, 300
Oral contraceptives: and eye, 323
Orbit
  cellulitis, in children, 39
  fracture, four incisions for, 347
  Graves' disease of, 32
  infraorbital fold in atopic dermatitis, 40
Oxygen therapy: retinopathy after, in prematurity, 249

P

Pain
 chest, in postoperative ophthalmic patients, 346
 eye, symptom of, 364
Painful ophthalmoplegia: in diabetes, 313
Palsy
 double elevator, 60
 VI nerve, benign recurrent, in children, 59
Paralysis: of cranial nerves III, IV and VI, 306
Paresis: oblique, masked bilateral superior, 60
Pars plana vitrectomy: in diabetic retinopathy, 231
Pemphigoid: ocular cicatricial, 89
Perimetry: in occipital lobe infarction, 298
Phagocytosis: and pigment epithelial cells, 362
Phakic eyes: epinephrine distribution in, 360
Phenylephrine: for pupillary dilation, blood pressure increase after, in prematurity, 363
Phlyctenular keratoconjunctivitis: tetracycline for, 83
Phosphorus-32 uptake: in eye tissue in melanoma, 222
Photochemical transillumination, 285
Photocoagulation, argon laser
 of neovascular membranes, 262 ff.
 of neovascular membranes
  choroidal, 264
  subretinal, 262
 of retina, electroretinography after, 365
 in retinopathy, diabetic, 252
Photographic screening: for strabismus and high refractive errors, in children, 46
Photography: fluorescence fundus, with retrobulbar administration of dye, 285
Pigment
 dispersion syndrome, 164
 epithelial cells, and phagocytosis, 362
Pigmentation: of nail after timolol, 155
Pigmented lesion: of lid and ocular melanosis, 86
Plastic surgery: fascia lata and sclera in, 24
Pneumoencephalography: of glioma of intracranial optic pathway, in children, 300
Polymyalgia rheumatica: eye complications in, 303
Precancerous melanosis: of conjunctiva, cryotherapy in, 87
Prematurity
 pupillary dilation in, blood pressure increase after, 363
 retinopathy after oxygen therapy in, 272
 retrolental fibroplasia in transfusion and, 273 ff.
 vitamin E for, 270
Preterm infant (see Prematurity)
Prostaglandin assay: of aqueous humor after intraocular implant, 322
Pseudophakic cystoid maculopathy, 257
Pseudophakos implant: and cataract extraction (in primate), 190
Pupillary dilation: blood pressure increase after, in prematurity, 363

Q

Queyrat erythroplasia: of conjunctiva, 88

R

Random-Dot E test: for screening, 69

Randot circles stereotests: for
  screening, 69
Reconstructive surgery: fascia lata
  and sclera in, 24
Refraction
  errors, high, photographic
    screening for, in children, 46
  near work and familial
    resemblances in, 70
Renal failure: and acetazolamide,
  324
Retina, 275 ff., 339 ff.
  atrophy, arginine-restricted diet
    in, 282
  degenerations, lattice and snail
    track, 281
  detachment, 275 ff., 340 ff.
    repair, and balloon buckle,
      340
    rhegmatogenous, vision and
      reattachment after, 275
    surgery, silicon and, fluid, 341
    surgery, visual acuity after,
      277
    traction, 234
  dialysis, pathogenic factors in,
    278
  fluorescent light damaging (in
    monkey), 372
  meridians, and eye torsion, 63
  nerve fiber defects in ocular
    hypertension, 160
  photocoagulation of,
    electroretinography after,
    365
  reattachment, and Na-
    hyaluronate, 339
  subretinal (*see* Subretinal)
  vein obstruction, glaucoma after,
    156
Retinopathy
  diabetic (*see below*)
  eclipse, 284
  after oxygen therapy, in
    prematurity, 272
Retinopathy, diabetic, 246 ff.,
  252 ff.
  circinate, argon laser
    photocoagulation in, 252
  discussion of, 246 ff.
  proliferative, 249 ff.
  coagulation of, 254
  course of, 250
  visual outcome in, 249
  serious, prevalence of, 248
  vitrectomy in, pars plana, 231
Retrabulbar anesthesia:
  topography, CT in, 354
Retrolental fibroplasia, 270 ff.
  new look at unsolved problem,
    271
  transfusion in, 273 ff.
  vitamin E in, in prematurity,
    270
Rheumatoid scleritis, 126
Rubeosis iridis: correlation with
  optic disc
  neovascularization, 251

S

Salicylate: in senile cataract, 183
Scanning: brain, of glioma of
  intracranial optic pathway,
  in children, 300
Sclera
  in lid retraction, 27
  use and fate of, in surgery, 24
Scleritis: rheumatoid, 126
Sclerosis: multiple, visual evoked
  potentials in, 297
Senile, 181 ff.
  cataract, diabetes and salicylate
    in, 183
  lens changes and diabetes, 181
Shearing intraocular lens: position
  of, 189
Shunt: aqueous-venous, in
  glaucoma, 169
Silicon: fluid, and retinal
  detachment surgery, 341
"Slipped muscle:" discussion of, 64
Sodium
  cromoglycate, 81 ff.
    in conjunctivitis, allergic, 82
    in keratoconjunctivitis, atopic,
      81
  hyaluronate, 336 ff.
    in cataract extraction, 336
    in keratoplasty, 337

vitreous hemorrhage and, 236
Sports eye injuries: prevention of, 369
Stereotests: for screening, 69
Stimulus deprivation amblyopia, 49
Strabismic amblyopia: contact lenses in, 51
Strabismus
  photographic screening for, in children, 46
  vergence eye movements in, dynamic, 61
Subretinal
  neovascular membranes, photocoagulation of, 262
  neovascularization, laser in, 265
Sunglasses: for protection from ultraviolet radiation, 372
Sutures: ophthalmic, evolution of, 376
Sweat gland origin: of lid tumors, 16

T

Temporal arteritis: eye complications in, 308
Tetracycline: for phylctenular keratoconjunctivitis, 83
Thermosclerostomy: vs. trabeculectomy, 139
Thrombosis: laser-induced endovascular, and vessel closure, 366
Thygeson's punctate keratitis, 122
Thyroid, 33 ff.
  myopathy, diagnosis and treatment, 36
  ophthalmopathy, lid retraction after, 27
  -related upper lid retraction, 33
Timolol, 145 ff.
  bronchoconstrictive effect, and obstructive lung disease, 143
  bronchospasm after, 153
  corneal anesthesia during, 152
  in glaucoma, 145
    low-tension, 149

  with other drugs, 146
  in intraocular pressure lowering, 147
  nail pigmentation after, 155
  penetration into aqueous humor, 150
  safety of, 151
  tolerability of, 151
TNO test: for screening, 69
Tolosa-Hunt syndrome: case review, 310
Tomography, computed, 298 ff.
  axial, in intraocular foreign body detection, 344
  of glioma of intracranial optic pathway, in children, 300
  in melanoma of choroid, 214
  in occipital lobe infarctions, 298
  in retrobulbar anesthesia topography, 354
Trabecular
  surgery in glaucoma, uncontrolled phakic open-angle, 133
  tightening with laser in glaucoma, 131
Trabeculectomy, 139 ff.
  in black patients, 140
  vs. thermosclerostomy, 139
Traction, 232 ff.
  retinal detachment, 234
  vitreoretinal, macular edema in, 232
Transfusion: in retrolental fibroplasia, 273 ff.
Transillumination: photochemical, 285
Transplantation, cornea
  (*See also* Keratoplasty)
  outcome of, 105
  preservation of cornea, prolonged donor, 110
Transposition: anterior, of inferior oblique, 57
Trauma (*see* Eye, injuries)
Tumors
  of choroid, nerve, 219
  lid, of sweat gland origin, 16
  optic nerve, transcranial enucleation in, 344

U

Ulcer: cornea, herpes keratitis after, 106
Ultraviolet
  risk factor and cataract, 193
  sunglasses as protection from, 372
Uvea (see Melanoma, uvea)

V

Vein
  aqueous-venous shunt for glaucoma, 169
  retinal, obstruction, glaucoma after, 156
Vergence eye movements: dynamic, in strabismus and amblyopia, 61
Very low birth weight: retrolental fibroplasia and transfusion, 274
Vessel closure: and laser-induced endovascular thrombosis, 366
Viruses (see Herpes)
Vision
  central, after retinal and macular detachment, 275
  impaired, genetic counseling for parents of children with, 367
Visual, 296 ff.
  acuity
    after cataract surgery before 6 months, 196
    normal, evaluation of, 67
    after retinal detachment surgery, 277
  disturbances due to glasses or lenses in cataract with lens extraction, 71
  evoked potentials in multiple sclerosis, 297
  field defects, chiasmal, screening for, 296
  function, good after congenital cataract surgery, in newborn, 349
  outcome in diabetic retinopathy, proliferative, 249
  pathway, compressive lesions, contrast sensitivity in, 302
  prognosis in keratopathy, with keratoplasty, 109
  results after penetrating keratoplasty, 108
Vitamin E: in retrolental fibroplasia, in prematurity, 153
Vitiliginous chorioretinitis, 225
Vitrectomy: pars plana, in diabetic retinopathy, 231
Vitreoretinal traction: macular edema in, 232
Vitreous, 235 ff., 370 ff.
  fluorescein in, pharmacokinetics of, 370
  fluorophotometry and variability, 371
  hemorrhage, pseudo, 236
  surgery in macular pucker, 235
von Recklinghausen's neurofibromatosis: and iris hamartoma, 217

Disease–a–Month®

Edited by **Nicholas J. Cotsonas, Jr., M.D.,** *The Abraham Lincoln School of Medicine, University of Illinois.*

Each pocket–size, 50–60 page issue offers one original article on a single topic of vital importance written by an expert in the field.

Subscription: 1 yr. . . . $27.50   Binder . . . $6.95.

Now you can order by phone!

Dial toll-free **800-621-9262** Monday through Friday. (Continental U.S., Virgin Islands & Puerto Rico only.) In Illinois, call collect **312-726-9746.**

The Year Book of Pediatrics NEWSLETTER

Edited by **Frank A. Oski, M.D.,** *Professor and Chairman, Department of Pediatrics, State University of New York Upstate Medical Center, Syracuse.*

This 4–page monthly publication refers you to clinically significant pediatric articles published the previous month.

You'll receive a variety of editorial comments including recommendations and precautions; new developments and recommended articles for reading.

Subscription: 1 year. . . . $26.50.

---

detach and mail

Enter my subscription to the periodicals checked below:

	1 yr.	2 yr.	binder*
Current Problems in Surgery	$ 33.00	$63.50	$6.95 (each year)
Current Problems in Pediatrics	33.00	63.50	6.95 (each year)
Current Problems in Cancer	38.75	73.50	6.95 (each year)
Current Problems in Cardiology	38.75	73.50	6.95 (each year)
Current Problems in Ob/Gyn	38.75	73.50	6.95 (each year)
Current Problems in Diag. Radiology	32.00		6.95 (each year)
Pediatric Newsletter	26.50	52.50	N/A
Disease–a–Month®	27.50	51.50	6.95 (each year)
		(price includes storage box/binder)	

Illinois and Tennessee residents will be billed appropriate state sales tax. Prices in Canada slightly higher but billed in Canadian funds. International prices also slightly higher. A small additional charge will be made for postage and handling. All prices quoted are subject to change.

Name _____ Acct. No. _____
(Please print including middle initial)

Address _____

City _____ State _____ Zip _____

YEAR BOOK MEDICAL PUBLISHERS
35 EAST WACKER DRIVE, CHICAGO, ILLINOIS 60601
TIMES MIRROR

Printed in U.S.A.   PAYB

Detach and mail today

You already have enough to read—
So why are we suggesting you read these too?

Because nowhere else can you find periodicals offering these special advantages—

- ✔ *original* articles on a *single* topic
- ✔ convenient *pocket-size* format
- ✔ written by experts in the field

←——————— *except* in these ———————→

NO POSTAGE
NECESSARY
IF MAILED
IN THE
UNITED STATES

BUSINESS REPLY MAIL
FIRST CLASS   PERMIT No. 762   CHICAGO, ILLINOIS

POSTAGE WILL BE PAID BY ADDRESSEE

YEAR BOOK MEDICAL PUBLISHERS
35 EAST WACKER DRIVE
CHICAGO, ILLINOIS 60601

Detach and mail today

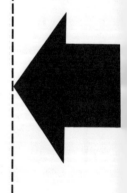